Rhode Island's
Civil War Hospital

Rhode Island's Civil War Hospital

Life and Death at Portsmouth Grove, 1862–1865

Frank L. Grzyb

Foreword by Robert C. Rubel

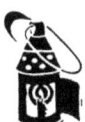

McFarland & Company, Inc., Publishers
Jefferson, North Carolina, and London

LIBRARY OF CONGRESS CATALOGUING-IN-PUBLICATION DATA

Grzyb, Frank L., 1946–
Rhode Island's Civil War hospital : life and death at Portsmouth Grove, 1862–1865 / Frank L. Grzyb ; foreword by Robert C. Rubel.
    p.   cm.

Includes bibliographical references and index.

ISBN 978-0-7864-6861-4
softcover : acid free paper ♾

1. Portsmouth Grove Hospital (Portsmouth, R.I.) — History. 2. Military hospitals — Rhode Island — Portsmouth — History — 19th century. 3. Medicine, Military — Rhode Island — Portsmouth — History — 19th century. 4. Rhode Island — History — Civil War, 1861–1865 — Hospitals. 5. Rhode Island — History — Civil War, 1861–1865 — Medical care. 6. United States — History — Civil War, 1861–1865 — Hospitals. 7. United States — History — Civil War, 1861–1865 — Medical care. I. Title.
E621.G79   2012   973.7'76 — dc23   2012014923

BRITISH LIBRARY CATALOGUING DATA ARE AVAILABLE

© 2012 Frank L. Grzyb. All rights reserved

No part of this book may be reproduced or transmitted in any form or by any means, electronic or mechanical, including photocopying or recording, or by any information storage and retrieval system, without permission in writing from the publisher.

On the cover: (inset) Patient Franz Robert Jaeger of the 5th Regiment, New Hampshire Volunteer Infantry (Dr. Stephen Altic, D.O.); Drawing by J. Baker and J.M. Taylor, Jr., 1864. Front cover design by Bernadette Skok (bskok@ptd.net).

Manufactured in the United States of America

*McFarland & Company, Inc., Publishers
Box 611, Jefferson, North Carolina 28640
www.mcfarlandpub.com*

For my grandchildren
Andrew and Adela
and life's quest for knowledge

Table of Contents

Acknowledgments — viii
Acronyms and Abbreviations — xi
Foreword by Robert C. Rubel — 1
Preface — 3

1. Present-Day Portsmouth — 5
2. Nineteenth-Century Medicine — 7
3. Genesis: Early 1862 — 14
4. A Shaky Beginning — 19
5. The Pen Is Mightier Than the Sword — 30
6. Shelter and Rations — 41
7. Hospital Guards — 52
8. Liquor, Trouble and Discipline — 61
9. Hospital Volunteers and Benefactors — 68
10. New Arrivals: Unanticipated Problems — 73
11. Angels of Mercy — 80
12. Late 1862 and 1863 — 90
13. 1864 — 123
14. War's End: *Glory, Glory, Halleluiah* — 134

Appendix A: Hospital Guards — Rhode Island Volunteers — 161
Appendix B: Roll of Honor — 164
Appendix C: Map of Cypress Hills National Cemetery — 170
Notes — 171
Bibliography — 184
Index — 191

Acknowledgments

This book would not have been possible without the help of some wonderful people from diverse age groups and backgrounds. There were writers, historians, doctors, researchers, librarians, students, memorabilia collectors, decedents, retirees, friends and neighbors, and even innocent bystanders swept up in my insatiable quest for more definitive information. Some were already my acquaintances while others were unknown to me. Upon reflection, the rewarding part of tackling such an endeavor is not only the strengthening of long-term relationships but adding new friends as well. For this I am immensely grateful.

The list of contributors is long, and hopefully I have not forgotten anyone. Yet, there is always that fear. If I missed crediting someone, the oversight was not intentional. Having reached a ripe old age, I have more senior moments than I care to reveal.

The following people helped me research my topic and assisted me in presenting this work in a more thorough and professional manner:

Ken Garthee, who can empathize with the entire military hospital experience, having lived through it as a patient during the Vietnam Conflict, for his tireless research assistance helping to reassemble several bits of information scattered over time and place, expert photography, help with digitizing numerous photographs and illustrations, assisting with on-site visits, and more than anything, much-needed moral support;

Matthew Garthee, Ken's son, for the recreation of a hospital diagram that will greatly enhance the reader's ability to comprehend the narrative;

Dr. Stephen Altic, D.O., an invaluable source of information, for allowing me to use his vast collection of research material, period images of the hospital and its patients, and for answering numerous questions while sustaining his busy medical practice. Until my arrival on the scene, Dr. Altic considered the hospital his own special project. That he is willing to share his passion and multitude of amazing finds with a much larger audience is something for which we should all feel grateful;

Robert C. ("Barney") Rubel, a friend and fellow author, for reading the initial draft and providing worthwhile comments and corrections along with a thoughtful foreword that captures the true essence of this work;

Russell DeSimone for rekindling my love of history and for his continued professional advice;

Thomas Greene for graciously opening his home and providing more insight about the hospital through patient letters, historical documents, and photographs;

Glenn W. Russell Jr., for help with correcting soldiers' names and regiments for the "Roll of Honor" and for providing additional information about soldiers' military and civilian records, burial locations, and cemetery photographs;

Robert Grandchamp, Civil War author and historian, for all his leads and for allowing me to quote from his works. His research skills and writing talents are unsurpassed for a gentleman so young. He is a rising star in the field of Civil War literature and one to watch;

Virginia Grzyb. If you want to gain respect as a writer, marry a former high school English teacher, now an adjunct professor. Without her skills, I would still be floundering in a sea of incoherent sentences and punctuation mishaps;

Matthew Grzyb. My son's education paid off not only for him, but for me. Matt did almost everything I could not do using his proficiency in word processing and spreadsheet preparation. If you think it is easy teaching an old dog new tricks, ask my son;

Dr. Katie Grzyb, DVM, my daughter, for taking time away from her busy schedule to help find gravesites at a national cemetery and also for her continuing words of encouragement;

Kenneth S. Carlson, a tireless, hard-working state employee at the Office of the Secretary of State, A. Ralph Mollis State Archives Division. Ken has always made himself available whenever called upon. He is truly a state asset;

Mark Dunkelman, for allowing me to quote from diary entries previously published by the Rhode Island Civil War Round Table and for putting me in touch with some fascinating people who share similar interests;

Peggy McGuire for granting permission to quote from her great-great-grandfather's letters and for use of his photograph;

Lyman John Brooks, Lou Cirillo, Tom Cottrell, and Leo Kennedy for allowing access and permission to reproduce photographs;

Fred Swarz, "Mr. Portsmouth," who cleared up some misconceptions I held about a particular house in Portsmouth with an addition built from lumber retrieved from Portsmouth Grove Hospital;

Henry Rodrigues for providing an article about the hospital he thought interesting and I found most useful;

Jim Garman for his books, photographs, and wisdom about the town of Portsmouth;

Dr. William Condon, VMD, John Finnegan, Carol Hutchinson, Noreen Kissell, R. Lee Parks, John Pimental, Ed Poulin, Richard A. Rupp, and George A. Thurston for their patience, understanding, interest, help, and hospitality;

Staff members at various historical societies, presidential libraries, university libraries, military libraries, and museums such as Bertram Lippincott III and Megan Delaney of the Newport Historical Society; J.D. Kay, Lee Teverow, and Jordan Goffin at the Rhode Island Historical Society; Richard C. Malley and John Potter of the Connecticut Historical Society Museum and Library; Ray Battcher of the Bristol Historical & Preservation Society; Marjorie Gomez O'Toole at the Little Compton Historical Society; Cheryl

Schnirring from the Abraham Lincoln Presidential Library and Museum in Illinois; Laura Anne Heller from the Dickinson Research Center, National Cowboy and Western Heritage Museum in Oklahoma; Karen Drickamer of Gettysburg College, Musselman Library Special Collections and College Archives in Pennsylvania; Jeremy B. Dibbell of the Massachusetts Historical Society; Margaret Hrabe from the Albert and Shirley Small Special Collection Library, Alderman Library of the University of Virginia Libraries; Roland Goodbody from the Milne Special Collections and Archives Department, University of New Hampshire Library; John Varner of Auburn University Libraries; Kristin L. Strohmeyer from Hamilton College; Wayne Rowe, Danielle Brazil, and Jamil Radae of the U.S. Naval War College, Henry E. Eccles Library; Richard J. Ring and Jordan Goffin of the Providence Public Library, Special Collections (C. Fiske Harris Collection on American Civil War and Slavery); Sarina Rodrigues Wyant and other staff members at the University of Rhode Island, University Libraries; Robert Pimentel and Sue Rousseau, from the Portsmouth Free Public Library; Marlene L. Lopes, from Rhode Island College James P. Adams Library, Special Collections; Patricia Redfern at the Warren Public Library; Lisa Long, the Redwood Library; Ann Amaral, Gail Shepherd, Pat LaRosa, and Patrick F. Murphy from the Newport Public Library; Susan Aprill at the Kingston Public Library in Massachusetts; and Kathleen Pratt of the Cotuit Library, also in Massachusetts.

Most of the photographs published in this book, the majority of them for the first time, were taken during the Civil War and credited to a gentleman named Joshua Appleby Williams. No one knows for certain how many images were taken of Portsmouth Grove's hospital grounds, its staff, patients, and visitors, but what first appeared to be only a smattering of photographs turned into a much larger assemblage. Though staged, the images paint a vivid picture of the medical facility. Williams originally owned studios on South Touro Street and fashionable Bellevue Avenue in Newport, Rhode Island. A house he occupied there in 1876 still stands and continues to bear his name. Without his images, this work would have been incomplete. I salute the memory of Joshua Appleby Williams and honor his noble profession.

A final word regarding photographs: there were simply too many to publish. Near the closing stages of this project, the flow seemed endless. With limited space, many interesting period shots and patient images could not be included; a shame indeed. Should this book spark additional interest, a comprehensive photographic collection of the hospital may be warranted.

Again, to all, my heartfelt thanks.

Acronyms and Abbreviations

AU—Special Collections & Archives, Ralph B. Draughon Library, Auburn University, Auburn, AL.
ALPLM—Abraham Lincoln Presidential Library & Museum, a Division of the Illinois Historic Preservation Agency, Springfield, IL.
AWOL—Absent without leave.
BUA—Brown University Archives, John Hay Library, Brown University, Providence, RI.
CHS—The Connecticut Historical Society Museum & Library, K. Nolin, Civil War Manuscripts Project, Hartford, CT.
FSH—Fairfax Seminary Hospital, Alexandria, VA.
GAR—Grand Army of the Republic.
HCL—Hamilton College Library Special Collections, Clinton, NY.
HGH—Hammond General Hospital, Point Lookout, MD.
LCP—The Library Company of Philadelphia, Philadelphia, PA.
MHS—Massachusetts Historical Society, Boston, MA.
MOLLUS-MASS, USAMHI—Military Order of the Loyal Legion of the United States—Massachusetts Photograph Album Collection, the U.S. Army Military History Institute, Carlisle Barracks, PA.
MSC&AD/UNH—Milne Special Collections and Archives Department, University of New Hampshire Library, Durham, NH.
NARA—National Archives and Records Administration, Washington, DC.
NDN—*Newport Daily News*, Newport, RI.
NHS—Newport Historical Society, Newport, RI.
NM—*Newport Mercury*, Newport, RI.
PG—Portsmouth Grove, Portsmouth, RI.
PPL—Portsmouth Public Library, Portsmouth, RI.
RIC—Rhode Island College, James P. Adams Library, Providence, RI.
RICWRT—Rhode Island Civil War Round Table.
RIHS—Rhode Island Historical Society, Providence, RI.
RIMJ—*Rhode Island Medical Journal.*
RISA—Rhode Island State Archives; officially named the Office of the Secretary of State, A. Ralph Mollis State Archives Division, Providence, RI.
RLA—Redwood Library and Athenaeum, Newport, RI.
ROTC—Reserve Officers' Training Corps.
SC/ML, GC—Special Collections/Musselman Library, Gettysburg College, Gettysburg, PA.
URIL—Special Collections, University of Rhode Island Library, Kingston, RI.
UVL—Special Collections, University of Virginia Library, Charlottesville, VA.
VA—United States Department of Veterans Affairs, Washington, DC.
WSUL—Wichita State University Libraries, Department of Special Collections, Wichita, Kansas.

Foreword
by Robert C. Rubel

The Civil War was a cataclysmic and transformational event in American history, the effects of which are still being felt. It is still the case that more Americans were killed and wounded in that conflict than in any other we have fought. Despite the relatively recent shock of the 9/11 attacks, and the small but seemingly endless drip of casualties from Iraq and Afghanistan, it is almost impossible to conceive of the trauma, both physical and psychological, that the Civil War inflicted on Americans, both individually and collectively. The vast literature of that conflict depicts the carnage at Shiloh, Antietam, Gettysburg, Cold Harbor, and so many other battlefields, and both histories and novels of the period tell us much about the soldiers themselves. Indeed, the emergence of Civil War reenacting provides many with an even deeper insight into the lives of soldiers and civilians of that age.

However, as is true for any event of such magnitude, there remain gaps in the historical record and so very many stories that have not been told. In many cases, these gaps and untold stories are oversights of professional historians, whose focus is on the central and prominent events and characters. Not infrequently, the gaps are filled by amateurs, people who, for various reasons, stumble upon and are drawn into these narratives. This book is a case in point. Portsmouth Grove Hospital has been, to this point, an obscure footnote to the dramatic sweep of Civil War history. However, its story, and the stories of the doctors, nurses, patients and guards that gave it life, give us a new perspective on the individuals and society of that time. Portsmouth Grove Hospital was on the periphery of the war, but for that reason, its story is all the more interesting because it gives us a unique look at the interaction between the army and civil society in those years.

As its title indicates, the heart of this book consists of the experiences of common soldiers whose wounds and diseases brought them to a secluded corner of the nation's smallest state. Through their eyes, we see not only the confines of a hospital, but also Civil War New England. We are brought to feel the barbarities of Civil War medicine, but also the yearnings for peace, freedom and family. It is through the previously untold stories of these forgotten souls that we gain new insight on Civil War Americans. Knowing more fully what happened to a soldier after he was wounded in battle or took sick on campaign, we can read the famous histories of the Civil War with fresh eyes.

It was said of the Marines at Iwo Jima in World War II that uncommon valor was a common virtue. We observe in this narrative that compassion, patriotism, charity and perseverance were common virtues displayed by so many of the men and women involved with Portsmouth Grove Hospital. Despite the failings of Civil War medicine, the deficiencies of planning and supply, and the derelictions of a distant army bureaucracy, the doctors, nurses and patients were able, over time, to create a place of recovery and recuperation for those men maimed and sickened by the war.

While this is a local history of a single Union army general hospital, it is, in many respects, universal and reflects well on Americans. It is worth the time to read.

Robert C. ("Barney") Rubel is dean of the Center for Naval Warfare Studies at the U.S. Naval War College in Newport, Rhode Island.

Preface

The Civil War story that lies ahead has little to do with famous battles, star-studded generals, brilliant strategies or, for that matter, which side won or lost the "whole shebang," as veterans who served would say. In a much deeper and personal sense, this offering is about man's ultimate struggle for survival, the essence of what happens to those seriously wounded in combat or beset by life-threatening illness. What follows is also a story about those who guided soldiers through the healing process: to cope with death all around; to fight the fevers; to heal the wounds; to instill the desire to live; and all too frequently, to defeat the emptiness of boredom and homesickness. It is the saga of the Portsmouth Grove Hospital in Rhode Island.

I'm not the first to face this question, nor will I be the last: "Where will you go to find the details to write the story?" I was asked one morning during a gentlemen's breakfast by a friend figuring it to be a daunting if not near-impossible challenge. "Oh, it's out there," I said, "You just have to keep looking." A simple answer, I admit, but one that was true enough. When researching history, it's much like the radio waves and television signals that leave our planet and travel through the infinite universe. History is there, somewhere; it just needs to be rediscovered. Luckily the peripherals of this story had already been uncovered; maybe even many of the specifics. What I managed to find was the chocolate and vanilla icing that add flavor to incidents previously recorded. Not to belabor the point, the reader at his or her leisure can read the sources listed in the bibliography. Mysteries do not abound, just diligent detective work networking through people and visiting places and conversing with those whose job it is to retain American history. And thank God for personal computers and the Internet. What a magnificent tool to aid present-day researchers and writers that was not available a few decades ago.

I wish I could remember the first time I learned about the hospital. I can't. A carpetbagger to Aquidneck Island, I must have read something about the place at the local library while skimming through books on Aquidneck Island history; and, believe me, there is plenty to swamp the most avid amateur historian. A Civil War addict, not just a buff, I was intrigued by what I read; but it was never my original intention to write a book about the hospital. Getting along in years and with no person forthcoming to write about these forgotten souls who passed through the hospital gates—some only one way—and more importantly, strongly believing that the plight of these soldiers needed to be remembered, I decided to draft a short article for inclusion in a Civil War magazine. The story soon became long and mushroomed into a reasonable-sized manuscript, then into the book you are now reading.

Did I find everything I was looking for in my research? Hardly; I would be naïve and foolish to think I cornered the market on all the photographs and stories that surround this place. But I do believe that someday others will add more insight: more pathos, comedy, additional historical information than I was able to uncover. The past is out there, somewhere, locked away in attics and old trunks, in historical societies and museums, or in private collections yet to be accessed.

A final word: to make the reading easier to comprehend, I've corrected punctuation and spelling errors within veteran and family correspondence without changing the writer's intent. I felt it necessary and in the reader's best interest. In several instances, missing periods and commas along with phonetic spelling made reading extremely difficult. I also changed the spelling of contracted words (e.g., to-day, some-one, can-not, head-quarters, etc.) to the more modern combined version while leaving all the slang intact to retain the flavor. Oftentimes common nouns were capitalized in letters and when read seemed a nuisance. Capitalization of these words has been removed. Lynne Truss, author of *Eats, Shoots & Leaves,* would have had a field day highlighting and correcting some letters I reviewed. Though the literacy rate in America in 1860 was among the highest in the world (90 percent), many Civil War soldiers could barely read or write. Yet they tried their best to express their thoughts and feelings; and considering their educational shortcomings, as you will soon see, they did a commendable job in conveying their message.

Chapter 1

Present-Day Portsmouth

Time flies over us but leaves its shadow behind.
— Nathaniel Hawthorne,
The Marble Faun, 1860

Nestled in the smallest state of the Union, near the northwestern tip of Aquidneck Island not far from Newport and Middletown, lies a twelve-acre stretch of land in the affluent community of Portsmouth. Formerly called Portsmouth Grove, the area currently encompasses a myriad of nautical businesses like boat manufacturing, sail design, fleet maintenance, and maritime outfitters all crammed along a maze of short private roads. The complex also hosts a large mooring on the western harbor side that includes 340 boat slips often jammed to capacity in the summer when yachtsmen look for berths close to the historic and bustling city of Newport.[1]

Maritime businesses have flourished here since the U.S. Navy deeded a large parcel of land back to the town in 1978. But land and building preservation was never a paramount concern to the military, especially during World War II. Except for its proximity to Narragansett Bay, a person would be hard-pressed to call this area picturesque, with its plethora of storage sheds, concrete block structures, rusted galvanized-aluminum buildings, and short- and long-term boat storage facilities scattered throughout the area along a few access roads.

During the summer months the Newport Dinner Train rambles through the area as passengers peer out the windows at vegetation and what little wildlife remains. The railroad's maintenance yard is also located here, next to an abandoned stone railroad trestle from yesteryear. Positioned to the east are many trees indigenous to the area, species far too numerous to mention. The thick and impenetrable underbrush, miscellaneous species of weeds including enormous cattails, along with a slow-draining ditch, cause the eastern area of the complex to appear more like an Egyptian marshland than New England countryside. A quarter acre of mowed grass adjacent to the main paved road serves as an undesignated dog run. Barely visible along this stretch are a few truncated roads cutting through heavy foliage that are now fenced and chained as briar dangles along the entire pathway. The grounds are in startling contrast to a mid–nineteenth-century description of "a twinkling brook bordered with elder bushes in full bloom, with occasional wild roses peeping out from the grass."[2]

Yet, to the northeast and up the ridge lies a town-owned campground that offers enjoyable hiking experiences along tree-lined paths that straddle small ponds and a dam. In a clearing, and as an added convenience, picnic tables are arranged for families who frequent the grounds. The aesthetics of the hilltop are in stark contrast to the valley below.

Melville Boat and Marina District, as it is known today, is still considered off the beaten path by most locals. To an even greater extent, what happened on these grounds nearly 150 years ago has long since been forgotten. Mother Nature and endless development in the name of prosperity have sadly erased Portsmouth Grove's brief but important contribution to our country's Civil War effort ... or have they?

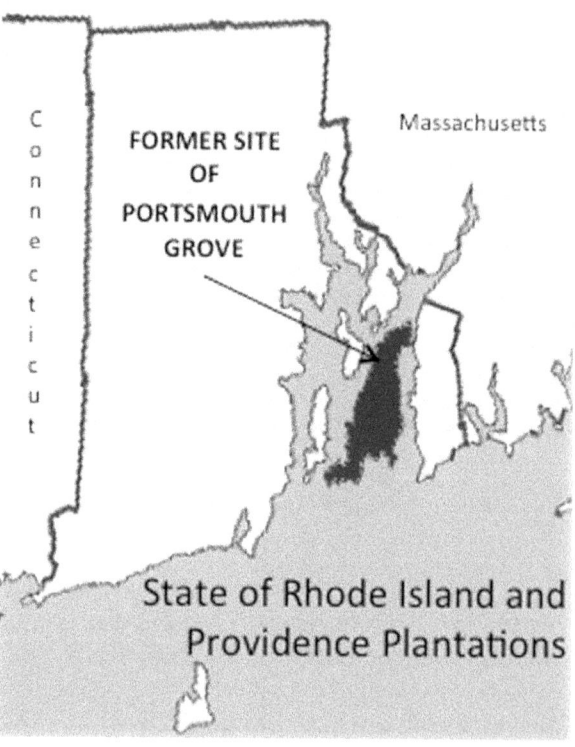

A former district of Portsmouth, Portsmouth Grove is now known as Melville. Aquidneck Island is highlighted in black.

Chapter 2

Nineteenth-Century Medicine

He's the best physician that knows the worthlessness of the most medicines.
— Benjamin Franklin

Military hospitals during the Civil War were first established in Washington, D.C., and the surrounding areas of northern Virginia because of their proximity to the battlefields. At the time, Civil War hospitals were classified into two major categories: field and general. Field hospitals were temporary quarters set up close to battlefields and used to address the immediate needs and the stabilization of soldiers recently injured in battle or disabled by illness. Usually they were established within a civilian-owned structure like a warehouse, mill, or hotel that had been leased or confiscated for use by the army, depending on the urgency of the moment. Hospital tents were also erected for use when no other permanent or semi-permanent structures were available.

Early in the war, surgeons in field hospitals were often accused of only worrying about surgical cases and not the sick. Critics—and there were many—complained about poor nursing care and patient diets that were neglected, or at best, limited.[1] Poor nutrition resulted in malnutrition, and malnutrition led to disease, sickness, and all too often, death.

General hospitals, so named because admissions were not restricted to men of any particular military unit or post, were much more permanent in nature and located hundreds of miles from the stresses of the battlefield.[2] Though they provided long-term health care for the sick and wounded, as harsh as it sounds, general hospitals had a primary objective: to return as many soldiers back to the front lines as quickly as possible. Yet, many a man felt lucky being cared for in a Northern army hospital where the cool air proved therapeutic and rejuvenating, except during the frigid months of winter. Private Stephen O. Rogers, Company I, 36th Regiment Massachusetts Volunteer Infantry was one of several who wrote home with such thoughts about his experience: "I feel fifty percent better.... New England air is having a renovating effect upon me." He concluded, "My diarrhea is entirely checked and my food digests better than it did two weeks ago."[3] But even the best laid plans go awry. General hospitals were still considered notorious breeding grounds for disease.[4]

A period account boasted "50 hospitals ... in the Washington, D.C., area alone with 12 more under construction."[5] Upon analysis, the estimate appears extremely high. In reality, working hospitals may have been less than half the reported number. Why the discrepancy? The estimate may have been skewed in the way hospitals were counted. Converted hotels, churches, town halls, taverns, mills, barns, and temporary wooden structures built for short-term patient care were probably included in the tally. A more reasonable estimate was that of Noah Brooks, an assistant secretary to President Abraham Lincoln, and a person in the know, having lived in Washington, D.C., during the rebellion. He said: "At the height of the war there were twenty-one hospitals in and about Washington."[6] With unforeseen sick and horrendous battlefield casualties, hospitals were stressed to the limit, no matter what the actual tally.

According to Page Smith in his book *Trial by Fire*, by the end of June 1863, "Out of every 1,000 men in the army there were 91 in army general hospitals and 44 in field hospitals," of which the largest percentage were sick rather than wounded. After battles the gap would close, but only for a short while.[7]

Though unintentional, after First Bull Run and into the better part of 1862, a majority of general military hospitals were disorganized, with patient care bordering on barbaric. Plans drafted before hospital construction were made in haste; logistic elements received only passing consideration, and sometimes not at all. The problem began immediately after the initial battles when a macabre harvest of sick and wounded descended upon hospitals in mind-boggling numbers. Qualified doctors handling the enormous influx of patients were in the minority and adequate medical facilities were nearly nonexistent.

A sad scenario of the war was that far too many general hospital physicians were granted military commissions to practice medicine through political favoritism, usually by state governors, and most of these appointees possessed little or no formal medical school training. "It is much to be feared," said Samuel Wiessell Gross, M.D., in his book *A Manual of Military Surgery*, published in 1861, that "from the rapid manner in which our volunteers have been hurried together, many medical men, old as well as young, have already been admitted into the service utterly unfit for the office." In the same breath, Gross warns of "charlatans and unworthy men" who found their way into the profession.[8] As casualties mounted, so too did the demand for doctors and surgeons. Grossly unqualified men calling themselves physicians easily found their way into Northern general hospitals either as military officers or contractors, the latter given the title of acting assistant surgeon, while wearing the uniform of a first lieutenant and receiving the same pay. Some came because of patriotism; others because they lacked a profitable private practice. Though it was the government's intention that "none but men of the best talent and of the highest education ... be received into the public service," a stringent certification process for military doctors was sadly lacking.[9]

After the war's first shots were fired at Fort Sumter, the Federal government had only 98 physicians on its rolls. At war's end, there were 13,000.[10] As for the physicians considered well qualified during the war, the medical techniques practiced and the remedies they employed were highly suspect and, at times, unintentionally cruel, even deadly. James M. McPherson, in his book *Battle Cry of Freedom: The Civil War Era*, quotes an Illinois private as saying, "Our doctors know about as much as a 10 year old boy."[11] And in his book *Civil War Soldiers: Their Expectations and Their Experiences*, Reid Mitchell cites a Union soldier as saying, "I had rather risk a battle than the hospitals."[12] Neither opinion serves as a resounding testimonial to the skills of Civil War–era military doctors. Medical care assessments by soldiers like those listed above were in the majority, and it is no wonder men on each side of the conflict labeled doctors as nothing more than "quacks" and "butchers."[13]

Early in the war, general military hospitals lacked not only qualified doctors but competent administrators. A hospital was controlled as follows: a senior surgeon or surgeon-in-charge would supervise a staff of assistant surgeons. The senior surgeon would usually visit the wards daily, but sometimes only when needed. Loose government recommendations — more like suggestions — stated that hospitals should be clean, well-ventilated, and not especially crowded. That left considerable leeway for the engineers who designed and built the hospitals and the staff who would administer them. Record keeping would normally be the responsibility of assistant surgeons, but this duty assignment differed depending on the wants of the surgeon-in-charge. Stewards would assist the surgeons and provide medicines as prescribed by the doctor. They also performed clerical and storekeeper duties as assigned. Not to be forgotten, nurses would assist the assistant surgeons and work with stewards. But most nurses, especially during the first few years of the conflict, were nothing more than general housekeepers.[14]

Besides the commanding officer, who was accountable and responsible for the entire workings of the general hospital, assistant surgeons (ward physicians) cared for as many as 75 to 100 patients (sometimes fewer, sometimes more, depending on patient load and medical condition). As for added staffing, in a 1,000-bed hospital there would normally be 20 ward masters, 5 or 6 cooks, twice as many assistant cooks, 10 to 15 handymen spread between carpenters, blacksmiths and plumbers, the same number of storeroom workers, a few dead-house and burial yard attendants, several clerks in the administrative office and library, and 3 for the officers' quarters and mess. Every hospital had at least one chaplain who not only served as a spiritual advisor, but as a counselor, morale and recreational officer and, in some cases, a librarian and mailman.[15]

Assistant surgeons visited patients in the morning when most of the work was accomplished. Normally, they were met at the hospital door by the ward master and soon joined by the ward nurse and perhaps a steward. Afternoon visits were also performed, but with less frequency, depending on the condition of their patients. Convalescents who could rise were expected to jump to attention, salute, and remain standing until the gesture was returned — military tradition was not abandoned at the door. Patient beds were arranged about four feet apart on each side of the ward such that two were between each pair of windows. Here the assistant surgeons would walk down the center aisle, "examining wounds, changing dressing, prescribing drugs and changes in diet." When completed, the doctor would depart and the ward master would be back in charge.[16]

Though procedures to visit patients were fairly well established and observed, patient care by Civil War doctors was regarded as a frightening adventure of drug experimentation and voodoo medicine. Depending on the type of stomach wound, treatments consisted of a plug of opium or a concoction of mercury and chalk called "blue mass."[17] Before the war, Abraham Lincoln was said to have taken blue mass in pill form to relieve constipation but abandoned its use because it made him depressed. No wonder. The pill had 120 times the level of mercury now considered acceptable for an adult.[18] Opium was also used to treat pneumonia, along with whiskey, quinine and mustard plaster.[19] Those suffering from typhoid fever and nausea were given a dose of ammonia, while others with less serious symptoms a dose of creosote.[20] Morphine as a painkiller was also frequently prescribed.

A word about opium, morphine, and other painkillers; when taking them orally, either in pill form or as a solution, soldiers quickly became addicted to the substances. By the time the war ended in 1865, many veterans were full-fledged addicts. The final irony: there were no federal controls on these addictive medications and a soldier could buy them over the counter without knowing the lasting effect of such powerful and potentially lethal drugs.[21] Not until 1906, when accurate labeling of patent medications was enacted by the Pure Food and Drug Act, did citizens become more knowledgeable about the contents of the remedies they consumed. By then, it was too late for many disabled Civil War veterans who had suffered from drug dependency for years.

Then there was the scourge of diarrhea and dysentery that proved so deadly to many a brave soldier regardless of what side held his allegiance. According to one account, chronic diarrhea "was characterized by prolonged, severe, daily diarrhea with frequent liquid or unformed stools, accompanied by weight loss, severe weakness, and wasting, often progressing to emaciation," while dysentery included all the above and the passing of blood.[22] Diarrhea and dysentery—called the "quick-step" by soldiers and the "alvine flux" by doctors— were common afflictions that could turn deadly not simply because of the illness but also because of the cure. Highly dangerous and misunderstood toxins along with blatant medical quackery became a lethal combination as arsenic, mercury, calomel, strychnine, turpentine, lead acetate, and silver nitrate were routinely prescribed. As Dr. Gross stated at an anatomy and surgery lecture, "In chronic or frequently-recurring intermittent and neuralgic affections, arsenic forms a valuable, and, indeed, in many cases, an indispensable addition."[23] For burns, he extolled the application of "white-lead paint, such as that employed in the arts, mixed with linseed oil to the consistence of very thick cream, and applied so as to form a complete coating." At the time of these pronouncements, Dr. Gross was Professor of Surgery in the Jefferson Medical College of Philadelphia.[24] Dr. Gross is not meant to be singled out, as many of his preparations were indeed legitimate cures. What is true is that most doctors during the mid-to-late 1800s prescribed the same useless and sometime dangerous remedies.

In reviewing a list of medicines in the army supply table, it is a wonder that patients survived the treatments. One prescription called Hydrargyri Chloridum Mite consisted of mercury, sulfuric acid, sodium chloride, and distilled water. The mixture was used for cleansing wounds but was withdrawn from the army's pharmacy supply table in May of 1863.[25] No reason was given for the medicine's withdrawal.

Those lucky enough were administered Spiritus Frumenti, Spiritus Vini Gallici, or Vinum Album, more commonly referred to as whiskey, brandy, and sherry wine.[26] Spirits used for medicinal purposes, especially whiskey, were mixed with several ingredients like quinine, eggnog, or punch. In a concoction more reminiscent of a cocktail than a prescription, cinnamon, cloves, and nutmeg were the main additives. The panacea was called "Spiritus Lavandulae Compositus."[27] But usually alcohol was administered undiluted. In George Worthington Adams's book *Doctors in Blue: The Medical History of the Union*

Army in the Civil War, Adams describes alcohol as "the sovereign remedy of the Civil War, rivaled only by quinine." His assertion would be difficult to argue. Adams tells of a 16-year-old soldier, a patient in a St. Louis hospital, who was administered "36 ounces of brandy a day" to keep him alive. No mention is made of the outcome. If the soldier did pass away, did he die because of his original illness or alcohol poisoning? In another case, a patient in a Virginia hospital "was given 48 ounces of eggnog and two or three bottles of porter every day for several weeks."[28] Writing home to his parents, a soldier said, "I continue to have my ale, and I think it does me good. It is strengthening and gives me a good appetite and that is what a person needs if he has got to live on hospital rations."[29] The ale was prescribed. Records show alcohol consumption was in vogue medicinally and, as shall be seen in a subsequent chapter, recreationally as well.

Pills in every conceivable size, color, and mixture were also prescribed regularly. A soldier whose hospital recovery and exploits will be revealed to a greater degree in a later chapter wrote home to say, "I am taking no medicine now except a pill every night. One man in my room has nothing but a rupture and the doctor gives him one pill every night. Another had a slim stroke and he gives him taregonic. I have faith to believe we shall all get well double-quick under such treatment." He ended the letter writing boldly: "'Pill' for a lame back, Pill, Pill, Pill, Pill."[30]

Wounded soldiers fortunate enough to survive the first week's ordeal only passed the initial test for survival. Injuries to limbs (fingers, hands, toes, and feet) were feared because of the high probability of infection. This was the case with or without amputation, though operating with unsterilized surgical instruments significantly accelerated the risks of gangrene and other infections. Victims of stomach wounds fared worse. Such wounds were looked upon as the kiss of death.

Doctors had few tricks in their medical bags to deal with infections. Although several medical professionals during the war did associate the dangers of infections with operations, few reasoned why. A Union medical cadet during the war, W.W. Keen, later a leading surgeon at the turn of the century, writes what almost sounded like an apology for the harsh treatment patients had to endure during their risky recovery. While reminiscing, he tells of unsanitary operating techniques: "The silk with which we sewed up all wounds was undisinfected. If there was any difficulty in threading a needle we moistened it with ... bacteria-laden saliva, and rolled it between bacteria-infected fingers."[31]

But there were a handful of doctors beginning to understand that cleanliness—cleaning surgical instruments and changing sponges—significantly lessened the risk of infection.[32] Pioneers like Surgeon Middleton Goldsmith emphasized the need for cleanliness even ahead of proper ventilation. He said, "The cry of the hospital builders is air, air, ventilation, ventilation! If such people had seen as much of great hospitals as they have of books, the cry would be water, water, cleanliness, cleanliness!"[33] But his cry fell upon deaf ears, at least initially. Several years would pass before infections would be studied in detail and sanitary procedures and antibiotics developed to fight them.

While thumbing through history books, readers often experience their first glimpse of the realities of war as they gaze at photos of Civil War amputees who lost limbs on the battlefield and were leaning on crutches or lying on bare ground. There seems to be a morbid fascination about seeing such carnage. What was usually not visible, however, were images showing the aftereffects of infections like hospital gangrene that proved to be more ghastly and disturbing than battlefield wounds. Hospital gangrene is a serious bacterial infection that at first progresses gradually as an ulcer and then accelerates swiftly, much to a patient's horror. When the dreaded disease first appears roughly three to four days after infection, the individual may notice "a black spot the size of a dime."[34] As the disease passes through several different stages that varies according to type (wet, dry, or gas), so does its appearance. Pus discharge, swelling, a "black-green-purple-yellowish" discoloration, dead skin and muscle tissue, along with fever are symptoms of the most common type.[35] Even without being close to the patient, one can easily detect the presence of gangrene in a hospital ward, as a patient's infected wound expels an unmistakable and distinct "sickening-sweet stench" that overwhelms the nostrils.[36] The disease is also extremely painful.[37] Once the infection enters the bloodstream, the patient's chance for survival diminishes significantly, though according to one account, nearly 75 percent of patients who underwent amputation surgery during the Civil War survived.[38] Another surprising fact: only four cases of hospital gangrene were reported in 1861. In late 1862, the numbers would increase dramatically as two epidemics suddenly surfaced at hospitals in Frederick, Maryland, and in Philadelphia. Hospital gangrene remained a significant medical issue for the balance of the war.[39] Today the disease has been all but eradicated except where poverty still plagues developing nations.

Tetanus, more commonly called lockjaw, is caused by the bacillus tetani. During the war, doctors attributed the disease to many causes: the exposure to hot or cold air; drafty air; bone splinters; bandages; poor cleansing of wounds; and even injuries caused to nerves by surgeons probing open wounds. What is known today is that the bacillus is often found in soil contaminated by deposits of horse manure which had carried the bacteria in horses' intestines. The illness is not transmitted from stepping on a rusty nail, as many believe, unless the nail was first contaminated on the ground. Surprisingly, tetanus was not very common during the war, as most battles were fought on land "untouched by the plow or prepared with manure for planting." But worries about contracting the disease were prevalent among soldiers because of the reported high mortality of 89 percent.[40]

There were other illnesses to fear, such as erysipelas, osteomyelitis, and pyemia, a disease with a higher fatality rate than tetanus. Blood poisoning was said to have taken the lives of "over 97 percent of those afflicted."[41] Facing the risks of illnesses or injuries, solders not only fought heroically on the battlefield but on operating tables and in hospital recovery wards as well.

Despite all the bad news, there were some effective medicines and treatments. Hailed as a wonder drug, quinine helped to prevent as well as cure malaria.[42] Unfortunately quinine was prescribed for illnesses where its use was dubious at best. As one soldier claimed, "This is the cure-all in the army (but ends up the kill all). I have taken a large quantity of it but will take no more if I know it."[43] Then there was bromine. Bromine treatments directly applied under the wound to cure gangrene achieved astounding results in many documented accounts, though some doctors in the twentieth century felt that "the disease has a tendency to spontaneous recovery."[44] Confederate surgeons discovered an even simpler, though disgusting, cure for gangrene. When the doctors were denied bandages while confined with their patients in a Union stockade in Chattanooga, Tennessee, they found that maggots would eat only the dead tissue, allowing the wound to heal without further treatment.[45] Was this the spontaneous recovery process mentioned above?

There were successes, some professionally documented, and others claimed but without corroboration. But the sick and wounded, unless incapacitated in the field, preferred their own home remedies and held them in higher esteem than those prescribed by military physicians.

In fairness to the good and conscientious doctors—and there were many—all relied on basic medical knowledge of the time and the severe limits that it imposed: sterilization of surgical equipment was unheard of; wounds seeping pus were considered a positive sign, which is why many doctors of the time called it "laudable pus"; disease prevention and control were only beginning to be understood; sanitation in and around campgrounds was appalling; sources of drinking water were usually contaminated because they were located near open latrines; diets were of poor quality and variety; and pneumonia caused by exposure to the elements was gravely misunderstood.

There were other concerns. As cited in Kuz and Bergtson's book *Orthopaedic Injuries of the Civil War*, and extracted from a circular of the Surgeon General's Office, a doctor said, "Operating, as I did, upon men whose vital force had been diminished by scorbutus and malaria, and exhausted by transfer from a distance, I had little hope of successful results."[46] At best, medical care provided by a doctor during the Civil war was elementary; at worst, savage.

Chapter 3

Genesis: Early 1862

The real war will never get into the books.
— Walt Whitman,
"The Real War,"
Specimen Days, 1882

In Rhode Island's capital city of Providence, casualties were beginning to mount at the Marine Hospital, so much so that the small hospital building was deemed inadequate to handle future patient estimates and their projected medical needs.[1] Expansion, if considered, was judiciously ruled out. With backs against the wall, politicians in Providence knew something had to be done and done quickly. On May 19, 1862, the surgeon general of the U.S. Army, William A. Hammond, authorized Governor William Sprague of Rhode Island to "provide suitable hospital accommodations for wounded and sick soldiers."[2] Governor Sprague hastily commissioned a team to investigate an appropriate location along Narragansett Bay. Within a month, property known as the "Portsmouth Grove Estate" in the rural town of Portsmouth was selected by state officials as the most advantageous because of "accessibility and reasonableness of terms."[3]

A former vacation resort, Portsmouth Grove Estate was a sprawling expanse with a wharf said to be capable of handling 800-ton vessels and a railway along with depot. Categorically, it appeared to be an ideal location for supply and logistics and also for patient convalescence. Governor Sprague submitted the state's recommendation to the Federal government and the site was duly accepted, though some deemed the fortress at Fort Adams in Newport a more economical and sensible choice.[4] Whether the right choice, this is where the hospital complex would ultimately be built.

Covering slightly more than twenty-three square miles of land, Rhode Island's second oldest community, Portsmouth, occupies the northernmost tip of the island. Also included as part of town are the small islands of Prudence, Patience, Hope, and Hog. North to south, Portsmouth measures approximately ten miles long and is relatively narrow, at its widest only three miles across in the southernmost sector.[5] Purchased on March 24, 1638, by William Coddington from the Narragansett Sachems, the town was founded on a compact by 100 families from Boston, nearly all of whom were Puritans. A year later seeking religious freedom, Anne Hutchinson arrived from Providence with some of her followers. William Coddington's influence soon diminished. Undaunted, he and his main followers moved to the southern end of the island, and there they founded the town of Newport. In 1640, after reconciliation, both groups formed what became known as the Rhode Island Colony. By 1647 five towns made up the United Colonies, with Portsmouth the most populous. Portsmouth, however, would not hold the distinction for long.[6]

In his book *History of Newport County, Rhode Island*, Richard M. Bayles describes Portsmouth as having "beautiful rolling hills with sufficient elevation to secure a dry and healthy condition of atmosphere." The land, he says, "is clear of trees or forest growth ... [with] beautiful views of the water on either side, the numerous islands, the jutting peninsulas, the rambling coves and the distant hills of the mainland shores greet the eye from almost every point."[7] As for the lack of trees, it is mentioned in several accounts that while the island was occupied by the British during the Revolution, their soldiers chopped and burned every available tree for warmth and cooking. This is an exaggeration to some degree, but not entirely untrue, as engravings of the island during the period picture the area as a beautiful but semi-barren expanse.

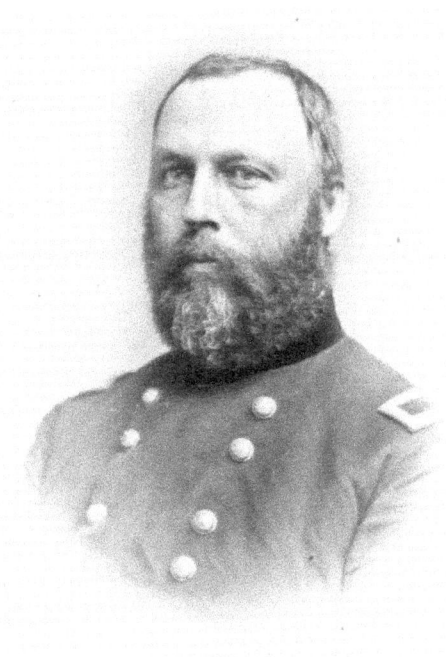

Surgeon General William A. Hammond, U.S.A. (courtesy Massachusetts Commandery Military Order of the Loyal Legion and the U.S. Army Military History Institute, Carlisle, Pennsylvania).

To the west, Portsmouth is bordered by Narragansett Bay, and diagonally to the north, the town of Bristol is visible. To the east flows the Sakonnet River, where striking views of Tiverton and Little Compton can be seen, especially during sunrise. The lands to the north offer a pristine view of Mount Hope and its bay. As for the south, the border is landlocked with the neighboring community of Middletown.[8]

Paying the ultimate compliment, Bayles offered a descriptive view of Portsmouth by saying, "This town is probably second to no other in the New England states."[9] Many residents agreed wholeheartedly with this assessment. Julia Ward Howe, author of "The Battle Hymn of the Republic," summered here with her family in a house at Lawton Valley, only two and a half miles from the future site of Portsmouth Grove Hospital.

Since its establishment and into the mid–twentieth century, Portsmouth had been predominantly agricultural, with a sizeable amount of acreage under cultivation. Residents of the town prided themselves as being self-supporting, as evidenced by the crops they grew: "potatoes, corn, oats, barley, hay, apples, peaches, strawberries, pears and garden vegetables."[10] The abundance of produce would prove a blessing to patients arriving at Portsmouth's doorstep from southern battlefields in the early summer of 1862 and those to come the following three years.

From inception, Portsmouth never had what remotely resembled a town center, and even today the town's small business enterprises are spread out along a single stretch of roadway, making it nearly impossible to identify its true center. An unsuccessful attempt was made in the colonial days to develop the center of town. The village was called Newtown. Initially the design and development of the area proved to be an ambitious undertaking, and in the process, Portsmouth made little effort to hide the fact that the primary motive was to design roads and adjacent property in a similar fashion to that of Newport. In reality, and not surprisingly, the plan and its subsequent implementation proved impractical. Perhaps the most insurmountable obstacle was the lack of a large waterfront harbor comparable to that in Newport. This deficiency proved costly and served as the ultimate death blow to the vision.[11]

There was one area, however, where Newport depended on Portsmouth's economy. As Newport grew rapidly, so did its demand for agricultural products. With an abundance of cultivated land, Portsmouth became the city's main supplier of produce.[12]

No discussion about early communities in New England would suffice without mention of stone walls, which marked all three communities on the island. None held a monopoly; walls built from split shale or solid boulders were everywhere. Constructed by farmers to mark boundaries, protect gardens and orchards, and retain cattle, they were built to last. Wooden fences were also constructed and hedges planted as well to act as barriers and enclosures. As fences and hedges became victims of the harsh and diverse New England elements, stone walls survived for generations. In letters home, soldiers traveling in steamers along Narragansett Bay commented about the island's charming countryside, making particular note of the hills, valleys, pastures, and stone walls that dotted the landscape.[13]

As the population of Portsmouth grew arithmetically between 1800 and 1860 (adding about 50 inhabitants per decade), Newport's population exploded exponentially; at least it seemed that way.[14] Compared to Portsmouth, Newport had long since been a city, and in the colonial days served as Rhode Island's capital. Newport became one of the principal trading ports in North America during the eighteenth century. Much of its growth can be traced to slave trading, in which Newport merchants played an active role. In contrast, Portsmouth, with its deep-rooted Puritanical views, chose not to participate.[15]

There is another development that greatly enhanced Newport's metropolitan image and added to its stature. In 1845, Secretary of the Navy George Bancroft helped establish the U.S. Naval Academy in Annapolis, Maryland. Because the border state of Maryland had many Southern sympathizers during the early stages of the war, Bancroft, a lifelong summer resident of Newport, persuaded members of Congress to move the military establishment to Newport. The former Atlantic House Hotel in the center of Newport was leased and used as the educational and training center during the remaining war years.

By 1862, Portsmouth's dreams of urbanization had long since dissolved, and inhabitants reconciled themselves to the fact that the town would remain small.

That being the case, soldiers destined for Portsmouth Grove Hospital who eventually recovered sufficiently but not completely from their wounds or illnesses would have to seek merriment elsewhere: in Newport and Providence, or in the neighboring state of Massachusetts, where cities like Fall River and the booming metropolis of Boston seemed more appealing. These locations offered more lively entertainment better suited, at least in the soldiers' minds, to their needs. Two brothers stationed at the hospital in 1863 visited Portsmouth on pass; they returned to the hospital in four hours. One wrote home to his mother telling her about their sightseeing trip, commenting on the beautiful scenery and the surrounding ocean. By contrast, one of the brothers had traveled to Providence a few weeks earlier and had remained there on pass for 40 hours.[16] In short, while anointed as an ideal location for patient recovery, Portsmouth had little to offer in the way of personal enjoyment for a recovering soldier other than makeshift drinking establishments typically found in other Civil War era communities that catered to military transients.

Not to be forgotten, Middletown, mentioned briefly above, was a small community sandwiched between Portsmouth and Newport. Like Portsmouth to the north, in the 1800s much of Middletown's land was used for farming. For the most part, Middletown, as did Portsmouth, served as a pass-through for those traveling by land or rail onto the island with Newport as their final destination. The travelers were looking for cultural treasures and other offerings and adventures not found in either of these two small island communities.

Interesting to note, the Rev. Obadiah Holmes, a distinguished ancestor of Abraham Lincoln, is interred at the Holmes Family Burial Ground in Middletown, a tranquil setting far from the beaten path. His remains were laid to rest 180 years prior to the establishment of Portsmouth Grove Hospital. By European standards, the island was young; by American standards, the settlement was showing its age. Of further interest, Edwin Booth, celebrated Shakespearean actor and brother of Abraham Lincoln's assassin John Wilkes Booth, built an estate along the Sakonnet River in Middletown where he vacationed for several years. The views from this location remain as fresh and spectacular as they were then.

Collectively the three communities of Newport, Middletown and Portsmouth were known as Aquidneck Island, a name that remains in vogue today. Aquidneck is an old Indian word translated by English settlers to mean *Isle of Peace*.[17] For many of the sick and injured soon to descend upon the island, the name was fitting; for others, finding peace would prove difficult if not impossible to attain.

The transfer of the Portsmouth Grove Estate for hospital use was officially recorded on May 15, 1862; but it would not be until the first of June that Captain William W. McKim, an assistant quartermaster in the United States Army, stationed in Boston, would sign a lease with the current owners of the property at a reported cost to the government of $3,000 a year.[18] The contract had a clause that allowed an annual option for renewal.[19] The clause proved to be a wise decision as the war dragged on. On the sixth of July, the U.S. Army Hospital, Portsmouth Grove, Rhode Island, was officially established. A brief description of the area's logistic capability is found in *The Medical and Surgical History of the War of the Rebellion (1861–1865)*: "The grounds were bordered at the east by the Old Colony and Newport Railroad, on which was a station with a side track ... and a good wharf on the water-side."[20]

It now became the responsibility of the Quartermaster Department to issue the required contracts to build the semi-permanent barracks and hospital buildings.[21] But somewhere along the line, there was a massive disconnect. Unquestionably the sheer number of casualties hospital personnel would have to care for was never imagined. But there was more. The vast scale of the Portsmouth Grove endeavor and the immediacy of arrivals were either poorly conveyed by the Quartermaster General's Office in Washington, D.C., or misconstrued by upstate bureaucrats and the quartermasters in both Providence and Boston. The learning experience would prove costly, especially to the first invalids who arrived.

Chapter 4

A Shaky Beginning

A hospital is no place to be sick.
— Samuel Goldwyn

General George B. McClellan believed that to defeat the Confederacy the Union army would have to seize the capital city of Richmond. In the early months of 1862, he set about devising a plan to do just that, but took precious months that caused President Abraham Lincoln to say to a White House war counsel, "If General McClellan does not want to use the Army, I would like to borrow it for a time." Although frustrated by McClellan's past and present military inactivity, what Lincoln called "the slows," he gave his endorsement, but not without reservation. In truth, he had devised his own plan of attack. But at the last minute, and in a show of support, Lincoln acquiesced in favor of his general. At his current stage of frustration and with his patience running thin, he would have agreed to almost any offensive by the general that would move the army toward victory.[1]

President Lincoln was not the only person in the administration having reservations about McClellan's ability to fight; Secretary of War Edwin Stanton also had his doubts. Whereas Lincoln was forthright with his concerns and discussions with McClellan, Stanton proved the opposite. In one breath, Stanton showed his support for the general by telling McClellan's chief engineer, General John Barnard, "General McClellan ... ought not to move until he is ready." Then, but a few days later in front of a group of legislators, he openly criticized McClellan by telling them he wished the general "sacked and replaced." He also told Senator Orville Browning, a Lincoln friend from Illinois, that the "general ought to have been removed long ago."[2]

McClellan's strategy was simple and appeared well thought out, but even the simplest plans can go awry. He would attack Richmond, Virginia, by circumventing Confederate Major General Joseph E. Johnston's troops near Manassas Junction. He would transport an estimated 100,000 men down the Chesapeake Bay to the mouth of the Rappahannock near Fort Monroe, where he would march them northwest across the peninsula to the heart of the Confederacy in Richmond. An integral component of the plan was McClellan's strength in numbers moving at speed so that Johnston could not rally his men in time to defend the capital.

Like an omen, the weather turned ugly and McClellan marched his troops through a quagmire of rain and mud, making dirt roads all but impassable. Then another problem arose: his maps were suspect. And that was not all. McClellan's reconnaissance convinced the general that he was vastly outnumbered; this was not the case, but the misconception was helped along by Confederate brigadier general John B. Magruder's tactics of deception. In one instance Magruder marched a regiment through a clearing, not once, but several times to make it appear he possessed superior numbers.[3] Furthering the ruse, he constantly moved his artillery positions. McClellan was befuddled. In reality, the North had a distinct advantage in troop strength.

On May 3, 1862, and lasting nearly the rest of the month, McClellan dug in for a "protracted siege," first near Yorktown, allowing Johnston to bring down 60,000 troops.[4] McClellan planned to attack on the fifth, but before he could, Johnston took the initiative. In the morning, the Confederates had vanished. Brash and flamboyant, McClellan declared a victory. Though claiming to be pursuing the enemy, McClellan continued to stall. As the days dragged on, battles were fought, but on the last day of May near a crossroads called Fair Oaks (Seven Pines, as the Union army called it), McClellan met his match, physically for his troops and psychologically for himself. The Union army lost a thousand fewer men in battle that day than the Confederates, who sacrificed 6,000, but the damage to McClellan's command ability and decision making were seriously eroded. After the smoke cleared, General Johnston was replaced for the same reason General McClellan would be several months later. General Johnston's replacement was Robert E. Lee.[5]

General McClellan's campaign was yet to end as he continued to operate in reverse gear. After fighting a series of battles in late June that came to be known as the Seven Days' Battles (June 25–July 1), McClellan kept falling back southward, "retrenching," as he preferred to call it, instead of retreating. Most baffling, and what solidified Lincoln's suspicions about his field commander, was that although the Union army had proved victorious in all but one of the week's conflicts, McClellan would not feel safe until he arrived at Harrison's Landing on the James River, where gunboats and supply lines would quell his fear. Historians continue to argue whether Robert E. Lee could have been defeated much earlier in the war when the Confederates launched a frontal, some say suicidal, attack at Malvern Hill against the likes of 230 Union cannons. For Lee, the outcome proved disastrous; for McClellan it would be another missed opportunity. With Lee's troops in disarray, he may have been able to march north and capture Richmond. But he did nothing of the kind.[6]

Private Alfred Luther, a resident of Warren, Rhode Island, serving with Battery C of the 1st Regiment Rhode Island Light Artillery would have the misfortune of participating in the only battle the Union lost that week: Gaines' Mill. After President Lincoln's call for troops to squelch the rebellion, Luther was the first to enlist from his hometown — whether for patriotism or a sense of adventure can only be speculated.[7] Before fighting in the Seven Days' Battles, he saw little action as a ninety-day recruit in Battery B Rhode Island Detached Militia, where the only act he witnessed was his own men in a chaotic retreat from the battlefield at First Bull Run. His three-year reenlistment with the 1st Regiment Rhode Island Light Artillery would be a chance for payback, or so he envisioned.

On the morning of June 27, Luther awoke from what little sleep he could muster during the previous night after participating in the Battle of Mechanicsville.[8] On a day already hot and humid, the Union army of 35,000 would face a reinforced Confederate force of 60,000, in one of the few times during the war where the South's fighting force mustered such a large manpower advantage. All day the cannonading and gunfire were ferocious. During the afternoon, Luther's battery repelled repeated charges on the Union's right flank, during which several officers had their horses shot out from under them. An eyewitness described the Union soldiers as "men working with the courage of desperation."[9] Firing was at point-blank range while smoke from cannon fire shrouded the few Union artillerymen still standing. A final cavalry charge by an overwhelming force of Confederates managed to bring the Union men to their knees. During the fury and while serving as the "No. 1" man of the battery, Luther was severely wounded attempting to load a 10-pound rifled gun when the cannon prematurely discharged before he could pull his arm away. The wound was massive, breaking three bones and shredding his hand and forearm just below the elbow. Standing near the powder flash, he also suffered severe burns to his face and eyes.[10]

A surgeon's headquarters was established at an old farmhouse on a hilltop not far from Grapevine Bridge where Luther was carried. Scattered around the farmyard underneath the shade of cherry trees, the wounded waited their turns to be, as a soldier described it, "hacked and maimed by the surgeon's knives."[11] Sometime during the day, Luther's arm was amputated three and a half inches below the elbow joint.[12] Shortly afterward, the Confederates overran several Union positions and the old farmhouse where Luther and the other wounded soldiers lay in agony. That day the Confederates captured a thousand prisoners, along with much-needed supplies and unspent ordnance to use in future engagements against the North. The losses to the Union were so severe that the Union victories during the week could not outweigh the losses of men, equipment, and horses during that single day's battle.[13] Alfred Luther was no longer just a critically injured soldier; he was also a prisoner of war. His rise from the ashes and his fight for survival will be discussed in a subsequent chapter.

Not all Northern men wounded in battle met the same fate as Luther, as many eluded capture and made it safely back to the rear. But the rear quickly became a sea of anxiety as rumors swirled that the Confederates were preparing to overtake the position. Fearing the makeshift hospital area would be overrun, officers decided to transport the invalids to a more stable and less dangerous location. The evacuation of the sick and wounded commenced immediately, but not without difficulty. The patients were to be loaded onto either of two steamers, the *America* or *Atlantic*, and transported to a new hospital up north. The time was none too quick as a Confederate advance on the retreating ranks at Yorktown was expected shortly. As the army fled the possibility of being overrun, buildings were abandoned and non-essential supplies were left in heaps at the dock. The wounded were brought to the ships half-starved, several barely clinging to life, while a majority of surgeons were still on the battlefields tending to the recently wounded. Making matters worse, nobody was authorized to take charge of the men.[14] Dr. Francis L. Wheaton, who commanded several field hospitals, assumed the responsibility for moving the patients out of harm's way, first to Fort Monroe and then to Rhode Island, a judgment call debated by some historians for years to come. The question was and still remains whether he conducted the evacuation without official orders.[15]

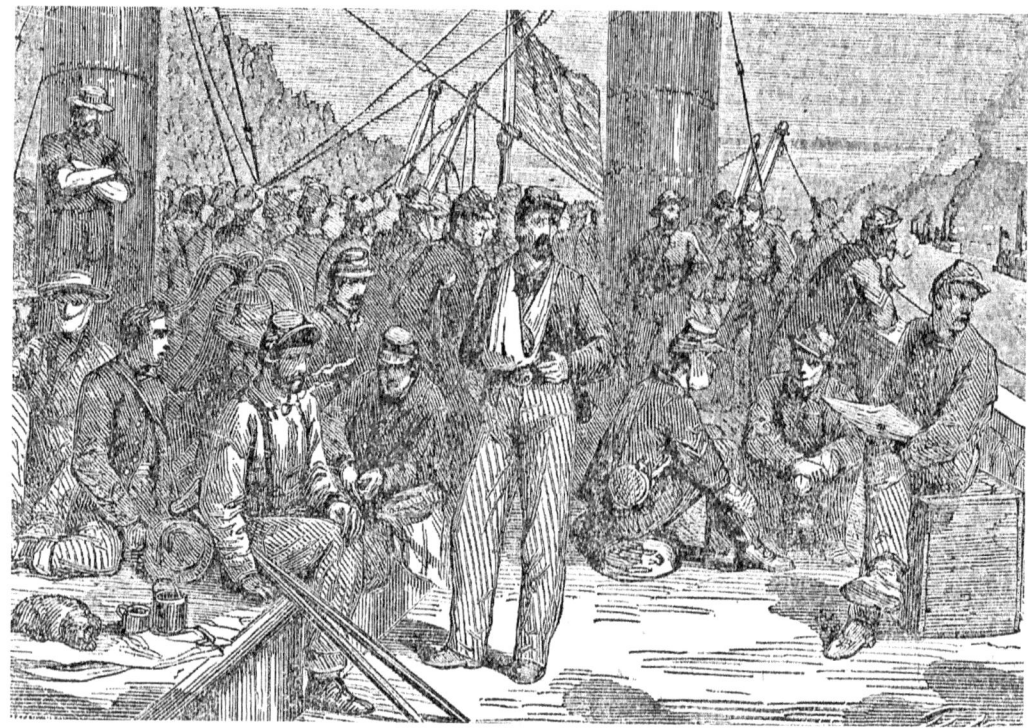

Battlefield casualties crowded on the upper deck of a hospital steamer while being transported to a hospital (*The Boys of '61* by Charles Carleton Coffin).

Private William S. Dennett, Company B, U.S. Engineers from Saco, Maine, had spent a month at a field hospital called Camp Winfield Scott after being "placed in a small log Negro shanty on a shelf built with poles and sticks" that was situated roughly "three or four feet from the ground against the logs of the hut." He would remain within the austere confines of the 8 x 10 foot area with two other "very sick men," a soldier with severe diarrhea and another with an undisclosed illness and raw bedsores on his back. They would wait there until the Fourth of July, then be placed aboard the *Atlantic*. Dennett, too, was seriously ill with "typhoid or camp fever." Dennett remembers his doctor calling it "malarial typhoid fever."[16]

On board the steamer there were "no stores, no beds, no hospital stewards, no food, no stimulants," as a nurse later described.[17] Perhaps her assessment was an exaggeration, but one not far removed from reality. The disparaging scene would have been a recipe for disaster had it not been for the U.S. Sanitary Commission. But even they had their hands full with all the confusion and panic rampant at the docks. During the chaos, only a few meager provisions were loaded on board. With a bit of foresight, Dennett was fortunate. He sold his revolver for $12, and as he explains, "With the money, I went to the sutlers and bought 'Boston' crackers and other 'dainties' from time to time which, I have no doubt, saved my life for we had nothing but salt meat and very poor hardtack to eat in the hospital."[18] The same could be said for the voyage.

After the remaining invalids were on the *America*, the boat departed for Rhode Island late on the afternoon of the Fourth. Because of *Atlantic*'s larger displacement and resultant hull depth, the loading of the second steamer would have to be accomplished by ferrying passengers in a smaller transport from the wharf to the *Atlantic*, moored in deeper water. This necessity slowed the process considerably and the *Atlantic* was unable to depart Yorktown until the following morning.[19]

The vessels carried 1,724 patients (all enlisted men), including 60 to 70 Confederate prisoners, 9 surgeons and 108 male nurses.[20] The captain of the *America* was given strict orders to rendezvous with the *Atlantic* in Newport Harbor without making contact with the shore before proceeding in tandem several miles up Narragansett Bay to their final destination. Several correspondents would write that the weather was fine and the passage went without incident, other than the passing of Pvt. Eliza Smith, Company B, 101st Pennsylvania Infantry, who died on Independence Day on board one of the vessels before departure and was buried in a Yorktown cemetery, and Pvt. Isaac T. Sherwood (37th North Carolina Infantry), a Confederate, who died the following day during passage and was buried at sea.[21]

Aboard one of the vessels, junior medical officer Dr. George M. Sternberg not only served as a physician but also a patient, having contracted typhoid fever at Harrison's Landing. His first experience as an assistant surgeon was at First Bull Run, where he was captured during the Union rout by the Confederates. Somehow, Dr. Sternberg managed to escape. His medical knowledge and practice would be severely tested during the following months.[22]

While at sea, the surgeons along with their staff looked after the immediate needs of the patients.[23] The doctor-to-patient ratio was roughly 1:192, an alarming statistic in anyone's mind. With depleted numbers, surgeons had to rely heavily upon their stewards and nurses, assigning them countless duties throughout the ships. The accommodations at the time were described as "immense" but measured against today's standards were dreadfully crowded. When a nurse was allowed on board one of the transports, she saw men crammed into every conceivable space; in staterooms, on floors, in passageways, and on every deck. When similar steamers from Yorktown laden with their human cargo of pain and suffering docked at large port cities like Baltimore and New York, they created an immediate sensation.[24] Nobody could have imagined the extent of injuries and illnesses. Citizens from Newport, Middletown, and Portsmouth, Rhode Island, would soon get their fill.

On Saturday morning, the fifth of July, Lt. Governor Samuel G. Arnold of Rhode Island notified Mayor William Cranston of Newport that the hospital ships were on their way.[25] Having been forewarned by dispatch from Yorktown, Aquidneck Islanders had no idea when the transports would arrive, so citizens kept a sharp lookout at the entrance of Narragansett Bay. The first sighting of a convalescent ship came a little after dawn on Sunday morning, July 6.[26] Not long afterward and contrary to orders, an officer on the steamer *America* (misidentified in the papers as the *Coatzacoalcos*) stopped in Newport shortly after daybreak. Dr. G.C. Striebling was in command of the ship. A prior plan by officials to provide a tugboat assist to such vessels was immediately put into effect. Departing around 9 A.M. and traveling ten miles north, the first ship from hell arrived at Portsmouth Grove around 10:00 A.M.[27] According to Thomas Coggeshall Jr.'s account, the weather was brutally hot, "92 in the shade," and one of the island's warmest days so far that summer.[28] The heat would soon intensify but not solely because of the scorching sun.

There would be no oration or ribbon-cutting ceremony by politicians, as only a single high-level dignitary from the state was in attendance to receive the sick and wounded. But an estimated crowd of 1,800 citizens (the island's population in 1862 was about 14,500), including local physicians, did descend upon Portsmouth Grove. They came by foot, on horseback, or as drivers and passengers in omnibuses, coaches, buggies and express wagons.[29] Some came under sail.[30] Whether for personal curiosity or a genuine desire to offer assistance, they arrived en masse. By noon all the horses at the livery stables in Newport were said to be taken.[31] Regrettably, the people who came to help were in for a rude awakening. As the situation began to unfold, matters quickly went awry. Except for a resort hotel, there were no buildings, whether permanent or temporary, to house the massive number of invalids. Destitute of facilities and medical supplies, the area lacked nearly everything a patient required for proper medical care, even by mid–nineteenth-century standards. Except for shade trees in the grove, there was no escape from the relentless summer sun and humidity during that first day.

Tensions between the military and civilians escalated when Dr. Striebling refused any assistance with the unloading of patients, though he did allow several locals on board to comfort the sick and wounded.[32] The only aid that could be offered (and eagerly accepted) was "lemonade and cool water."[33] Later, a citizen reported that he witnessed a patient expire while writing a letter to his parents, stating that he expected to recover shortly.[34] Dr. Striebling remained steadfast. No patients were allowed to disembark until the *Atlantic* sailed into port. The citizens were enraged, but there would be neither negotiations nor a resolution to the matter. Losing patience, most of the crowd dispersed without incident before the *Atlantic* arrived about 4:30 P.M. The anchor was dropped sometime after 5 P.M.[35]

The first to be brought ashore were the dead, and coffins had to be "hastily prepared" for a "decent interment."[36] Thomas Coggeshall Jr. from nearby Middletown visited the site that day, arriving just before sunset, when the weather would have been a tad cooler. He stayed an hour or two before returning home.[37] What he witnessed that evening probably remained with him for years to come. In a letter dated July 9, he describes the scene: "I saw them carry seven dead bodies up from the shore that was taken out of the steamer. They were in rough pine board coffins and they carried them up above the house to the east of the woods and left them standing there on the ground as there had been no graves dug then."[38] Coggeshall surmised that the seven remains would be buried the next day. He was mistaken. Soon after he departed, graves were dug and the dead were buried that night, aided by the illumination of a lamplight. Officiating at the solemn occasion was the Rev. George W. Chevers, rector of St. Paul's Episcopal Church in Portsmouth. The ceremony was witnessed by Lt. Governor Arnold, his wife, Surgeon Wheaton and members of his staff, a Mrs. Borden Chase, and a contingent of soldiers. Those in attendance must have felt that the nocturnal scene was more reminiscent of a tomb robbery than a sacred burial rite. Three more deceased would be buried in similar fashion the following night.[39]

Though the first phase of unloading the invalids was completed, over 1,650 still remained onboard. Those unfortunates had to wait decidedly longer before catching their first breath of fresh air. If they survived, it would be the first clean air they inhaled in over a week.

Dr. Wheaton, an 1826 graduate of Brown University Medical School and a member of the 2nd Regiment Rhode Island Volunteers, commanded the *Atlantic*. Upon arrival, Dr. Wheaton would become the first commanding officer at Portsmouth Grove with the official title surgeon-in-charge. Possessing impeccable credentials, with service during the Mexican War and later as Rhode Island's surgeon general for four terms, he appeared an excellent choice for the difficult assignment.[40] But he learned quickly that his physician skills and organizational abilities would be severely tested as he confronted casualties of enormous proportions with an intolerable and nearly impossible patient-to-doctor workload. Soon his concerns would swell. Dr. Wheaton and his wards had arrived at a hospital totally unprepared for this level of casualties.[41]

The drama now unfolding at Portsmouth Grove was not an aberration; it had been and would continue to be the rule. As more hospitals sprouted in the north due to basic necessity, the same sins would be repeated. Whether through negligence, malfeasance, disorganization, miscommunication, or all of the above, army general hospital startups were not a picture of sound management practices or well-oiled machines. The absurdities that had taken place on the steamers while at sea were only a precursor of things to come.

With the hasty departure from Yorktown, neither vessel carried sufficient tents or hospital supplies. Even food rations were meager. During the voyage, men ate only hardtack and salted beef, a diet acceptable to hardened soldiers but not prescribed or beneficial for the sick and wounded. A young man later told a reporter that on board the *Atlantic* he witnessed a feverish and starving comrade who seized a piece of raw pork and devoured it only to die within a half-hour.[42]

The soldiers now arriving at Portsmouth Grove came from the earliest battles of the Peninsula Campaign. Adding insult to injury, the casualties had not had their wounds tended to in days.[43] They were a frightened, dirty, half-starved, stinking mess of soldiers, many barely clinging to life.

As stated earlier, the first day at Portsmouth Grove was an inauspicious beginning as only 40 sick, a few of the wounded, and the dead were unloaded. Some citizen volunteers were later allowed to carry tents and other meager supplies off a vessel, but only after "sharp talk" between the two parties.[44] The next day, the pace of patient disembarkation improved, but not to the satisfaction of the local citizens. Accounts differ about the time it took for all the patients to be landed, some saying 48 hours and others 4 days.[45] Four days seems accurate according to the date of Thomas Coggeshall Jr.'s letter in which he says, "I heard last night that they had landed most all of them."[46] Though many soldiers could walk down the gangplank, several had to be carried off the ship on litters or, if these were unavailable, with blankets. Until given permission to disembark, men roasted between decks where the lack of oxygen caused stifling conditions and putrid odors continued to make them sick. Patient illnesses varied: typhoid fever along with diarrhea being the most prevalent, to the more severe, festering wounds and infections caused by unsanitary and non-sterile amputations.

Typhoid was an extremely common disease during the war and a savage killer of men. The disease is transmitted by the ingestion of feces through contaminated food or water. The bacterium travels on its deadly mission throughout the body in a four-stage process, with the third stage being the most dangerous. During this stage, a patient's fever can reach 104 degrees Fahrenheit and no vaccine to combat the disease had yet been discovered.[47] A brief article noted that "perhaps one-quarter of noncombat deaths in the Confederacy resulted from this disease."[48]

Of interest is an account written in Geoffrey C. Ward's book *The Civil War: an Illustrated History*, by a Union chaplain who served in the Peninsula Campaign. He writes about "a great secesh army of wood ticks…. Few [are] so happy as not to find half a dozen of these villainous bloodsuckers sticking in their flesh."[49] Perhaps some illnesses and fever associated with other known diseases resulted from the bites and latching-on of these eight-legged parasites.

When night fell, those in less serious condition were still lying on litters or bare ground, covered by only a blanket as tents and tent posts were difficult to find. While some tents were furnished, many patients were incapable of raising them, even those less feeble, and as one newspaper reported, "although out of danger, they are very far from strong."[50] The more serious cases were placed in large hospital tents that would accommodate about 20 men each, south of the former hotel in what one correspondent described, in terms usually reserved for a vacation travel guide, as "cooled by the prevailing southwest winds."[51]

William Dennett, a future ward master at the hospital, would write that he was "glad enough to escape the horrible scenes onboard ship."[52] Other veterans of the infamous voyage surely felt the same. Later during the week when a local newspaper reporter asked the medical staff about deaths that occurred a previous day, the response was blunt, sarcastic and unsympathetic: "There's one over there in that tent that ought to be dead, he's been long enough about it."[53]

Four men died the first afternoon of the first full day. All were privates. They were Samuel E. Clift, Company D, 61st Pennsylvania Infantry; Abraham Irving, Company D, 37th North Carolina Infantry; Peter Cristy, Company K, 5th Michigan Volunteer Infantry; and Abraham Evans, Company K, 37th North Carolina Infantry. Of the four, two would be buried that night and the other two the following day. The Grim Reaper favored neither Union nor Confederate soldiers as an equal number of lives were sacrificed. Tragically, though ten soldiers had been laid to rest, another ten would suffer the same fate by the end of the week.[54]

On the second day, local citizens, most of whom were ladies, took the afternoon steamer *Perry*, destined for Providence, and disembarked at the hospital wharf laden with bread and butter, cordials, preserves, wine, and other foodstuffs needed for convalescence. A report that officers appropriated much of the food for use at their quarters is probably true. This abominable situation wiped out what little morale remained within the lower ranks.

After the unloading of patients was completed, some semblance of order prevailed. Some time during the first week's turmoil a cemetery was cut deep into the grove. The burial yard would predate by twenty-two months the first veteran burial at what would later become America's most hallowed ground: Arlington National Cemetery.

When deaths occurred, which were frequent during the first month at the hospital, a funeral detail was selected and went about its ghastly work of digging the graves, placing the bodies in wooden caskets, reading a Bible passage if clergy was available, then lowering the coffin with the remains into the ground for eternal rest. The graves were then covered with Rhode Island soil and properly marked with head and foot pieces provided by the hospital carpenters. The headboard listed the deceased's name, company, regiment, state from which he had mustered, and the date of death.[55]

After Private John Robinson, Company F, 88th New York Infantry died on July 8, a fellow soldier inscribed on his headboard, "*He never turned his back on an enemy or on a friend.*"[56] The tribute did not last, as the wooden marker weathered and disappeared in time.

Another brave soldier, Private Albert H. Stone, a native son from Scituate and a member of Co I, 2nd Regiment Rhode Island Volunteers, seemed to be recuperating after a bout with typhoid fever; so much so, he was seen walking the hospital grounds. Seven days after Private J. Robinson's passing, Stone suffered a relapse from which he never recovered.[57]

On July 22, Private Frederick Wolfe, Company E, 72nd Pennsylvania Infantry died. His memorial service is well documented in a letter to the editor of the *Newport Daily News* and affords the reader an opportunity to review the exact proceedings. Pvt. Wolfe was wounded at Fair Oaks in Virginia. After a difficult struggle of nearly two months, he died. At 4 P.M., his remains were placed in a coffin, dressed with an American flag, and carried in procession upon the shoulders of men from his company and brigade. Stopping in front of the main administration building, the mourning group was joined by the Pawtucket Guard (on duty that week), surgeons, clergymen, and many patients. "Under martial plaintive music," the procession moved to the grave. Upon arrival, the mourners formed a square around the grave, after which scriptures were read and prayers said by the Rev. Dr. Jackson of Newport. When the Rev. Jackson finished, a hymn was sung. Then Dr. J. Spaulding moved to the head of the coffin and "solemnly and fervently" committed the remains to the Almighty. Gathering at the side of the coffin, a three-round salute was fired on command by a rifle squad. Shortly after, the band began to play and the procession proceeded to the main hospital area before officially being dismissed. Pvt. Wolfe was well liked and many tears were shed during and after the funeral.[58] A widow, mother and sister at home in Philadelphia would soon learn of their tragic loss, a heartbreaking scenario played out every single day during the deadly conflict.

Eventually a small white picket fence would be erected around the cemetery, with premises described by a soldier "to be very pleasantly located." "Headboards to each grave with the names of the men buried," he commented further.[59] During the next three years, the graveyard would be consecrated with the remains of Union and Confederate soldiers on a fairly regular basis—sometimes weekly, sometimes daily, and sometimes multiple times each day.

Patients died so frequently at the hospital over the next three years that the matter became commonplace among the men. Corporal George H. Peck, a member of the Hospital Guards—Rhode Island Volunteers and a resident of Bristol, Rhode Island, noted the following in his diary:

- June 27, 1864: "Five soldiers buried, one of them a rebel."
- July 8, 1864: "Four more buried, and they are still dying."
- July 18, 1864: "[More] buried in the yard."
- Aug. 5, 1864: "One corpse went away in [rail] cars this afternoon."
- Aug. 14, 1864: "[A soldier died] under the operation of amputation."

- Aug. 30, 1864: "Two corpses sent away today, one in the boat, a sergeant, and one [a] private in the cars."
- Oct. 19, 1864: "Four buried today."[60]

As noted, not all who died at Portsmouth Grove were buried in the cemetery. After notification of a loved one's death, if the family desired, the body would be removed from the dead house or disinterred if the remains were already buried. Depending on the distance to the deceased's hometown, some remains were shipped by boat while others were placed on rail cars—railroads nurtured a thriving side business hauling caskets containing the remains of the war's fatalities. Bodies transported in this manner were embalmed to survive the journey, greatly lessening the risk that the remains would putrefy en route. Embalming, a technique substituting preservation chemicals for body fluids, had been employed in Europe some fifty years previous and was a less expensive means of preparing bodies for shipment than the packing of remains in ice and sealing them in metal containers. Some of these containers were so elaborate they were designed with a see-through window so the family could view the face of the deceased at the funeral ceremony. Deceased officers were the usual recipient of such elaborate preparations. It is fair to assume that relatively few bodies transported from Portsmouth Grove were embalmed and those shipped within the state were probably not subjected to the technique unless requested by a surviving family member.[61]

Most of those who died from Rhode Island were brought home, as was 47-year-old Private Elijah Pomeroy, Battery G, 1st Regiment Rhode Island Light Artillery, who passed away in Ward 7 on September 12, 1862. His remains were transported the following day, possibly by rail car, then by a horse-drawn hearse, to his family on Oliver Street in Providence, with burial services conducted on the Sabbath. He left a grieving widow and five deeply scared children.[62] Another local was Private Samuel S. Whiting of Company A, 12th Regiment Rhode Island Volunteers, who was severely wounded in the wrist at Fredericksburg and died of complications thirty-three days later. His remains rest at First Cemetery in his hometown of East Greenwich, Rhode Island.[63]

The hospital did not look much like a hospital, as Dr. Cyrus Bacon, Jr. could attest after seeing the grounds for the first time. Dr. Bacon, Assistant Surgeon, U.S. Army, originally served with the 7th Michigan Volunteer Infantry before being assigned

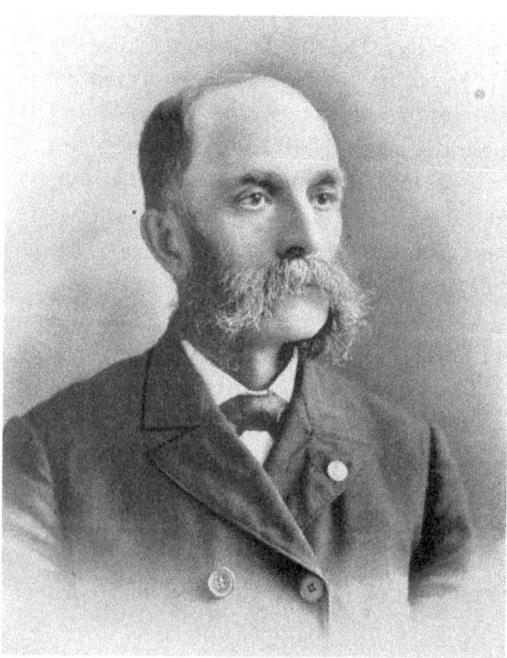

Through his diary, George H. Peck provided a wealth of information about the inner workings of the hospital, especially the hardships faced and the questionable antics of some of the guards (*Representative Men and Old Families of Rhode Island* by anonymous editors).

to the Rhode Island hospital. In his diary, he notes that in early July when he first saw the hospital complex, it consisted of a "hotel with the small outbuildings of sheds, saloons, swings, bowling alley, bathing houses. Tents are being rapidly pitched for the sick. Necessarily slow...." On the following day Dr. Bacon complained about the summer heat. He added "I am so unwell.... Can eat but little. Took my blanket and lay out in the shade part of the afternoon." He noted that men arrived from an artillery company stationed at Fort Adams in Newport volunteering their services. Not mentioned in his account were sailors from the frigate *Constitution* who brought tents, but not enough to shelter several hundred invalids.[64]

In the meantime, to assure order at the hospital, on July 12, Francis L. Wheaton, as the surgeon in charge, drafted a brief note to Brigadier General Edward C. Mauran, the adjutant general of the State of Rhode Island, asking for a detail of fifty men along with a lieutenant and six days of rations. The request proved timely. Two days later, a Confederate prisoner attempted an escape. According to a newspaper account, the Confederate arrived at the dock dressed in civilian clothes but was immediately recognized and apprehended before he could board the steamship *Perry*. This action may have precipitated Dr. Wheaton's writing a similar note requesting men five days later. In the same letter, he asked for relief of the present company. Similar requests would follow into the month of August.[65]

By now the grounds looked like a mass of off-white canvas tents except for the former hotel and stables. As the *Bristol Phenix* astutely pointed out in its Saturday morning edition of July 12, "The tents are arranged in long rows on the lawn in front of the house with wide streets running east and west, presenting the appearance of quite a village."[66] The house (the former resort hotel) was turned into officers' quarters and then an administration building. Portsmouth Grove had become a tent city and the complex would remain unchanged for some time.

Unofficially, the hospital was called Wheaton after its first commanding officer.[67] Previously, a hospital in Yorktown held the same name. When the name was changed to Portsmouth Grove Hospital is anyone's guess, but it probably happened within the first month of the hospital's existence; the reason why will soon become self-evident.

Chapter 5

The Pen Is Mightier Than the Sword

To the press alone, chequered as it is with abuses, the world is indebted for all the triumphs which have been gained by reason and humanity over error and oppression.
— James Madison,
Report on the
Resolutions, 1799

Watching one steamer moored just off the wharf, several citizens witnessed a surgeon and his staff "deliberately" eating dinner in the shade of an awning on the quarterdeck. Later, adding insult to injury, the officers relaxed, smoking cigars.[1] The locals were appalled. Wasting little time, the citizens of Aquidneck Island complained to their representatives. Matters quickly escalated and finally reached Washington. Concerned by the reports, the War Department sent an officer to investigate the accusations.

In the meantime, construction of wards had started, and a local branch of the U.S. Sanitary Commission was established, supplying the men with different foodstuffs not found in the regular hospital diet. Even so, when a reporter from the *Newport Daily News* was asked to check on conditions at the hospital, he was shown "tables lavishly prepared for dinner," but soon learned all had been a charade. A mother of a patient told the correspondent that her son "wishes the reporter visited the hospital more as we have enough to eat when you come."[2]

The press was a powerful force in the nineteenth century and had a significant influence on public opinion. Within days of the steamers' docking, the *Newport Daily News* went on the offensive with a tirade written and published to stir the hearts and minds of the local citizenry. The effort was a resounding success. On July 9, under "Local News Items—The Sick and Wounded at Portsmouth Grove,"[3] the newspaper presented its case against the establishment by asking several searing questions and voicing numerous condemnations directed against the obvious: the federal government, the state of Rhode Island, and the surgeon-in-charge, Dr. Francis L. Wheaton. Although names were omitted, the thinly veiled accusations made the culprits easy to determine and identify.

The journalistic assault was presented in two-plus columns and sectioned by paragraphs listing each concern separately. The first, "Who's to blame?," vented against those responsible for packing some 800 soldiers into a steamer during an oppressive summer month by describing it as "an outrage upon humanity."[4] The correspondent writing the article had factual evidence that invalids were left to go without food and that wounds were not dressed for days.

While castigating the men in charge, they praised the work of a lieutenant from a New York regiment, he too an invalid, who voluntarily "made large quantities of gruel and distributed it to the sick with his own hands." The soldier performed other merciful works as a steward, like doling out jellies to the more seriously ill and injured, a gesture that prolonged, if not saved, the lives of a dozen men.[5]

Not finding anyone accountable seemed especially disturbing to the newspapermen as they displayed their frustration by stating, "So the blame in all these matters will pass from the War Department down through every subordinate department and official, and phiz out like a railroad accident, with nobody to blame." But they offered a caveat: "No! The people will take this matter in hand, and the culprit though he may hope to escape in the din and smoke of strife and carnage; yet, rest assured, he will be brought to strict justice."[6]

That the *Atlantic* was unable to dock and disembark, its passengers did not miss the reporter's scrutiny. The newspaper criticized the use of only a small steamer, the *Sylph*, and a few scows to do the work of what should have been many. Conceding difficulties that needed to be overcome, the editorial went on to state, "Energy and system would have conquered them, and every man [would] have been landed yesterday."[7]

The second criticism dealt with the selection of Portsmouth Grove as the appropriate place to establish a hospital. Fort Adams in Newport was presented as "a more eligible and more economical place." The government already owned the garrison and a lease would not be required. Further, the fort included several acres of land situated along the bay that offered "invigorating breezes" and ample room for tents. A bakery was already on the premises with the capability to bake soft bread for the more seriously ill patients (also considered a highly sought-after food by many hungry soldiers, healthy or otherwise). Additionally, the barracks were plentiful and spacious. Easy access to large vessels and the proximity to a major port city (Newport) were distinct advantages. Why then was Fort Adams not selected? This is where it becomes interesting. The reporter answered the question thus: "But it was *too far south*. The people in the north[ern] part of our State are so thoroughly loyal that it seems to be unfortunate for anybody else to live in a southerly direction from them." As a final dig at upstate politicians and the lack of support for their southern Rhode Island constituents, they concluded: "We say, the ways of Providence, are inscrutable, '*they is.*'"[8]

The article failed to mention two major issues with using Fort Adams as a hospital. First, the dungeon-like atmosphere, produced by concrete walls and low ceilings, was damp and dingy, not at all conducive to recovery from respiratory illnesses. Second, no passenger or freight rail lines existed for miles. To make the location work, everything would have to be transported by dirt road or steamer.

Additional criticism in the article dealt with slow progress, not accepting aid from local citizens, and the reluctance to accept food, shelter and supplies to care for the invalids. Though an obvious and easy solution, the failure was reiterated in the strongest of terms. Earlier, hundreds of men from the city came to unload passengers. All were rebuffed until Surgeon General Wheaton's arrival. "Many of the returning men were able bodied and had there been more system or head [supervision], [they] might have been more useful in preparing accommodations," the newspaper attested. In the end, the opportunity was lost, as only a few citizens were granted permission to assist.[9]

The correspondent then turned his attention to the "secesh" prisoners. The newspaper noted that some had already died, and of those with whom he was able to converse, several felt mixed sentiments about their allegiance. Some despised their captors and were determined to fight on, while others felt the Confederacy had deceived them. Several expressed a pleasant surprise at how well they were being treated, at least thus far, and appeared grateful for all the attention. The correspondent seemed awestruck by two wounded Confederates. One prisoner was recuperating nicely from a clean gunshot wound that passed through his liver and right lung and exited out his back. The second, "a pitiable case," had his lower jaw shot away and was still in excruciating pain.[10] If he survived, he may well have become a social outcast, as the technology to perform major reconstructive surgery did not exist at the time.

Concluding the article, the newspaper issued another urgent appeal for food and clothing. Men of the 9th and 10th Regiment Rhode Island Volunteers responded by sending shirts, drawers, stockings, and handkerchiefs that were used on their campaign in and around the Washington, D.C., area. Now the citizens of Providence and the rest of the state were requested to answer the call.[11] And answer they did. A young soldier of seventeen was given a clean shirt from the clothing drive but didn't know how to thank the benefactor. The following brief conversation was reported to have taken place during the encounter:

> "But I have no money," said the soldier.
>   The citizen looked the young man in the eye and said, "Don't talk to me about money. We don't come here for money."

The soldier was said to have tears in his eyes while accepting the needed clothing without further comment.[12]

Food always seemed in short supply, but soft bread was in dire need. Give "bread, bread, bread," was the plea. A thousand loaves of bread were required every single day at the hospital to satisfy the appetites of the convalescents. Hardtack, a diet staple in the field, would no longer suffice, as the sick simply could not digest the hard cracker; and even if they could, they would not be sufficiently nourished to help with the recovery process. A call was also made for black raspberries to help those with "bowel complaints."[13]

Clean clothing continued to be desperately needed. Shirts, nightgowns, slippers, and undergarments were only a few of the items requested from civilians. A reporter noted that he witnessed several men bathing and later being "compelled to sit down and go through with the interesting amusement of picking off the vermin" before dressing.[14]

Waste sanitation and removal became a significant issue. Brass toilet pails were requested from the general public because they were constructed such that they left little odor. As most tents were lacking such pails, outhouses had been placed close to the abodes. The foul odor became even worse when lime was thrown on the slop to accelerate the decomposition; as a correspondent noted, it was "almost unendurable." The brass toilet pails would allow for the outhouses to be moved a greater distance away from the living quarters, thus eliminating much of the stench.[15]

On July 14, still seeing little progress at the hospital after an earlier visit, the newspaper continued its offensive. Acknowledging the difficulties of caring for the sick and wounded on the battlefield and in a hospital, especially in times of chaos and in such large numbers, the newspaper maintained that still "there is a vast difference in the qualifications of men for certain positions." Calling those who succeed under trying circumstances "magicians," the newsmen documented their concept of a managerial failure by saying, "Others ... when placed in such positions seem to be stricken with a paralysis of the few faculties which have been committed to their charge, and dwindle away into imbecility whereby the public interest committed to their keeping, suffer." Further, they said what others already knew: that far too many surgeons were entirely unqualified for the job. A bitter soldier told a reporter, "It seems as if the physicians do not care for a man after he is rendered unfit for duty by a wound or disease."[16]

Before leaving the hospital grounds, a correspondent felt privileged to meet a 61-year-old man from Pittsburgh, considerably senior to those in his outfit, by the name of David Miller. Miller served with Company I, 102nd Pennsylvania Infantry before being wounded at the Battle of Williamsburg. He seemed to be slowly improving yet weak, having suffered "from want of due care." A trusted nurse at the hospital, a Mr. Wood, washed the patient and placed him in clean clothes given for the occasion. The action seemed to have a resounding effect and revived the old gent. The soldier was so pleased that he offered all the money he had in exchange. "We think he will recover," the reporter concluded.[17] On a second visit, the same reporter saw that Pvt. Miller had been given a Bible from a Mrs. Mason, who inscribed it on the flyleaf. Again, Miller was greatly appreciative. A Mr. Seabury also presented Miller with a pair of glasses for reading. Four days later, the veteran soldier from Pittsburgh took a turn for the worse. Sometime that day it was reported, "He went to his home, where 'the wicked cease from troubling, *and the wrong are at rest.*'"[18]

Another correspondent visited the hospital at about the same time. He asked if he could assist with feeding the sick, but a group of invalids pointed to a man in the tent and said that "it was *too late.*"[19] With little hope for recovery, the man died soon after. The patients attributed his death to criminal negligence caused by improper care and inattention by the hospital staff.[20] Whether he could have been saved is anyone's guess, but the effort to keep him alive by those entrusted with the responsibility was unquestionably an utter failure.

Criticism about the intolerable situation was not confined to Aquidneck Islanders and its press alone. Across the bay, the *Bristol Phenix*, in consideration of information furnished by the *Providence Press*, revised its initial opinion of the situation, for which it had at first displayed a great deal of forbearance. "Reliable reports, coupled with a careful personal observation yesterday, lead us to belief that we formed a hasty estimate of the character and executive ability in our remarks relative to a certain high official ... and yet it seems incredible that one who is reputed to be so incompetent should have been suffered to hold so responsible a position for such length of time, especially when human life is at stake," the paper said. Not to prejudge further, the article concluded:

"We forbear further remark, waiting an investigation which we are assured will be sought for."[21]

Months earlier, Mathew Brady's horrifying photographs brought home the carnage of war to Aquidneck Islanders, just as they did within all communities, North and South. A northern reporter elaborated upon the point by saying, "Mr. Brady has done something to bring to us the terrible reality and earnestness of the war. If he has not brought bodies and laid them in our door-yards and among our streets, he has done something very like it."[22] But now the images became visceral and considerably more focused and personal. What locals saw were no longer horrifying photographs viewed by males and stored out of sight to protect the feminine eye; they were living, breathing human beings who inadvertently served as models for the photographer's camera. Citizens visiting the hospital — male and female — were faced with casualties of the dreadful war scattered throughout the grounds with bodies laid at the dooryard for all Aquidneck Islanders and visitors to see. With a crushing blow, the effects of war had unceremoniously come home to roost in the small rural community of Portsmouth and its former resort village, Portsmouth Grove.

By the end of the third week, the hospital was still without permanent facilities, adequate supplies, and sufficient food. Another call went out for bread and milk, milk being the top priority.

Clean clothing continued to be increasingly scarce. Stockings, drawers, shirts and pantaloons were requested from the general public along with a clarification: "secondhand ones will answer." There was no time for fashion statements. A soldier was given a change of undergarment, but was still without new pants. He could not make the change until new pants were found, as mites from his old pair would have quickly spread to the new clothes.[23]

Mattresses, commonly called bed sacks at the time, were in short supply. The ladies from Aquidneck Island, the rest of the state, and Fall River, Massachusetts, were asked to manufacture and contribute over three hundred without delay. The dimensions were specified as follows: "length six and one half feet; width three and one half feet." Pillows of the same quantity were also requested.[24]

Semi-permanent facilities were now under construction at the hospital, but few details about progress and completion dates survive. The first building erected was a barracks and was to be occupied by those without cots, or for those "occupying small tents."[25] It was never the government's intention to build permanent structures at the site. The facilities were to be "generally framed buildings of a simple character," to allow for rapid construction, as was the case for most general hospitals during the war.[26]

Civilian laborers performed most of the construction with some help provided by the more capable invalids. Yet a long road still lay ahead before patients were properly sheltered from the elements. The plan was to have a significant portion of the complex finished before the bone-chilling weather set in about mid–November.

Stumbling and fumbling remained the status quo, though not nearly as catastrophic as the two preceding weeks. Interestingly, the *Newport Advertiser* said that the sick and wounded were "getting along finely."[27] On what basis this was determined is uncertain, but based on several accounts, it was highly presumptuous. In the meantime, Dr. Wheaton set up a pass system to manage the "rush of visitors." The pass could be obtained from either civic or military officials, and for Newport residents, directly from Mayor William H. Cranston's office.[28] The policy may have been implemented for three reasons, one questionable and two legitimate: to deflect the harsh criticism of the townspeople of the poor handling of patients and lack of suitable shelter by restricting access and keeping visitors under close scrutiny; to monitor the diets of patients being given gifts of food deemed unsuitable for their recovery; and to keep civilians whose interest was nothing more than idle curiosity off the premises.[29]

There had been reports of deaths at the hospital attributed to improper food consumption provided by well-intentioned visitors. As Sergeant Whitman W. Bosworth explains, "There is a good many ladies come here to visit friends. They have to be escorted up to Headquarters by a guard and are not allowed to bring in *any* [Bosworth's emphasis] eatables whatever."[30] Bosworth, a member of Company I, 15th Regiment Massachusetts Volunteer Infantry, had arrived at Portsmouth Grove Hospital by an indirect route similar to those other invalids would take in the future. Captured by the Confederates on October 21, 1861, at Ball's Bluff, Virginia, he was sent to Richmond as a prisoner of war. During the battle his regiment lost over 300 men, with 44 listed as killed or mortally wounded. Soon he and other Union prisoners were released in an exchange for Rebels held by the North. Bosworth first spent time at Hammond General Hospital, located in Point Lookout, Maryland. After initial stabilization, he was transferred to Fairfax Seminary Hospital near Alexandria, Virginia, before being moved a short distance across the Potomac to Armory Square Hospital in Washington, D.C.[31] By the time Bosworth finally arrived at Portsmouth Grove Hospital, he may have been off his special diet.

Early on, Medical Inspector Vallum issued an order prohibiting the indiscriminate distribution of food, wine, or medicines at the hospital, so there remained considerable validity to Dr. Wheaton's argument. When visitors came to the hospital bearing gifts of food, the staff had no idea who brought what and which invalids were the recipients except by mere chance. This put the medical staff at an enormous disadvantage as patients requiring controlled diets could not be properly monitored for food intake. Men who were scheduled to eat twice or thrice daily were consuming improper food on an irregular basis, an unsound practice even for the healthiest of convalescents. The human digestive tract is simply not designed for snacking when it is operating inefficiently. However, the policy, as necessary as it was, did not always meet with patients' approval. Some felt that preventing citizens from distributing butter, eggs, and other produce directly to the patients, would result in shortages and compel the men "to purchase ... supplies from the sutler, at his own price."

Within days of the hospital ships' docking, sutlers pounced on the hospital grounds. As a correspondent noted: "We go down to the wharf, where, as the eagle smells the prey afar off, the tradesmen's boats have come with their merchandise of liquor, tobacco, papers, cakes, oranges and ham, and large crowds are hustling for the opportunity for an investment."[32] Sutlers were said to be charging 10 cents for a quart of milk, and 20 cents for a quart of berries.[33] For whatever reason, sutlers were not allowed to sell butter. Stephen Rogers received his in a box from a lady named Mary. "It is just what I have been wanting for we do not have any here," he said.[34] During the war years, butter seemed to be as precious as gold. Before First Bull Run in 1861, butter sold for 20 cents per pound. By 1863 the price of butter ranged from $2.00 to $4.00 per pound. But during 1865 the

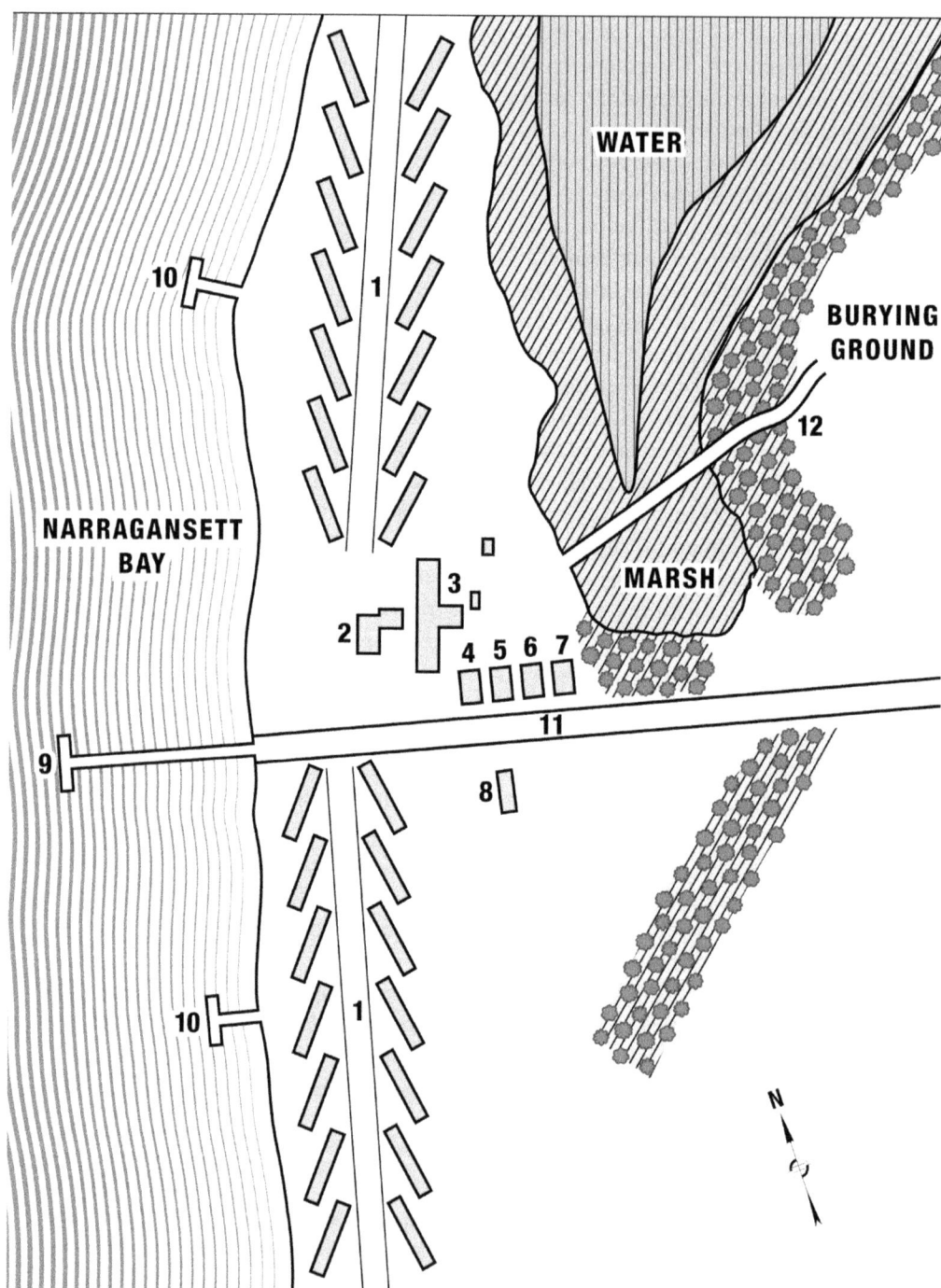

Hospital plan (1862). 1, Roadway; 2, Kitchen; 3, Administration; 4, Stores; 5, Subsistence; 6, Quartermaster; 7, Knapsack; 8, Special diet; 9, Landing; 10, Sinks; 11, Road to railway; 12, Embanked roadway across marsh leading to burial ground (redrawn by Matthew Garthee from original hospital sketch stored at the State of Rhode Island and Providence Plantations, Office of the Secretary of State, Archives Division, Providence, Rhode Island).

price of butter inflated astronomically to between $15.00 and $20.00 per pound.[35] Whitman Bosworth probably explained it best: "When I can get butter I live well.... That is all I ask for but they won't allow it to be sold here and I have to smuggle out a box once in a while by young women (wives of soldiers) and get it filled."[36] A week later, the topic was still on his mind; reiterating what he said in a previous letter, he then added, "We only have butter three times a week." When he was able to procure butter on the outside, it still became an issue. "They won't allow us to carry it in to the dining hall to eat," he said to his parents.[37] Having butter, or rather the lack thereof, seemed to be a general topic of discussion in many a soldier's letter during their stay.

In all, soldiers found sutlers repulsive for their price gouging, yet at the same time, a necessary evil. At 30 cents for half a cake of shaving soap, however, Whitman Bosworth had had enough. He wrote home to his parents saying, "There is plenty of it in Dad's cupboard." Within a short while, he received soap in the mail.[38] A member of Portsmouth Grove's hospital staff was quick to point out, and perhaps rightfully so, "God knows we have had enough of sutlers."[39]

When a group of citizens disembarked from a steamer and arrived at the head of the landing without a pass to visit patients with articles of favor, they were immediately halted by an officer who told them that they could go no further. The visitors were left standing under a burning sun for some fifteen to twenty minutes until they again yelled to the guard standing in the distance for admittance. The officer turned and is said to have replied, "We do not want you here at all."[40] Whether the men and women ever gained access to the hospital grounds that day is anyone's guess, though without a pass, it was unlikely. Those in attendance were so upset that they took the issue to the local newspaper in Bristol. Apparently, other than for family or someone important, there was "no suitable provision made by which passes for such persons can be obtained." The article concluded with a brief lament and a request: "In the name of humanity and of patriotism, we ask for a change."[41]

Thirty-five years later and into the next century, the citizens of Aquidneck Island continued to vilify Dr. Wheaton. There is little doubt he lacked a proficiency in public relations skills that may have calmed or even squelched the citizens' uproar. And, perhaps, Dr. Wheaton was abrasive with his pompous and inflexible military approach during his first few weeks of command. But the question remains: did he deserve the ruthless condemnation cast upon him by the newspapers? Arguably, his duties and responsibilities were Herculean and inherited after several misfortunes, most of which were out of his direct control.

While the press was attacking Dr. Wheaton's credentials, actions and indecisiveness, Bishop Thomas M. Clark of Providence drafted a detailed letter defending Dr. Wheaton and the disembarkation process. Bishop Clark said, "It is somewhat unfair that Dr. Wheaton should be held responsible for a transaction which was begun and finished while he was absent on the sea." The transaction he was referring to was the initial establishment of the complex and the preparation for arrival of patients, both of which were responsibilities of the federal government and the state of Rhode Island. Bishop Clark also offered any impartial observer a challenge: "I can only say that if he will stand by for a few hours and watch the operation [unloading of patients] he may be led to change his opinion."[42] But the blame game was now in full swing.

Not surprisingly, an investigation would follow. With New York State boys in residence at Portsmouth Grove, Governor Morgan sent down Dr. S. Oakley Vanderpool, surgeon general of the state of New York, on a fact-finding visit.[43] His final assessment was surprisingly positive and extremely supportive of Dr. Wheaton's efforts, so much so that his remarks immediately became suspect and reason for detailed scrutiny. "I found fine streets of tents, every man comfortable in bed, all well fed, the regular duty of each medical officer and nurse assigned, and a degree of personal cleanliness, creditable to the short period which had elapsed," he stated. Several men, including military colleagues and patients, came to Dr. Wheaton's defense. Oddly, it was a team of medical officers from Dr. Wheaton's staff who submitted the official report. They concluded: "With respect to the charges, which have been so maliciously and unjustly circulated ... they are without foundation."[44]

Far from a forensic audit, Vanderpool's investigative methods proved questionable and his lack of attention to detail, whether intended or not, resulted in a whitewash of the entire episode. To many, the investigation appeared nothing more than a farce. Immediately after Vanderpool's departure, the *Newport Daily News* tore at the jugular in its publication of July 16. "Why, a crowd of unimpeachable witnesses could be produced to show beyond a reasonable doubt — with a sufficient degree of certainty to hang any man before any intelligent jury of twelve honest men — that in four days after the arrival of the men at the Grove, there were not fine streets of tents and every man comfortable in his bed and all well fed," they exclaimed. Conceding that tents were erected, the correspondent advised, "The labor was altogether foreign to the government of the hospital which you are so highly extolling." As for being comfortable in bed, the correspondent said they were more like the family of the "old woman who lived in a shoe and had so many children she didn't know what to do." Continuing to tear apart the findings, the correspondent offered the following: "If they were all fed, it was not from food supplied by the parental hand of the government ... but because ... charity found a thousand ready hands to administer her alms for their relief." When Dr. Vanderpool relayed that he had talked with several patients at the hospital, the reporter did not dispute his claim. What was rebutted was how the questions were asked. "Why didn't you publish the fact, that when you asked these questions ... you were in uniform and unknown to them? Eh? Why didn't you? It makes all the difference in the world," the correspondent affirmed. And it does. Soldiers are usually tight-lipped when they know the possible ramifications of squealing on a superior officer. "Self-preservation dictated the answers which you received, Mr. Surgeon General, *and nobody knows it better than you*," the newspaper emphasized.[45]

The correspondent offered further evidence that four days after Dr. Vanderpool's visit, he personally visited the hospital at 10 P.M. and found 65 patients sleeping on the floor of the hotel lobby or on the ground. Taking a cynical approach, the correspondent suggested the beds these men had slept in while Dr. Vanderpool was performing his inspection were either lost or stolen. Discounting the idea that they were lost, the newspaper suggested, "The police may be put on the track of the rogues who stole them." The article then suggested that Dr. Vanderpool come again, this time with a magnifying glass "'*blessed*' by a certain high ecclesiastic that they will be sure *to tell the truth* and not deceive you."[46]

Within days of Vanderpool's unconvincing report, Dr. Wheaton was called to Washington. Rumors circulated throughout the hospital about the reason for his sudden departure. A story circulated in the *Providence Evening Press*, provided by a Washington correspondent and first published in the *New York Times*, reporting that the U.S. Surgeon General sent a recommendation to Secretary Stanton for Dr. Wheaton's dismissal.[47] What the newspapers didn't know may have afforded Dr. Wheaton at least a smattering of compassion from the newspapers and the civilian populace. On August 9, Dr. Wheaton was examined by several physicians and found to be suffering from severe varicose veins in the right leg above and below the knee. How debilitating the illness was was open to conjecture. But for Dr. Wheaton, a senior man in the service at age 58, his only recourse was to petition Surgeon General Hammond for a 60-day leave of absence to recuperate and/or to save face.

In the meantime, Dr. Benoni Carpenter, originally from Providence,

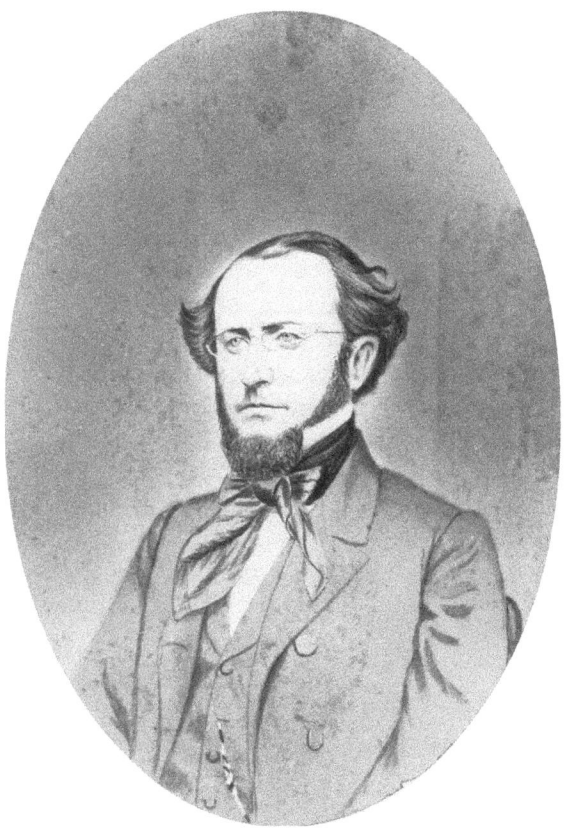

William Cranston, Mayor of Newport, was a tireless advocate for patients at the hospital (courtesy Newport Historical Society, Newport, Rhode Island; catalog number 2010.1).

was placed in temporary charge of the hospital. In the short time he served, the patients found considerable favor with him. Naming a temporary replacement came none too soon as the local newspaper reported, "There was an almost universal desire experienced by the soldiers that Dr. Wheaton may never be permitted to return among them."[48] Yet, a few weeks later, Dr. Wheaton did return to the Grove and his post. Though quickly and quietly exonerated of any wrongdoing, the stigma of the U.S. Surgeon General's recommendation, if true, the harsh press coverage, and the citizens' indictment remained upon his shoulders. The die was cast. By month's end, Dr. Wheaton was relieved of command and whisked away faster than a hummingbird flaps its wings.[49] Dr. Wheaton was officially discharged from the service on September 12, 1862.[50]

The now-vacant post was offered to Dr. James Harris, but for some reason, he declined the appointment.[51] The position was then tendered to Dr. D.J. McKibben, Brigade Surgeon of Volunteers from Philadelphia, who was mustered into the service on April 22, 1861, a few months before First Bull Run. He accepted the difficult assignment that had previously overwhelmed and hastily consumed the first surgeon-in-command a week shy of a month. During Dr. McKibben's brief tenure, additional barracks were erected in anticipation of casualties expected by late summer. Under Dr. McKibben and his successors a more permanent and better-organized hospital would emerge.[52]

While the hospital was under construction, it is important to note the patriotic atmosphere that infused Aquidneck Islanders at the time. War rallies and meetings were conducted nearly every month in each of the island communities and neighboring Bristol. These functions were looked upon with strong anticipation not only for the patriotic message, but for community bonding and their sheer entertainment value. The events were always well attended. During an afternoon rally in Newport headed by Mayor Cranston, an American flag was raised on the liberty pole under which was erected a speaker's rostrum "profusely decorated with the flags of various nations tastefully festooned in four triangular directions from the central point." Several hundred holiday-attired citizens heard the Naval Band play patriotic marches as the ship *Constitution* fired cannon salvos while moored in Narragansett Bay. Raised to a feverish pitch, the people's cry was loud and predictable: "WAR! WAR! WAR!"[53]

As the horrors of war persisted into months, then years, such sentiments would eventually subside. Unrelenting battlefield deaths and the numbers of those felled by disease had a way of bringing folks back to reality. Idealism became ancient history.

Chapter 6

Shelter and Rations

Mama always said, "Life was like a box of chocolates. You never know what you're gonna get."
—*Forrest Gump*, 1994

Near the end of July, the first large pavilion was completed. Those sleeping on the ground were immediately moved into the new ward. Although patients were now sheltered from the elements, many still lacked bed sacks (mattresses). Again, straw for bed sacks had to be requested from local citizens. Rheumatic aches and pains were beginning to surface with ever-increasing frequency and the medical staff attributed the complaints to patients' sleeping on the damp ground.[1]

By now the local newspapers were printing soldiers' letters from the hospital. The appreciation they felt for the citizens of Rhode Island was immense and their thank-you letters appeared regularly. A letter simply signed "Jerseyman" expressed most patient sentiments of the day when the writer thanked those responsible "for the kind and generous treatment which we have received at their hands."[2] Many specifically acknowledged the diligent efforts of the general staff, the hospital wards and nurses, while sometime naming names. In a diary entry, William Dennett expresses his gratitude by saying, "We were very kindly treated by the people at Portsmouth Grove who visited us in great numbers every day bringing nicely prepared food and dainties, clothing and doing all they could to make us comfortable."[3] No letters were found praising the commander.

During the first week of August, the *Bristol Phenix* reported the first mass discharge from the hospital. Eighty-two soldiers departed to rejoin their respective regiments.[4] While the newspapers published new invalid arrivals (by steamers or railroad), they were lax in reporting departures of men back to their units. Discharges, apparently, did not appear as newsworthy as arrivals from the field.

With over 1,800 men recuperating at the hospital, daily food rationing became a massive undertaking. By the end of July, the following food supplies were consumed by the patients and staff on a daily basis:

600 lbs.— Pork
1,650 lbs.— Fresh beef
1,800 lbs.— Hard bread
800 lbs.— Rice
72 lbs.— Coffee
13 lbs.— Tea
270 lbs.— Sugar
22½ lbs.— Adamantine candies
50 lbs.— Soup
2 sacks— Salt
3 gals.— Molasses
1,000 lbs.— Potatoes

Not all rations were government issue. Many foodstuffs, at least in the early months of the hospital's existence, came from the local populace as unconditional donations through fundraising activities or stockpiles from the U.S. Sanitary Commission.

A glimpse of how men were served their meals survives in letters to their family from nurses Georgeanna M. Woolsey Bacon and Eliza Woolsey Howland: "At the beating of the drum the 'convalescents' form in line, and march, by wards, into the long hall where three lines of tables, each 250 feet long, are set."[5]

Though meat staples like pork and beef were reputed to be of the highest quality, seriously ill patients experienced a difficult time digesting the meat, especially when dealing with the effects of typhoid fever. As for their attempts at consuming hard bread, it was just that; hard. A patient's digestive system simply could not tolerate a coarse diet without creating additional health risks. A good example is highlighted by Private John F. Austin, of Company K, 7th Regiment Rhode Island Volunteers. He had suffered a head wound, "a little scratch" in his opinion, caused by a spent bullet while fighting at Fredericksburg. After leaving Carver General Hospital in Washington, D.C., he found his way to Portsmouth Grove Hospital.[6] There, in a letter to his wife Emily, he complained of only getting bread to eat, which made him sick.[7] Soft bread for invalids was the bakery item prescribed by hospital dieticians. Why hard

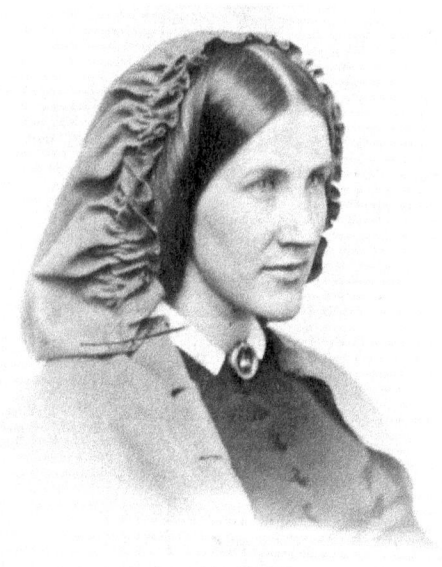

Georgeanna Woolsey Bacon was a close friend of Katherine Wormeley. They worked together on hospital steamers during the Peninsula Campaign. For several months, Ms. Bacon provided nursing care at Portsmouth Grove Hospital before returning home to Connecticut (courtesy Massachusetts Commandery Military Order of the Loyal Legion and the U.S. Army Military History Institute, Carlisle, Pennsylvania).

bread was served instead of the softer kind is pure speculation, but it may have been easier to bake.

There were other dietary issues. Men with typhoid fever or those with simple fevers quickly dehydrated and were in great need of fluids. When available, they were given lemonade or a sip of diluted wine every hour or two to quench their thirst.[8]

Hospital food was never considered a gastronomical delight during the Civil War, and even today, many still think of it as bland. Too many times the nourishment was only a single-course meal, and unfortunately for the recovering soldier, the cooks had a difficult time getting that right. Rarely did a man receive the best of nutrition, even those on special diets. Some food was so tainted it was unfit for human consumption. Portsmouth Grove had its problems, not unlike other general hospitals. George Peck's meticulous record keeping enlightens the reader about the quality of food served. Commenting on the reconstituted turkey served a day after Thanksgiving, he writes, "With what turkeys were left were used for soup — defined as 'spoiled dish water.'"[9] On a New Year's Day, he writes about turkey again: "Owing to the length of time they had been kept, [they] were not any too fresh."[10] Though men enjoyed potatoes, they were not always up to par. "Very poor potatoes for dinner," read one of Peck's accounts.[11] This would not be his last criticism. Several times he used the words "rotten" or "spoiled" to categorize the inedible servings.

Breakfast was no feast either. Cold meat and boiled potatoes were served all too frequently for the men's liking, but the most common and mundane meal, whether breakfast, lunch or dinner, was soup. "Everlasting soup today for both meals," Peck laments.[12] The plea for variety fell on deaf ears. When served sub-par meat on one occasion, he notes, "Today for grub, fresh beef soup and white bread by name if not by nature."[13]

Meal portions were also skimpy. As Stephen Rogers said: "They don't give me enough. The victuals are placed upon each one's plate and he only has what they put upon it."[14] Yet, a year earlier, Private Seth H. Alden, Company E, 16th Regiment Maine Volunteer Infantry, and now a patient in Ward 19, tells his sister, that "I have just been down to breakfast ... [and] I had as much as I could eat."[15] Two different times, two different opinions, that could be attributed to food shortages later in the war, or to nothing more than a fresh batch of uncaring cooks.

Not all meals were unpalatable. Some of George Peck's favorites included fried meat, "quite a rarity," and as he noted, "codfish hash that tasted first rate."[16] Whether breakfast, lunch, or dinner, the diet menu usually consisted of a single course with coffee, tea, or cold water. A year previous, a nurse at the hospital was quoted as saying, "The meals in our hospital were nicely served and well cooked."[17] After she and her fellow nurses left the hospital in late 1863, food quality and its preparation took a decided turn for the worse. Not that the food was always terrible; it only seemed like the cooks intentionally prepared it that way.

Cooks received the most complaints, as far as George Peck was concerned. Something as simple as soup preparation seemed to be an extreme challenge for the underachievers. As Peck tells it, "[I] reckon the cooks will learn to make soup by the time they are discharged."[18] The food quality was so poor that the men took up a petition to have a cook removed.[19] Apparently nothing was resolved as no mention was made in Peck's diary about a replacement. Yet for William Dennett, the food was an improvement over what he was served back in December of 1861 while quartered in Washington, D.C., near the Capitol: "It is a fact that dogs would not eat the food provided for us," he said.[20]

The hospital patients probably didn't know it, but if a particular source can be believed, at least one civilian cook hired under government contract was paid $150 a month, a tidy sum of money at the time.[21] In comparison, Surgeon John Hill Merrill of Battery H, 1st Regiment Rhode Island Light Artillery, in a letter home from the field to his wife Mollie, stated that contract assistant surgeons were paid "$1,200 pr. year at the most."[22] If both numbers are accurate, some contract cooks were paid considerably more than contract assistant surgeons. Apparently good cooks were worth more than bad or inexperienced surgeons.

Earning an attractive salary while cooking so poorly has to be considered a gross misappropriation of public funds. Yet even the most accomplished cooks with proven recipes and track records could do little with spoiled or sub-par ingredients.

Employing sarcasm, George Peck writes about his dinner experiences while at the hospital. "When we eat we are highly gratified to have a commissioned officer stand over us all the time we are at the table. It looks as though they wanted to give us half enough to eat and then stand and hear us to say something that they can punish us for," he said.[23] The incendiary comment proved prophetic: "Corporal O'Keefe was put under arrest by Sergeant Blackman for finding fault with the rations and telling him a little too much truth." Hours later, the captain released the corporal.[24] Sarcasm seemed to be the only way to deal with the issue, providing a bit of comic relief. In a similar incident, Peck refers to a skimpy meal along with a major discovery: "Salt meat and beans today ... one fellow found a square half-inch of pork, which created a good deal of curiosity."[25] And for an especially forgettable breakfast, he writes, "We had meat saltier than two oceans and bread and coffee that smelt as though it had been through a fish heap and the same for dinner with the addition of potatoes."[26] Finally, in an entry about breakfast and supper, he writes about "what the cooks called 'French bubble cum rubble'" [a concoction yet to be identified], and concludes with what he had for dinner that evening, "soup of course."[27]

Peck was not the only soldier to employ sarcasm in describing the meal selections. Whitman Bosworth wrote home about a great Thanksgiving supper he had experienced the previous night of August 6, 1863, that "consisted of a bowl of tea, a slice of dry bread, and about a double handful of whorled berries." Rhetorically, he asked them, "Don't you wish you could have some?"[28]

Since January, Bosworth had been used to eating bad food. While a patient at Hammond General Hospital, he said, "Our grub of late has been rather poor. For breakfast I get a piece of dry bread and a cup of coffee (the latter I should judge was made by boiling up the dirty warm water with the neck or wing of a chicken in it) ... [and] for supper, a slice of bread and cup of tea or rather dye."[29]

Even in a mess hall within a hospital setting there was little peace to be found among men who had been at war suffering from wounds or illness and then having to be confined for weeks, even months at a time. According to George Peck, on April 22, 1864, "A row occurred in the hospital mess hall and someone unknown stabbed a Negro in the forehead but not dangerously. He [the black soldier] drew a pistol but was stopped from using it."[30] Did bad food have something to do with the argument? More likely, it was another issue: racism perhaps?

With nothing better for amusement, or more likely to show his displeasure over the meal selections and variety, George Peck numerically recorded each serving inside the back covers of his diary. The period monitored is over a 14-month span and although Peck may have missed noting some meals, his was a rather large and extensive sampling. The meal frequency follows:

>Soup — 178
>Beans — 56
>Meat Hash — 71
>Fish Hash — 8
>Beets — 13
>Turnips — 2
>Potatoes — 77
>Rice — 17
>Chicken and Turkey — 8
>Onion — 1
>Peas — 1
>Fresh Chowder — 4[31]

Soldiers today would have a difficult time surviving on the meager and occasionally spoiled rations that Civil War soldiers and convalescents had to tolerate.

As was to be expected, patients held out hope for that elusive package mailed from Mom and Dad back home. That was their biggest thrill, as it still remains for soldiers today. They were called "boxes," rarely packages, and the shipments contained as many food staples as would survive long and perilous journeys. Items like jam and tea were usually at the top of the list. One patient received brown bread and consumed it for dinner, probably sharing it with his friends.[32] In another instance, a nurse relates that a patient invited her to share "a banquet" from a box sent from home. The soldier was happy with the contents but said that all it lacked was "a little gin," to which the nurse replied, "It is very lucky for you that there was none or the whole box would have been confiscated." Unperturbed, the patient responded, "Confiscated, indeed! I'm none of your cream and chocolate men."[33]

Food was one issue; patient care was another. The U.S. Sanitary Commission, along with Aquidneck Islanders, played an important role in stabilizing, improving, and humanizing health care at the hospital.[34] But it was no simple task. The U.S. Sanitary Commission referred to the year 1862 as its "dark days" as all its resources "were put to the severest test," especially after the Peninsula Campaign.[35] But the self-criticism may have been unfounded. Their work after the latest campaign was credited with saving hundreds of lives; and if it had not been for the U.S. Sanitary Commission lobbying Congress in December of the same year, reforms within the Army Medical Department would not have been implemented as quickly. Two of the more noteworthy changes included the creation of a corps of medical inspectors and the building of pavilion-type hospitals.[36] By mid–May of 1863, the agency had become considerably more adept at providing for invalid soldiers' physiological and hygienic needs.

Back on the island, the Rev. Francis Tiffany of the U.S. Sanitary Commission lectured those willing to hear his message. With firsthand experience of the soldiers' plight at Portsmouth Grove, he was in Newport to raise funds for the hospital.[37] The agency was a godsend, as the government was financially strapped, having to support the massive war effort, its front-line soldiers, and the bureaucracy it created. For most of the war, military hospitals received only a paltry allowance from a cauldron of rapidly evaporating resources.

Many hospitals in 1862 and the remaining years of the war were built by a Philadelphia contractor. Astoundingly, the builders promised completion in 40 days from commencement. Even more remarkable, though missing the scheduled completion date, they were delinquent by only a few weeks. Whether this firm was the same government contractor that built the complex at Portsmouth Grove may never be ascertained.[38]

The wards for the hospital were to be built using the pavilion concept originally designed by Dr. John Shaw Billings of the Surgeon General's Office. The pavilion design was first used by the British in the Crimean War and also by the French in Algeria.[39] The buildings were to be constructed in line with government recommendations for general hospitals at the time but the standards were those of the U.S. Sanitary Commission's findings after extensive study for improving patient care in hospital settings.[40] Part of a report of July 31, 1861, by a group called the Hospital Committee recommended the following actions:

> If the present hospitals are to be occupied during the fall and winter months, some plan should be at once adopted and applied, by the competent authorities, to correct their architectural defects, to provide facilities for bathing and water closets, to introduce water on each floor, and to separate the dead-houses from the wards occupied by the sick. Measures should also be taken to improve their ventilation, and for their thorough warming in winter.[41]

Portsmouth Grove Hospital would be constructed accordingly. But after the pavilions were built, the addition of more and larger windows caused drafts, an unintended consequence of the design. Another problem arose during the winter months. The structures tended to be cold, the result of having to heat such a large open area. Still, they were a far cry from tents and the poorly constructed buildings invalids were previously subjected to.[42]

Now that the U.S. Sanitary Commission was involved, hospitals were situated near a water supply with ward buildings positioned and large windows placed to afford proper ventilation for all patients within. Good examples of this improved design included Lincoln U.S. General Hospital in Washington and Nelson Hospital, Camp Nelson, Kentucky, each of which had sequential ward buildings situated as an inverted "V."[43] Hicks U.S. General Hospital in Baltimore, Maryland, conformed to the U.S. Sanitary Commission recommendations and spread its buildings over the grounds in the shape of an open fan. Portsmouth Grove Hospital employed a similar staggered design.

In a nurse's account, the walls of a pavilion were said to be plastered, but a patient reported that it was of little consequence against the wind and cold. Whether other pavilion walls were plastered is uncertain but it can be assumed that most, if not all, probably were, as indicated by a letter drafted from Jane Stuart Woolsey to her cousin Margaret. In the postscript she writes, "All the barracks are to be plastered, large bathrooms and steam washhouse to be built immediately." As for insulation, that too was likely provided, as Jane states in the same letter when describing her own quarters: "The outer walls are double and filled in with paper shavings (I believe), and this, with large stoves, will keep us warm, perhaps too warm some fine windy midnight." But to her displeasure, "they don't keep out voices," she said.[44]

There would also be a two-story dispensary, 25 by 40 feet, a cookhouse, a commissary department, a quartermaster office, a knapsack depository, and a steam engine room. Also planned was a two-story building, 25 by 30 feet, for women nurses. A one-story 12-by-18-foot brick building was intended for use as a dead house.[45]

As construction progressed, most patients were assigned a bed along with a mattress stuffed with fresh straw. Clean linens were issued as frequently as possible as long as the laundry could keep up with patient demands. On each patient's bedpost was placed a bed-card which listed the soldier's name and pertinent data about diet, diagnosis, and treatment.[46] The skimpy information required at the time, and deemed adequate then, is a far cry from today's exacting medical notation standards.

Ten feet north of the dock, plans were drawn to make a longer wharf that would expand thirty feet farther into the bay than the original. This would allow for the berthing of larger government transports. To ease the unloading process, a derrick was added to the design.

The original request for the wharf came in a letter requisition by way of Dr. D.J. McKibben of Portsmouth Grove to General L.B. Frieze, the Quartermaster General in Providence. In turn, General Frieze wrote Captain McKim in Boston with the specifications. "The wharf [is] to be built of oak timber and in the most substantial manner giving fifteen (15) feet of water at low tide," he writes. Two sinks (40 by 50 feet) standing on piles were also requested. General Frieze added that the "parties offer $5,250 [for] drilling piles and arranging the foundation," and he further stated that "the wharf is to be arranged for the wharfing of large steamers." General Frieze asked that the plan be accepted immediately so the contractor could order the timber. He ended his letter by saying, "Please telegraph at once."[47] Surprisingly, the general did not stipulate why the wharf and sinks were required, which immediately raised eyebrows in Washington and would soon lead to a bureaucratic nightmare back in Rhode Island.

The first negative feedback on the wharf request arrived by letter from the Assistant Quartermaster's Office to General McKim. He said, "The plan of wharf seems to be a very intelligent one, but until some evidence of the necessity for constructing a wharf is offered, or some official represents that the interest of the service is required for its construction, I do not feel authorized to assume the responsibility."[48]

Dr. McKibben quickly penned a return letter on August 23, 1862, which outlined the reasons why the wharf and sinks were urgently required. "A man narrowly escaped serious injury this morning after the arrival of the steamer 'Perry' by the giving way of the wharf timbers — the stones are insecure — and the boats arriving after dark with bread and fresh beef will surely result in loss of life from this cause." He continued: "The delay, if from motives of economy, is not well founded." In addressing the larger problem of the patient unloading process from large government transports, he simply said, "As it is calculated, U.S. transports with sick and wounded can discharge such in a few hours there being sufficient water to admit them at the proposed wharf, rather than the slow, insecure, and expensive one of lightening with tugs. Surely no valid reason can be given for delay in constructing latrines for a general hospital."[49]

On the 27th, McKim wrote General Montgomery C. Meigs at the Quartermaster General's Office in Washington for approval to construct the wharf and latrines. The response arrived in a letter formatted in short abrupt paragraphs. "Do not build any wharf at the hospital camp without estimate, and report of its necessity approved by the Quarter Master General," the letter stated, with the following paragraph providing a lecture: "Keep all expenses as low as possible. Surgeons in charge of hospitals, who do not see the infinite other necessary expenditures of the government, are not good judges of the propriety of spending money on temporary hospitals. Requisitions are made for constructing steam apparatus wharves as though each temporary hospital was a permanent town, where wharves and machinery were to continue in use for years."[50]

Along the way, the wharf and latrines did get built, though no evidence was found in the files at the Office of the Secretary of State, A. Ralph Mollis State Archives Division in Providence, Rhode Island, that documents the final approval for construction. The matter, however, was still not finished. On October 11, General Meigs notified Captain McKim of his concerns about the spending taking place at Portsmouth Grove. He told McKim that he was sending Mr. Edward Clark, "an architect of intelligence and with some idea of economy to examine this hospital." The inspection, if it happened, probably ended in McKim's favor. Today, after reviewing all the requisitions and letters, it's no wonder General Meigs expressed concern. Timber, plank, washing machines, wringers, cypress tables and Windsor chairs (all stained a dark color), large kitchen kettles, miscellaneous kitchen supplies, coal for heating, stoves, clothing, food, medical supplies, and sundry items were all requisitioned in a short period of three to four months.[51] The red flag had to be raised even though most, if not all, of the requirements were warranted. No one doubted there was a war to finance, but hospitals had to play second fiddle when victories needed to be won in the field. In a sense each officer was right with his argument. General Meigs had a huge financial responsibility and needed to supply the ravenous appetite of a fighting army. Captain McKim, conversely, had the utmost concern for the medical needs of his patients. The matter would continue as give-and-take for the duration of Portsmouth Grove's existence.

To secure the grounds, there was talk of constructing a thirteen-foot-high fence to surround the complex, but no records or photos exist to substantiate its completion. The fence, if built, was to encircle the patient pavilions "to prevent the men from wandering off from their wards without permission and give them sufficient room for exercise."[52] The reason sounded more like the justification for building a penitentiary, not a military hospital.

By damming a spring a quarter mile north of the hospital, a reservoir was to be created for a large water supply.[53] Situated some seventy feet — some accounts say eighty — above a ridge, the water would flow downhill through 4-inch iron pipes. The piped water was not only intended to be used for drinking, but by diverting the line through a steam plant, the water could be heated for cooking, bathing and laundry. The contract had been awarded to a gentleman named N.M. Chaffee and the material used was supplied by the Hope Iron Foundry. But the facilities project did not go as intended, and it had nothing to do with the plans or the labor to excavate, lay the pipe, or connect the plumbing. Material was the number one reason for delay. Whether from a lack of supply filters or simply through defective material, a problem always seemed to manifest. In one shipment, the wrong size pipe was sent, 3-inch instead of 4-inch. In another, three lengths of 4-inch pipe had to be replaced because they were either cracked or broken, "as to be entirely worthless."[54] Although the situation was rectified by the end of September, water and waste pipes were still not working properly.

To heat the water, a large steam plant had to be installed on the premises. Near the end of November when the boiler system was first tested, several defects were found. Brigadier General Frieze in Providence was advised of the problem by letter from the hospital administration. Six faults were noted:

1. A large leak was found at the rear manhole;
2. A large pipe hole was left unplugged;
3. A kettle leaked;
4. A cold-water feed pipe had leaks in one of the T-joints;
5. The steam gauge was defective; and
6. Faucets used to feed the kettles with cold water all leaked in the joints.[55]

Mr. Hudson, the installer, was asked to remedy the situation, which he presumably did. Only a few days after Mr. Hudson's departure from the hospital, two branch steam pipes leading to the kettles sprung leaks near the seams, proving that the workmanship was of marginal quality at best.[56] Mr. Hudson may have been called back to rectify the matter, but no correspondence exists in the archives to support that assumption.

Steam energy was also intended to be used to power a circular saw in the carpentry shop and a steam pump in case of emergency to extinguish fires.[57] Although far from flawless, the piping system was an ingenious yet uncomplicated engineering marvel.

Seven hydrants (also called fireplugs) along with appropriate piping were requisitioned, but the hydrants arrived with the valve incorrectly positioned at the top. On return of the hydrants in early October, it was noted that "New York City hydrants for 3 inch 'T' pipe" were required. Those that had been delivered would freeze in the harsh New England weather because of the placement of the valves. After Washington approved the new requisition, Providence advised the hospital that the new hydrants would be delivered with valves installed on the bottom so they could be partially buried in the ground to avoid freezing temperatures.[58]

For the convenience of the hospital, patients and staff, Portsmouth Grove was authorized its own post office. Edmund Cole was appointed its first and perhaps only postmaster.[59] Soldiers' morale depended a great deal upon the letters they received from family and friends. Those literate were usually prolific letter writers, not only for their own needs but also for those who had yet to master the written word. During the final three years of the war, the post office remained an active enterprise, bringing much cheer to the men.

On August 17, 1862, some six hundred former patients of Portsmouth Grove Hospital recently deemed fit for duty were returned to the army and shipped back to the field by U.S. transport. Rumors abounded that any day another thousand patients would arrive at the hospital, a number that proved to be extremely high.[60] By September, the hospital was prepared for much of the onslaught as the necessary buildings were completed. The hospital was now operating on a budget estimated at fourteen hundred dollars a day.[61]

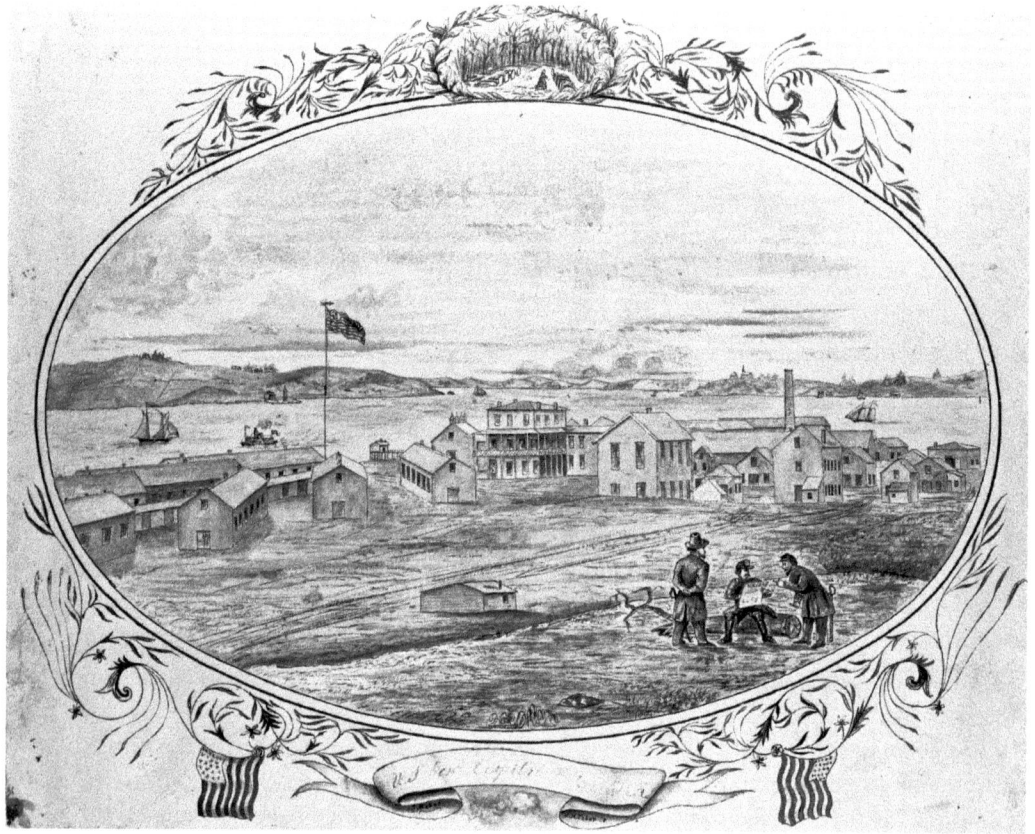

A period drawing of the hospital grounds by J. Baker and J.M. Tabor, Jr. Note the rudimentary image of the burial yard at top center (State of Rhode Island and Providence Plantations, Office of the Secretary of State, Archives Division, Providence, Rhode Island).

But satisfactory medical care and adequate facilities were not realized before far too many men would sacrifice their lives.

Although the hospital seemed like a never-ending construction project, most of the hospital wards and ancillary buildings were finished by late summer. *The Medical and Surgical History of the War of the Rebellion (1861–1865)* described how the complex appeared when finally completed:

> The hospital was built on low ground on the eastern shore of Narragansett Bay, eight miles north of Newport and twenty-three south of Providence. The grounds were bordered on the east by the Old Colony and Newport railroad, on which was a station with a side-track for the use of the hospital. There was a good wharf on the water-side at which vessels of 800 tons could discharge, but which could not be reached by the large steamers generally used for the transport of the sick. The extension of the wharf was therefore frequently recommended. The grounds comprised about twelve acres, the largest diameter north and south, parallel with the bay. They sloped gradually from the centre, to the beach on one side and a low marsh on the other. About the middle of their length was situated the administration building, formerly a summer hotel, with, on either side of it, a series of fourteen pavilions, each series constituting a division of the hospital [fourteen served as surgical wards, while the other fourteen were reserved for patients with illness or disease[62]]. A main

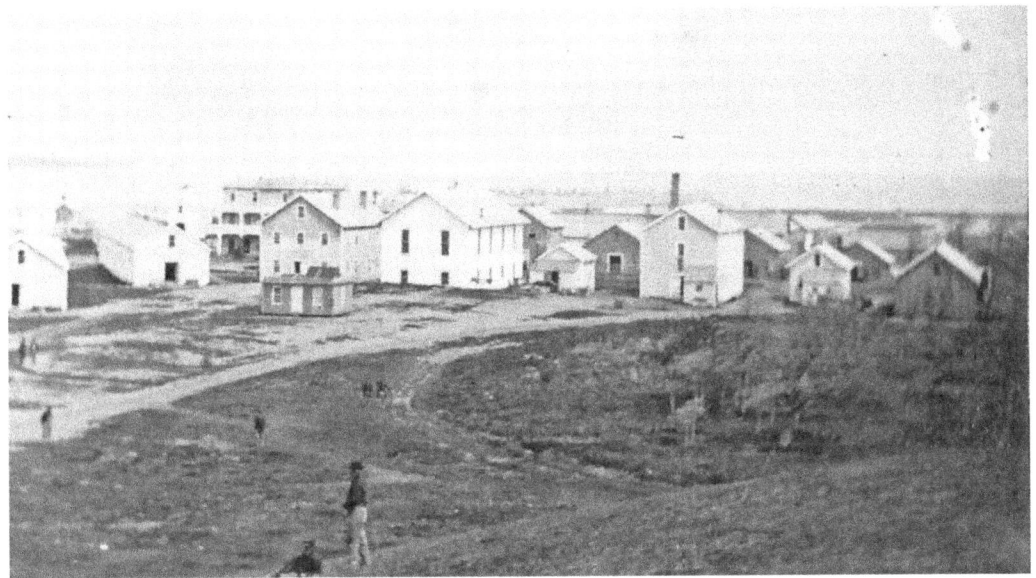

In this view, facing west toward Narragansett Bay, hospital buildings are seen in the distance. Photographer J.A. Williams took several images from this position (author's collection).

avenue, 50 feet wide, ran north and south from the administration building, and along the sides of this avenue the pavilions were placed obliquely like the feathers on an arrow. A covered corridor with sliding-doors to close in winter, facilitated communication between the wards and other buildings. The pavilions were 160 × 25 × 11 feet and 19 feet 11 inches to the ridge. A space 15 feet long was partitioned off as high as the plate for bath-room, lavatory and water-closet at one end of each and for wardmaster's and nurses' rooms at the other; the remaining length of 130 feet accommodated 56 beds with about 59 feet of area and 900 of air-space to each. A general mess-hall, barracks for the guard, laundry (*with separate drying room*), bakery, chapel, blacksmiths' shop, carpenters' shop, stables, etc., were subsequently added to the establishment.[63]

Not mentioned in the above description, an icehouse was added to the establishment, and also a building for the sutler to ply his trade.[64]

Chapter 7

Hospital Guards

But who is to guard the guards themselves?
— Juvenal, *Satires*, VI, l. 347

From inception, military police were deemed necessary at the hospital "to preserve internal order and prevent intrusion from without."[1] The Newport Artillery Company, an active militia stationed at nearby Fort Adams, was detailed to the hospital. Upon arrival, they pitched their tents on the south side of the grounds near a high hill where they bivouacked and cooked "picnic style," and ate their food "at the foot of a noble old oak tree."[2] The company remained there along with other details under the charge of Captain Christopher Blanding until relieved on November 15, 1862. Captain Blanding would soon take command of the permanent garrison force once they were recruited and mustered into the new unit.

One stipulation was imposed. Captain Blanding would not be allowed to recruit able-bodied men, but only those disabled by wounds or illness in the field, yet well enough to perform garrison duty. Both he and his lieutenants qualified by the rule. Captain Blanding was disabled by disease contracted in Georgia and South Carolina while serving with the 3rd Regiment Rhode Island Heavy Artillery. His lieutenants were walking wounded: Captain William S. Chace had been wounded in the face at New Bern, and Lieutenant John H. Hammond had been shot through the arm and leg in the Battle of Fair Oaks. The lieutenants served in Rhode Island units: the 4th Regiment Rhode Island Volunteers and the 1st Regiment Rhode Island Light Artillery.[3]

In Providence, the *Herald* and *Post* published a recruitment broadside endorsed by the state and authored by Captain Christopher Blanding. From a recruiting standpoint, the posting proved effective, and it took Blanding only a few months to fill the quota. And why shouldn't it have been that way? Rhode Island and bordering southern Massachusetts had a great many invalid veterans still capable of performing light duty, and with good jobs at a premium even during wartime, it was not hard to envision men knocking down the door at 10 Custom House Street. After all, who would not want to work in a "comfortable position and light duty," near home, with fully paid medical and hospitalization benefits and a bonus near the end of his tenure? Like many a "help wanted" advertisement, this one made some promises that proved too good to be true.

HOSPITAL GUARDS!

By an order from the War Department, His Excellency Gov. Sprague has been authorized to raise

A COMPANY OF INFANTRY!

To act as a Guard at

PORTSMOUTH GROVE HOSPITAL

The men will be enlisted to serve for a period of 3 Years or during the War, unless sooner discharged, and for this special service alone.

The above offers an excellent opportunity for a Comfortable Position and Light Duty in a new and independant organization, with the advantage of being near home. The men will have

GOOD RATIONS, COMFORTABLE CLOTHING,

And the Best of Medical Attendance, Free!

So that every soldier can have his entire pay for his family, and have the satisfaction of seeing it placed in their hands, in addition to his Bounty at the close of the War.

The non-commissioned officers will be selected from the best men.

Recruits preferred who are slightly incapacitated for active duty in the field, by wounds or otherwise.

Also 1 Drummer and 1 Fifer wanted.

Headquarters at No. 10 Custom House Street.

WHERE RECRUITS WILL BE RECEIVED.

C. BLANDING, Comd'g Guard.

As an enticement to enlistment, this broadside made guard duty look like an enjoyable assignment. Enlistees would soon learn the difficulties of dealing with unruly patients and harsh New England winters; no wonder they drank excessively and desertions were commonplace (courtesy Library Company of Philadelphia, Philadelphia, Pennsylvania).

The company was officially enlisted by the War Department under an order dated October 4, 1862, two months before their arrival at the hospital. They would be mustered in as the Hospital Guards— Rhode Island Volunteers and consisted predominantly of men from Rhode Island (see Appendix A). Their duties were similar to those performed at other garrisons. Under control of the commander, sentinels encircled the camp while prisoners were confined to the guardhouse.[4]

The cadre not only guarded Confederate prisoners but Union soldiers who awaited court-martial or were sentenced to serve time at hard labor for a military infraction. These invalid prisoners were segregated from the rest of the hospital population. According to one observer, it was not uncommon to see a ball and chain tied to a soldier's leg, and the unfortunates were not always Confederates.[5]

The hospital guards were also detailed to take Confederate prisoners to Governor's Island in New York Harbor after their convalescence. Such a trip was highlighted in George Peck's diary when he noted that Sergeant John E. Drohan from Fall River, Massachusetts, and Private William Davis of Providence, Rhode Island, escorted five Confederate prisoners to New York. The guards departed each fully armed with a loaded revolver, a musket, and a sword. In an entry dated the following day, Peck notes the safe return of the escort.[6] By mid-September 1862, thirty-eight Confederate prisoners were sent to Fort Monroe for exchange, accompanied part of the way by hospital guards. Guards also escorted Union soldiers who had recently recovered from illness or injury back to a predetermined transfer point. The duty was performed with some regularity and could be extremely unpleasant, especially when riding a boat on Narragansett Bay during a winter squall.[7]

On several occasions, guards were ordered to escort visitors in and out of the hospital grounds, sometimes with a sergeant.[8] In what appeared to be a ludicrous decision — especially to several guards — a minister who had just officiated at a burial service could not leave the grounds until escorted by an armed sergeant. In another seemingly senseless act, the captain was said to have stated, "He would not let Jesus Christ out of the lines," and in a direct reversal let the sergeants leave. George Peck's take on the event: the decision "thus makes them [sergeants] better than Christ."[9] Another soldier recuperating at the hospital made note in a letter to his cousin about the "pretty farms" that surround the area, "but we can't get to them [as] there is a heavy guard ... around the hospital."[10]

Once, George Peck was detailed along with a squad of privates to be at the train depot six times a day "to assist men coming back from pass and citizens coming in for visit." The additional duty, along with guard, went on for a few weeks until all men had returned from furlough. The duty did not make Peck happy; neither were the privates.[11]

Stephen Rogers found his return from furlough unpleasant for more than the obvious reasons. Two soldiers in his ward had died while he was on furlough enjoying the comforts of home: Thompson, who was a member of his company, and "a young man named Tupper." Their loss affected him deeply, as he expressed to his parents in a letter home: "There is no more toil and trouble. No more wearisome marches for them. They have gone to their rest."[12]

The hospital guards were now subject to regular inspections consisting of barracks, clothing, personal items, and muskets. Two sets of muskets were issued: one for standing guard and the other to be shouldered only for inspection and drill.[13] For obvious reasons, no one was allowed to have loaded weapons in the barracks except for officers, who were authorized to carry loaded pistols.[14] In preparation of a barracks' inspection, dry scrubbing of the floors was the accepted practice.[15]

On February 27, 1864, the men stood a knapsack inspection.[16] The sack was inspected to make sure all the needed supplies were included and that no contraband was hidden. Inspections were and always will be a way of life for all military personnel regardless of branch of service. Although disliked, they served their purpose. Inspections helped maintain a degree of cleanliness; they ensured men maintained their arms in working order; and they served as a stark reminder of who was in command.

Even in a hospital environment, the potential discipline problems within the Union ranks among men of different regiments were significant, not to mention men within their own ranks. Other problems surfaced. Guards had to contend with disease, a high desertion rate among their own company, and the hardships of bitterly cold weather from northwest winds that swept across Narragansett Bay. During the first winter, with frigid temperatures described as the "worst in decades," men were quartered in drafty canvas tents. Normal guard consisted of four hours on and two hours off, but in such severe conditions guards were relieved every hour usually with "trousers frozen stiff to the knee."[17] Even when the cold diminished later in the season, they still contended with puddles of slush.[18]

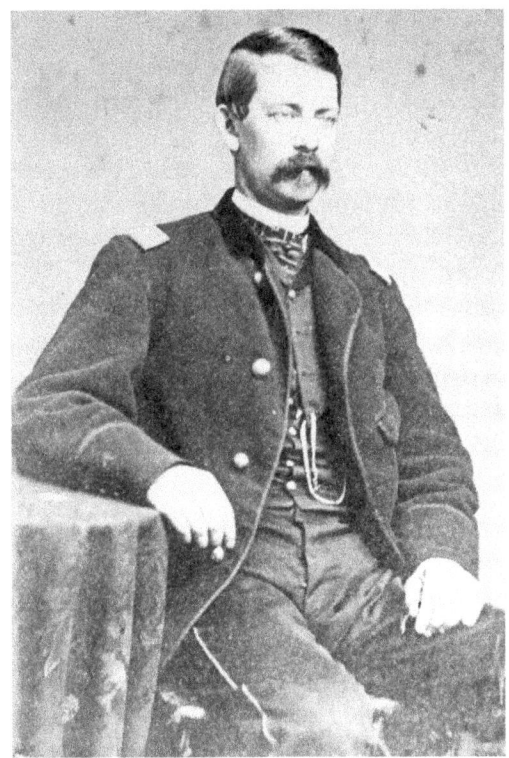

Lt. William S. Chace, second in command of the Hospital Guards—Rhode Island Volunteers (author's collection).

In the summer, there was another pervasive issue. George Peck described the adversary he contended with on guard duty during an early-August evening: "Mosquitoes are thick and savage."[19] One hundred and forty-five years later, the problem still exists on the island.

Staying bodily clean and keeping clothes unsoiled was another matter. With hot water pipes connected to all major buildings and a bathhouse, the guards had no problem washing themselves. They also took an occasional dip in Narragansett Bay, weather and season permitting. The recreational swim in the ocean was enjoyed immensely. Private Daniel Henry Austin, Company K, 81st New York Infantry (not to be confused with John F. Austin from Rhode Island) couldn't participate because of his wounded foot, but watched from "the big rock to see the boys enjoy a swim." While there, he observed what he called "sea poisoners," probably jellyfish whose painful sting even today threatens an occasional bather in the summer waters of the Atlantic.[20]

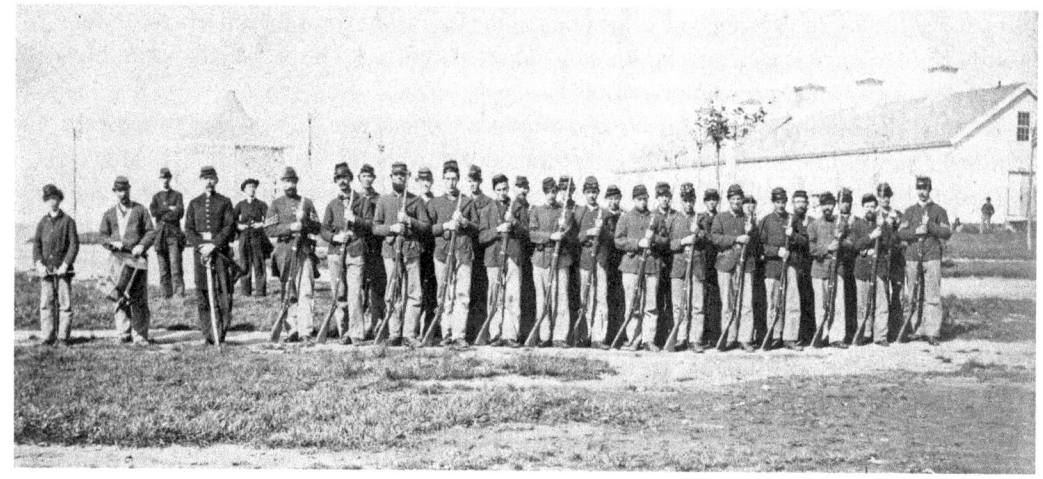

A company of Hospital Guards — Rhode Island Volunteers, one of two such images known to exist. Note the ward building in the background (courtesy Newport Historical Society, Newport, Rhode Island; catalog number P5725).

Though the hospital had its own laundry, the service was exclusive to the patients. Hospital guards had to wash their own clothes when deemed necessary or when they reeked and were ordered to do so.

Government-wide, an Invalid Corps was officially established in 1863, as part of which the hospital guards would soon be reorganized. As luck would have it, guards were required to wear the initials "IC" on their uniforms, which were intended to stand for "Invalid Corps" but were simultaneously used by the army's Quartermaster Department to mean "inspected and condemned." In 1864, when the army realized the negative connotation, the name was changed to the Veteran Reserve Corps.[21] The hospital guards at Portsmouth Grove must have breathed a collective sigh of relief.

Seth H. Alden heard about the Invalid Corps and had some testy opinions about its formation: "They are going to form a cripple brigade. I think that our government has got pretty low to have to scrape up all of the cripples." He then added, "They are going to enlist cripples besides." This action had touched a sore nerve with Alden, as he was doubly anxious to secure a discharge for his leg wound.[22] He felt that if he could obtain a discharge, the only way he would ever muster into the service again was if he was drafted. "Experience is a good teacher," he said, "and one has to pay pretty dear for his learning some times."[23]

Whitman Bosworth felt a bit differently. After reading his hometown newspaper, the *Webster Times*, and getting a glimpse of the men listed for conscription — men between the ages of 20 and 45 — he told his parents, "I would be willing to reenlist for three years if that would bring in that class." In addition he said, "Well I believe they have picked about the right ones and I wished they were obliged to go but those are the very ones that will pay the three hundred dollars." The $300 was the fee paid to buy a man's way out of the draft — commonly referred to as a commutation fee — making the entire process both inequitable and distasteful. During the Civil War, wealth bought a man's freedom from military service, regardless of what side the person was called to defend. By paying the fee and providing a substitute in the North, or, as a plantation slave owner in the South, having someone prepared to take his place, the affluent draftee was released from any future military obligations. Without money, property, and position, there was little a person could do to avoid conscription unless a serious health issue surfaced during the recruit's physical examination.[24]

A large percentage of substitutes who did enter the army held questionable allegiance, mostly to themselves and not to their country. In a letter written by one of Bosworth's friends, Sergeant Bryson writes that within Bosworth's company still in the field, of the nineteen conscripts recently received, seven had already deserted. All nineteen were substitutes.[25] In another letter, Sergeant Bryson advised Bosworth not to hurry back as there were only ten men remaining in his company.[26]

Conscription and the use of paid substitutes hit a sour note and matters came to a head as draft riots flared up in major U.S. cities throughout the North. Privy to newspapers, the soldiers at Portsmouth Grove Hospital were fairly well informed of the happenings. Whitman Bosworth talked about the riots in a July 1863 letter mentioning New York and Boston as trouble spots. Telling his parents about a report he read, he said "fifteen thousand in Newark, N.J., have risen to resist the draft. They say they are willing to be drafted if the government will throw aside the three hundred dollar exemption and make the rich men serve as well as the poor. I am afraid that three hundred dollars will make a great deal of trouble yet."[27]

The draft, along with the vehemently despised practice of allowing substitutes, was not the only matter bothering Bosworth. An acquaintance named Henry had just gotten home from the war and was "telling some tough *yarns*" [Bosworth's emphasis]. According to Bosworth, Henry "enlisted for three months but was sooner discharged without seeing any fighting. He thinks it is nothing but fun to be a soldier." With Bosworth's anger at its peak, he said, "I wish he could

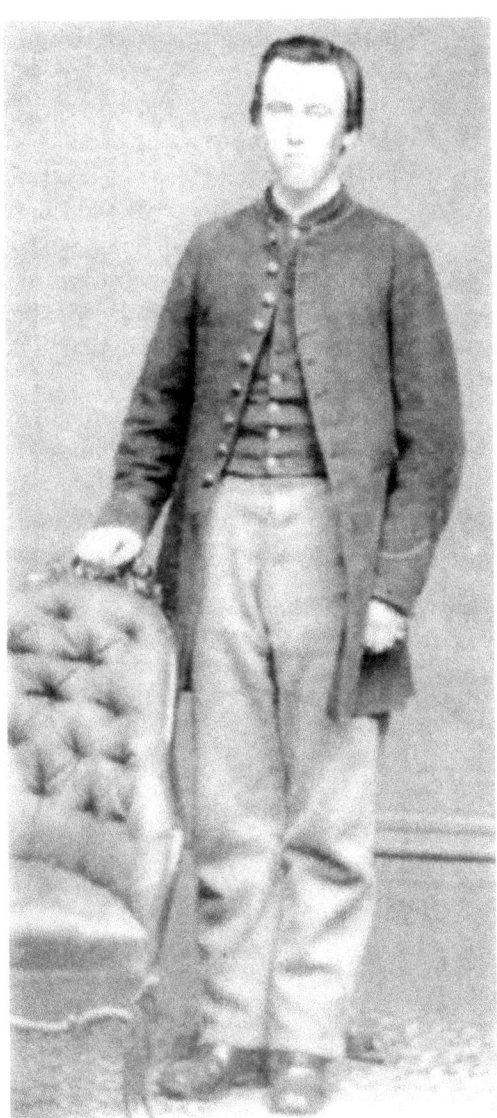

New York soldier John M. Lovejoy would write a deluge of letters to his cousin Cynthia from his hospital bed. Cynthia returned the favor. The correspondence would stimulate a romance, and after the war they would marry (courtesy Peggy McGuire, descendant of John Lovejoy).

serve in Virginia a few months. I think [he] would know what he was talking about better than he now does."²⁸

In spite of his present situation, John M. Lovejoy of Company G, 121st New York Infantry remained steadfast in his convictions. "I have the same patriotic spirit I had when I enlisted for I know our cause will conquer in the end, for we are in the right," he said. "But for one, I hope the end is near for I think it about time to stop the shedding of human blood. Many have fallen and many more will fall." Reflecting on what he had just said and now introspective, Lovejoy told his cousin Cynthia, "God only knows if we have seen each other for the last time, but I hope we may meet again on earth. If it was not for hope, the heart would break. And if it is my fate to lay down my life for my Country, I hope we may one day meet where hurting is no more and where the weary is at rest." Finishing his thought, he added, "I am determined to stand up boldly for the cause I am in wherever I may go hoping to come through victorious in the end."²⁹

Besides draft riots, braggarts at home, and the never-ending war, months earlier things had already gotten rather peculiar at Portsmouth Grove; and the circumstances had nothing to do with conscription, stolen valor, or patriotism. The unfortunate incident took place on February 28, 1863, and is documented in *The Medical and Surgical History of the War of the Rebellion (1861–1865)*. John Higgins, age 25, of Smithfield, Rhode Island, was confined in a cell after attempting to evade a guard while smuggling spirits into the camp. When confronted about his misdeed, he appeared inebriated. According to a postwar government account, the soldier was eventually released after spending four hours in the stockade. Immediately upon his release, he attacked the officer of the guard, striking him in the face. Protecting himself, the sergeant drew his sword, stepped back, and held the slightly elevated blade near his own right hip. Because of uneven ground, winter frost, and his physical condition, the prisoner slipped and fell on the point of the sword, then heavily forward unto the ground.³⁰ Here is where the story becomes suspect. *The Medical and Surgical History* provides details of the aftermath: "When picked up he was insensible and breathing heavily. After the blood, which had flowed copiously about his face was washed and dried, only a slight wound in the right nostril could be found. The officer of the day, an acting assistant surgeon, was summoned immediately. He could detect no other injury than the trivial one of the right ala nasae [nose]." The report continues: "The patient had been drinking heavily and it was felt, not unjust-

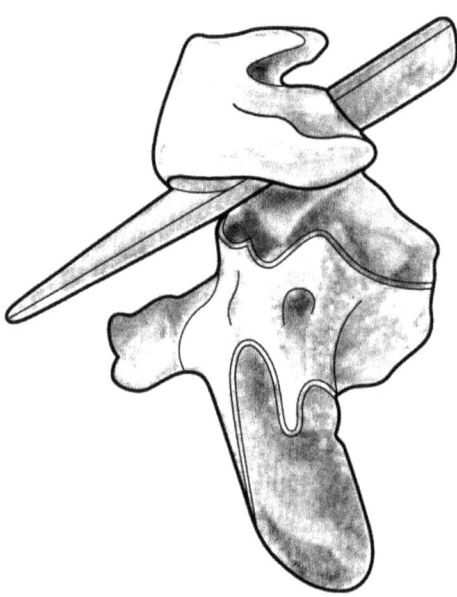

A post-mortem drawing (Specimen 1612) of the sphenoid bone showing a sword tip passing through the nasal cavity of a soldier who met his demise during a scuffle at the hospital. Was it murder, self-defense, or a tragic accident? (Digitized by Google Books.)

ifiably, that he was merely drunk, whereupon he was returned to the guard house. The next morning, still unconscious, he was removed to a ward, where he expired thirty-one hours after injury." Less than ten hours later, an autopsy was performed. The official report explained the cause of death as "a transverse fracture of the posterior clinoid process [fractured skull]," and added, "The specimen was forwarded to the recently organized Army Medical Museum."[31]

A conflicting account in *the Annual Report of the Adjutant General of the State of Rhode Island for the Year 1865* lists the death simply as, "Killed by officer of guard," but provides no details. Was it justifiable homicide or accidental death? A reporter from the *Newport Daily News* probably uncovered the true story after a brief investigation. The primary facts remain the same: a soldier runs the guard; he's confined but upon release is still unmanageable. The reporter concludes his story by saying the soldier "was instantly killed by the officer of the day who drew his sword and pierced him through the brain."[32] This account may not be the entire story, either, but appears to be the most plausible. The *Newport Advertiser* went on to chastise those responsible by saying, "It seems scarcely possible that petit officers, or those even of higher grade should be permitted to exercise with impunity such brutal authority within the precincts of an Army Hospital, remote from the seat of war."[33]

Now it was early August and an independent committee had just departed the hospital after conducting an investigation into cruelty to patients by resident doctors. Though the above incident may have played a part in the inquiry, there was another questionable episode that brought the high-ranking officials to Portsmouth Grove. Whitman Bosworth relates the accusation in an unaddressed letter most likely intended for and mailed to his parents:

> August 4, 1863
> There was an investigating committee here today to overhaul this institution and I will give you a brief sketch of the affair. About three weeks ago the doctor came in and found a man lying on his bed and for punishment he ordered the man a dose of castor oil and his clothes taken away from him. He refused to give up his clothes so they ordered him to be taken to the guard house, and he refused to go for he was a corporal and they have no right to put any non-commissioned officer in the guard house. Well the guards were about taking him along when the doctor interfered and soon commenced using a cane on his head. He went to the guard house and the next day some of the boys wrote a letter to the Adjutant General of the State of Maine and it was forwarded by him with another letter to the Secretary of War. There has been a great many letters written to Headquarters by the boys and they have at last taken notice of them.[34]

The second half of Bosworth's letter provides details of the hearing. The writing includes many run-on sentences, as if Bosworth was anxious to tell his story without forgetting any of the particulars. It reads:

> Well this committee first commenced on the doctor and after hearing their story called in a number of patients to hear their story and told them to tell all the particulars in regard to the management of this institution and not be afraid to bring up all the charges they could against the doctors for they should not be punished for it. So they sailed in and proved many a lie on different doctors. For instance, there is a very sick man in this ward and the doctor was sent three days ago and has yet to see him yet. The doctor said he visited this man twice or three times every day. The ward master and three nurses testified

that he had not seen him. Well the [illegible word] was spoken of and several said that the doctors put on more airs than Gen. McClellan did in front of Richmond. Every little thing was brought up and the doctors had to sit and hear them and there was some serious charges brought against them and are recorded and sent to Washington.

Bosworth concludes the letter by offering his opinion:

Probably there will be quite an overturn here soon. The doctors say this was all studied up before, for all the stories agreed. But this is false for no one knew anything about it until they were called in as witnesses and they were not allowed to hear each other's testimony.

I have mentioned but some of the many charges, but enough for now.

The outcome of the proceeding is not mentioned in any of Bosworth's remaining correspondence. Unfortunately the collection of letters only dates to September 9, 1863. Obviously there were additional letters written by him, as he survived the war. Whether they still exist and will surface to solve the mystery remains to be seen. Perhaps other soldiers' letters from Portsmouth Grove Hospital have yet to be researched and may provide the elusive answer.

Chapter 8

Liquor, Trouble and Discipline

'Tis not the drinking that is to be blamed, but the excess.
— John Selden,
Table Talk, 1689

Soldiers during the Civil War fondly referred to their liquor supply by many peculiar names and catchphrases: "nockum stiff," "busthead," "popskull," "tanglefoot," and "Oh! Be Joyful" were used most frequently, followed by "oil of gladness," "red-eye," "rifle knock-knee," "rock me to sleep, mother," and "sudden death."[1] Most spirits were home-brewed, of which a large percentage was of poor quality. That there were so many name variations attests to the frequency of alcohol consumption. As amusing as the slang sounds, liquor consumption and drunkenness were serious problems throughout the war, from privates to high-ranking generals. Even General Ulysses S. Grant was accused of overindulgence, not once but on several occasions. At the Battle of the Crater in Petersburg, Virginia, one of General Ambrose E. Burnside's commanders was so drunk from rum that he remained in his bomb-proof shelter (whether from drunkenness, fear, or both is still under contention) while Confederates annihilated his men. Even doctors got in the act. Jane Stuart Woolsey, a former nurse at Portsmouth Grove Hospital, tells of a visit to another hospital where she inquired of the whereabouts of the ward surgeon and at what time he made his rounds. "'Well 'm,' answered the ward master, 'that depends on how drunk he was the night before.'"[2]

Dr. Samuel David Gross recognized the problem of excessive alcohol consumption by soldiers and wrote about it quite extensively in his journal on surgery under a chapter titled "Military Hygiene." "Alcoholic liquors should not be permitted to be used except as medicine, and then only under the immediate direction of the medical officer," he said. In defense of his reasoning, he cited several examples of inebriated soldiers in the British army and the consequences that resulted because of their impaired mental state.[3]

At Portsmouth Grove Hospital, visitors were banned from giving spirits to patients, but within staff barracks, authorities may have looked the other way.[4] Clandestinely, however, liquor did find its way into the minds and stomachs of the patients. The method employed at Portsmouth Grove was simple and effective. A local merchant placed a full jug of liquor in a hollowed-out tree designated for such a purpose. One of the men would skirt the guard, run to the tree, take the full jug, leave the agreed sum of money and an empty jug, and depart a tad happier while attempting to evade the guard again upon his return.[5] How frequently and for how long this clandestine operation was sustained is anyone's guess, but in January 1865 a gentleman named Holloway was stopped from entering the grounds for being, as George Peck said, "too fond of selling liquor to the soldiers."[6] Could he have been the primary supplier?

Men on short-term pass found liquor easy to obtain, especially on the northern end of the island, where at least five or six establishments catered to the soldiers' devilish desires. Shanties selling liquor were also found along the railroad tracks near the hospital grounds. In one instance, "a poor Irish lady, the mother of a family, was badly beaten" at such an establishment after opposing a liquor sale to a convalescent soldier.[7] Who did the beating is unclear.

In short order, intoxicated soldiers from Portsmouth Grove were becoming a colossal nuisance in the town. One correspondent noted, "I now daily meet with soldiers in a state of intoxication along the road, and on Sunday last, an almost continual stream was pouring from the Camp in Newtown [the main business section of Portsmouth]."[8] The same correspondent noted "inferences" taken from his observations and why decisive action was needed to resolve the matter. "It will restrict the privileges of the soldiers," he said, as a few bad apples would contaminate the entire bushel. "It must tend to withdraw from the needy and suffering men the sympathy of our citizens," he continued, as folks would shy away from their benevolent works if having to deal with incorrigible persons. Noting that at time of war the country needed men of sound bodies and clear minds to overthrow the rebellion, he said, "It is a great wrong done our suffering country." And bringing the message home personally, he concluded, "It is also destructive both to the health and the morals of the men."[9] His logic is difficult to argue.

On August 12, 1863, the hospital guards were at it again. Two days later at 1 P.M., Whitman Bosworth returned to his ward and penned a letter to his parents recounting the recent disturbance at the hospital. After completing dinner — a skimpy serving of bread and water because he found the chowder difficult to digest — Bosworth added an addendum to the nearly completed letter using bold penmanship similar to a newspaper headline. He wrote:

Great Riot at Portsmouth Grove Hospital

Well I must tell you how the officers are frightened here. The outside guards are home guards, enlisted to do guard duty at this hospital. Well, some of them got quite drunk before yesterday and one of them came into the hospital to pick a fight with some of the patients. After insulting several, he came across a wounded man that would not stand his abuse and a free fight ensued, the guard getting roughly handled. The captain of the guard came down and took up sides with the drunken guard striking the wounded man across his old wound, breaking his sword and hurting the patient quite bad. Then the patients rushed in and used the captain roughly blackening his face and eyes quite considerable. Then the whole military force was called out to quell the fuss. There has been no fuss with the patients since, but the officers and guards are as scared as the patients would be in front of a rebel battery. The guard has been doubled and they have been kept under arms for two days and nights fearing an attack on the knapsack house where there is a quantity of old arms stacked. They put several men inside and barricaded the doors and windows.

Well, about one o'clock they heard a noise around the building and thinking someone was trying to get in, one of the men stuck his gun out of the window and fired in the direction of the noise and killed a dog.

Thus ends one of the most desperate riots ever recorded in the annals of history.[10]

The above is just one of many drinking accounts known to survive thanks to men like Whitman Bosworth and George Peck's meticulous letters and diary entries.

Peck in particular recorded a great many such stories. An interesting perspective about the seriousness of the problem is found in his diary, where he uses an assortment of euphemisms to describe the binge drinking that went on at the hospital. Peck, however, only mentions the overindulgence of men in his own company, while revealing nothing about similar problems among patients and medical staff. But there were drinking problems with these men also. Excessive drinking was pervasive throughout the compound, and as mentioned above, especially after men went on short-term leave. All the events listed below took place in 1864. On March 30, Peck writes, "McDermott drunk today and *saucy*. Put in the guardhouse."[11] And on a day in late April he notes, "Some of the men are rather *boozy* tonight."[12] In another entertaining anecdote he writes, "Last night, McDermott and McWilliams had a little bit of a row. Both a little *sprung*."[13] And when the boys in the Commissary Department were tired and sleepy one night in late May, they got into a tussle because they were "a little tight," he explains.[14] A week after the Fourth of July, Peck notes that four or five men in the company were drunk. No euphemisms were used here, just simple facts. And on August 29, he writes that the "boys stayed out over their passes and came in pretty well *corned*," while adding to the commentary, "One with his face in pretty bad shape, both eyes closed up and bruised." The men were later arrested and placed in a holding cell awaiting court-martial.

On September 1, 1864, to his own amazement, George Peck writes, "Co A is quite sober today" [Sunday].[15] With brevity he writes, "No one drunk." But three days later, he sings the same old tune: "Several men in the barracks drunk today."[16] Then on October 12, in an unusual twist, he notes, "Sutler White [is] in the guardhouse for being drunk." That incident must have been the last straw as orders were issued that day to stop all selling in the guardhouse.[17]

Coincidently, in Providence, a session of the Grand Division of the Sons of Temperance for the State of Rhode Island was holding its annual convention. The attendance was large, and as the newspaper reported afterward, the session was "a very *spirited* one."[18] No pun was intended, but the choice of words by the writer left something to be desired.

When Stephen Rogers, a patient in Ward 28, received an order from his surgeon to pick up a box at the post office, he was greeted by the officer-of-the-day. "All boxes had to pass an examination to see that no spirituous liquors are brought in," he explained in a letter to his parents. After inquiring what was in the box, Rogers mentioned several items, to which the officer responded "that there was enough to feed an army." Besides food, the box also contained undershirts, socks, and a vest, but no spirits.[19]

Over the months that followed, the hospital guards became more of a problem since most of the reported infractions on the compound were among themselves. Binge drinking was only one issue. Peck lists particulars more befitting a police rap sheet than a soldier's diary. Fighting, disobeying orders, disrespecting an officer, sleeping on guard duty, robberies, absent without leave (AWOL), and hiding contraband were nearly bi-weekly occurrences.

Those in authority had to wonder if more security was needed to control the unruly guards. The problem was that serious.

It is almost inconceivable that the following infractions took place on hospital grounds. Yet George Peck's accounts do not appear exaggerated or subject to idle imagination. Some infractions seem petty while others are considerably more serious. They are presented chronologically and verbatim to capture their full effect:

— Jan. 5, 1864: "A fight took place in the guardhouse today. Nobody hurt; cause, liquor."
— Jan. 25, 1864: "[John] Markey and [Wilson D.] Pierce in solitary confinement, the first for being drunk and the other for disobeying orders."
— April 29, 1864: "Flemming put in guardhouse today after staying over his pass. [John] Stewart confined tonight for absence without leave."
— May 26, 1864: "Creed put in confinement for grumbling."
— July 13, 1864: "Dr. Flowers was put under arrest today for trying to save a man's life and neglecting a trifling duty."
— July 13, 1864: "Corporal Russ [the] Quartermaster was also placed under arrest for sending a requisition without letting [Commanding Officer] Edwards see it."
— July 23, 1864: "[James] Ryder and Crofton put in guard house ironed and gagged. They were drunk when they were ordered to carry logs. They disobeyed [1st Lieutenant William S.] Chace's command. Ryder was struck on the back with a sword several times. He lunged at Chace but didn't connect."
— Aug. 29, 1864: Two men put in the guardhouse on August 29 were taken out for three hours and tied together "forced to wear a placard labeled 'drunkard' and marched up and down in front of the barracks."
— Sep. 25, 1864: "Two men arrested today for stealing money from the express office. The case is under investigation."
— Oct. 15, 1864: "Forty run the guard last night."
— Oct. 17, 1864: "Three of those who run the guard have been picked up and brought back. The Captain has put a veto on all passes until he finds out who lets the men out."
— Oct. 26, 1864: "[2nd] Lieutenant [John H.] Hammond and Sergeant [Horatio N.] Slocum were put under arrest and two privates [Michael] McDermott and Pierce put in the guard house."
— Oct. 27, 1864: "Three men are paraded on barracks for running guard."
— Nov. 7, 1864: "[Timothy] Collins found asleep on post at 7 o'clock." And in another entry for the same day, Peck writes, "Williamson escaped from the guardhouse tonight. Flemming being on guard at the time was arrested."
— Nov. 8, 1864: "[Bernard] Burns and [Thomas] Harper had a stand up fight," and as if the referee, he states, "About an even thing."
— Nov. 12, 1864: Creed again is put in the guardhouse for overstaying his furlough.
— Dec. 1, 1864: "A darkey confined in the guardhouse today. The first one ever in there." [No reason was given for the incarceration.]
— Dec. 10, 1864: "[Thomas] Duffy and [Ralph] Street had a fight. Duffy getting the worst of it. Searched Duffy's box and found two quarts of whiskey. Put him in the guard house."
— Dec. 10, 1864: "Pierce and [William] Gavin had another row about taps, but they were separated before they came to blows."
— Dec. 19, 1864: "Caught Collins asleep on post. Reported him to the captain who ordered him confined in a cell."[20]

So ended 1864, in what would be another tumultuous year for the hospital guards.

Intelligent men would think by now the hospital guards would have learned their lesson, but their behavior did not improve in the early months of 1865. On January 3, George Peck reported that Duffy was arrested and placed in a cell for selling liquor.[21] (Duffy, an Irishman from Pawtucket, Rhode Island, was a tough character, as his name appears many times for drinking and fighting, according to Peck's diary entries, but to his credit he managed to stay the course, unlike others who deserted. Duffy mustered out of service on August 26, 1865.) A week later, Duffy and [Edward] Pyers were arrested for selling liquor again.[22] Duffy had yet to learn his lesson and probably did not have any intention of doing so. Later that same day, a letter was read at morning roll which placed the entire blame for the "liquor trade" squarely upon the shoulders of the hospital guards. The admonishment may have been a bit late. Sometime within that day, Duffy and Pyers were court-martialed.[23]

On January 9, Dr. Cushing, acting as the officer-of-the-day, had a virtual field day arresting men. Six were sent to cells; George Peck fails to mention the offenses,[24] but based on his diary up to that point, one has to assume excessive drinking and fighting were contributing factors. Later in the month, Green and Collins were caught fighting, in what had now become one of the favorite extracurricular activities of the guards, running a close second only to inebriation. No mention is made whether either was incarcerated.[25]

Before George Peck's diary ends in late February, he tells of two additional incidents. On the ninth he writes, "One soldier captured trying to get back into the compound. Found with two quarts of whiskey, one in pants pocket, one in his [coat?] pocket," and on the following day he notes, "Pyers and Fleming had a little bit of a row in the guardhouse last night."[26]

The hospital guards paid dearly for their transgressions. According to John D. Billings in his profusely illustrated bestseller *Hardtack and Coffee*, published not long after the war, the most common offenses were drunkenness, absence without leave, absence from roll call, showing disrespect for superior officers, gambling, and leaving guard without relief.[27] Several hospital guards at Portsmouth Grove seemed to be guilty, at one time or another, of at least one of the above infractions.

The entire approach to discipline during the Civil War centered on the words *shame* and *pain*, though flogging ceased to be a remedy for bad behavior. In far too many instances, little good came from the corrective action, what is known today as corporal punishment. When released from incarceration, men waited for the opportunity to desert.[28] Like the fictitious Rhett Butler in *Gone with the Wind*, soldiers didn't "give a damn" and committed the same offenses time and time again.

George Peck tells of a soldier being released from the guardhouse and having his ball and chain removed after being in confinement for a year.[29] A sane man can only imagine the severity of his crime to justify such a long and cruel punishment.

From June 6, 1864, through January 19, 1865, when the diary was nearly complete, George Peck gives a ringside view of the punishments handed out at Portsmouth Grove. All at the receiving end were hospital guards. On June 6, he says, "Creed tied up by the thumbs today for insolence."[30] The following day he suggests, "Whitney is crazy again and the sergeant kick[s] and cuff[s] him round, which is shameful." The beating must have been bad, as two days later, Whitney was sent to Ward ll for treatment.[31]

Matters quieted down some; at least George Peck made no additional entries in his diary about disciplinary actions for two months. Then on September 1, he writes about two men, "one sentenced by Court Martial paraded in front of Headquarters, one on a barrel with a placard 'Absent Without Leave' and the other on the ground labeled 'drunkard.'"[32] On October 20, we read that Fleming was confined "and stood on a barrel at post one with 'drunkard' tied on his back for getting drunk and leaving post and going to his quarters." Three days later, we learn that Fleming was released in the morning, but not before his head was shaved. With relief, he writes in his diary: "No one drunk today."[33]

Before the year ended, (Michael) Haley and young (John) Smith, a resident of Portsmouth, would have more fisticuffs. "Haley got tied-up by the thumbs for two hours because of it ... Smith came off free," as Peck tells it.[34] And an entry written on January 19, 1865, simply states: "McDermott came back from Newport drunk and was confined after being gagged."[35]

In a chapter dealing with excessive drinking, rowdiness, and military discipline, the reader might think this an awkward place to include a story about children. Troubling as it sounds, it is appropriate. Maud Howe Elliott, in her book *This Was My Newport*, discusses an incident involving her and her friend at the hospital that deserves retelling. Though questioning its validity years later, she says, "It stands the clearest image in all the shifting picture of that day of days." Unbeknownst to her mother, 7-year-old Maud and her 8-year-old boyfriend decided to run away from home. Traveling less than three miles, they came upon the front entrance of the hospital. Two sentries "crossed their bayonets above the young couple's heads and proceeded to chaff them." Not seeing them as a security risk, the guards eventually let the children enter. Walking down the main road past hospital tents to the boat landing, they came upon an unpleasant scene, "a place of torture, where, in a small shed, a culprit stood with water falling drop by drop upon his head." Maud questioned her memory later in life and asked, "Was this a dream?" For those who are curious, Maud and her companion made it home safely that day after her frantic mother arrived in a horse-drawn carriage and took them home.[36]

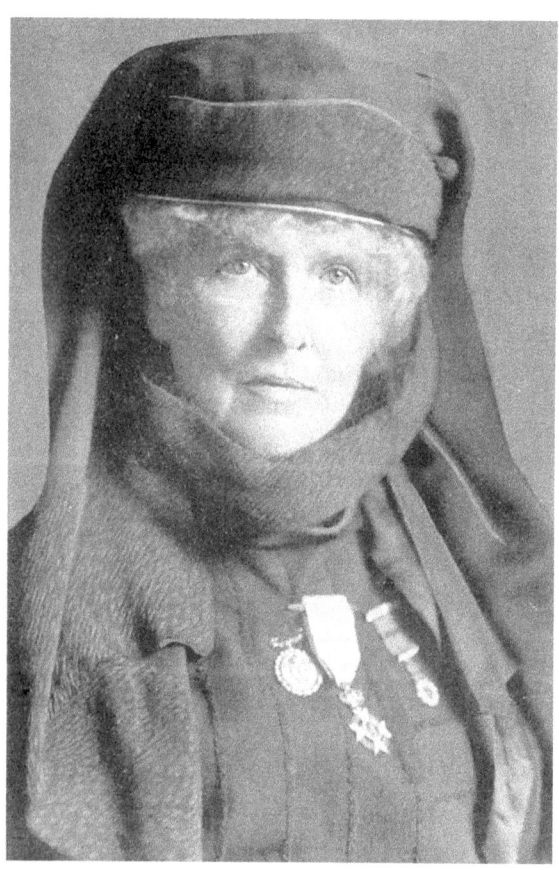

Maud Howe Elliott as she appeared later in life. Mrs. Elliott was the daughter of Julia Ward Howe, author of the "Battle Hymn of the Republic" (photograph by Bachrach).

On August 18, 1862, the Portsmouth Grove Hospital's patient load and staff were about to expand. Assistant Surgeon James Harris from the Marine Hospital in Providence was appointed surgeon at the new facility. Prior to his appointment at the Marine Hospital, he served with the 7th Regiment Rhode Island Volunteers. Because of the extensive scale of the Portsmouth Grove complex, all the patients from Providence were transferred to this new location. The hospital in Providence was disbanded but eventually reopened as a soldiers' home. During this period, 20 nurses from New Hampshire and Maine were ordered to Portsmouth Grove, each to be paid $13 a month for their services.[37]

Chapter 9
Hospital Volunteers and Benefactors

... it is the mutual duty of all to practice Christian forbearance, love, and charity towards each other.
— Virginia Bill of Rights,
Article 16, June 12, 1776

On August 28, 1862, a concert was held in Newport under the auspices of the First Ladies of Newport at Ocean Hall for the benefit of the sick and wounded soldiers at Portsmouth Grove Hospital. Signor A. Barili, a well-known Italian singer of the time, dedicated his services. The event was to be the social event of the season and Newport's privileged were expected to attend. After the concert, the event proved to be a resounding success, socially for the guests and charitably for the hospital.[1]

The hospital also had its own special benefactor, a Newport merchant by the name of Benjamin J. Tilley. Benjamin's store, in the commercial area of lower downtown Newport close to the waterfront on the corner of Touro and Thames Streets—now the site of a national retail clothing chain—was known without fanfare as Tilley's, as unpretentious as the man himself.[2] Benjamin Tilley made his living selling books, newspapers, and periodicals and advertised profusely in many local papers. Whenever possible, he distributed newspapers, periodicals and little gifts to the patients at the hospital. Despite his having to walk with a crutch due to disability caused by the scourge of an undisclosed childhood illness, he accomplished a great deal during his lifetime.[3] When the war seemed endless, Tilley became an enthusiastic supporter of former commanding general and now presidential candidate George B. McClellan. McClellan's platform of establishing peace with the Confederacy attracted Benjamin's attention and stirred his emotions, especially after he had visited patients with horrific battlefield wounds at Portsmouth Grove. Tilley became a staunch Democrat and served as an elected officer and campaign supporter for the local M'Clellan [sic] Club. In his early forties, despite his disability, he served two terms as a representative to the General Assembly of the State of Rhode Island, as a treasurer of the local chapter of the Freemasons, and a member of the Sons of Temperance.[4]

On the island there was barely a person who did not know and comment on Tilley's untiring and benevolent dedication to the invalid soldiers. For three years, and as long as his health permitted, he visited the institution several times each week. He also organized several clothing drives and raised donations to procure holiday meals for the invalids. When ingredients like jellies, lemons, oranges, and barberries were requested for making cool summer drinks for the patients, Tilley championed the cause. Donations were routinely accepted at his store, and sometime during the day he took time from his busy schedule to transport the proceeds to the hospital. Tilley became so well known and trusted that monetary contributions were mailed directly to him, as the letter below reveals:

> Mapleville, RI, July 11, 1864
>
> Mr. B.J. Tilley:
> My Dear Sir:
>
> Knowing you to be a friend to the soldiers, I enclose to your address six dollars contributed by the Mapleville Sabbath School from their Fourth of July fund. Will you please invest it for delicacies for the wounded at Portsmouth Grove?
>
> Yours, very respectfully, for the
> Mapleville Sabbath School,
> J.A. SMITH, Sup'd't[5]

The Thanksgiving and Christmas holidays were only surpassed by Tilley's preparations for Independence Day, for which he organized ceremonies, an oration, and much to the delight of the patients, evening fireworks. The dinner and events were paid for by subscriptions of the local citizenry championed by the efforts of Mr. Tilley.

Benjamin Tilley was so loved by patients at the hospital that one invalid presented him with "an elegant shell frame 10 by 15 inches, most exquisitely wrought of rare shells the whole work by his own hand." The newspaper article that published the above testimonial went on to conclude: "Mr. Tilley has done more than any other man in this vicinity for the soldiers."[6] Benjamin J. Tilley, a gentle and magnanimous soul, was undeniably the Walt Whitman of Portsmouth Grove Hospital.

Tilley was one of many who volunteered his time and energy to the needs of patients at the hospital; but most names are lost to posterity. One name, however, has surfaced: Charity Slocum. Little is known about her efforts except a brief testament that she was a constant visitor at the hospital.[7] As of this writing, no specifics have been determined. People like Benjamin Tilley and Charity Slocum helped, but there were other like-minded citizens in the area that contributed their time and energy.

Even when the hospital was operating at far less than capacity, medical supplies were scarce, as evident from a practice thought to be confined only to Southern belles of the Confederacy. Nurses at Portsmouth Grove resorted to tearing up their petticoats for use as bandages until their supply of undergarments was exhausted. Striking up the courage, nurses complained to the commanding officer about the situation; and later, after using his authority and perhaps ingenuity, he found bandages in a vastly depleted supply system.[8] But to alleviate this shortage, local newspapers printed several petitions by the Surgeon General of the U.S. Army requesting "a prompt response by all the women and children to furnish lint for the wounded soldiers."[9] Citizens picked or scraped lint from old garments and compressed them by hand into absorbent packing, then donated them to dress soldiers' wounds.[10] Even Dr. Samuel David Gross, in his book *A Manual of Military Surgery*, proclaimed the benefits of lint and recommended what type to collect: "The patent or apothecary's, as is it termed, is the best, as it is soft and easily adapted to the parts to which it is intended to be applied."[11] Good intentions aside, the treatment was highly unsanitary and caused numerous infections, many of which turned deadly. For the Union, the practice of lint collecting continued throughout the war with no one the wiser of the dire consequences. With the scarcity of cotton in the Confederacy because of the strangling Union blockade of Southern port cities, military and civilians had to make do. Used bandages, instead of being discarded, were washed in boiling water and reused. The cleaning process incidentally sanitized the bandages. As the war progressed, wound infections were far fewer for men of the Confederacy than those in the Union army.

On a cool late November morning in 1862, Portsmouth Grove received another 250 sick and wounded from Virginia. Whether advance notice was received so that hospital staff would be in readiness is uncertain. The new arrivals included men from local Rhode Island regiments.[12] The people on the island, however, were well prepared, giving food donations for the upcoming Thanksgiving holiday, in quantities estimated to last not one day but an entire week. The food assortment ranged from turkeys, chickens and geese to cases of wine, preserves, and pies. During one Thanksgiving season, the hospital guards were beneficiaries of forty turkeys sent by the ladies of Providence.[13] All

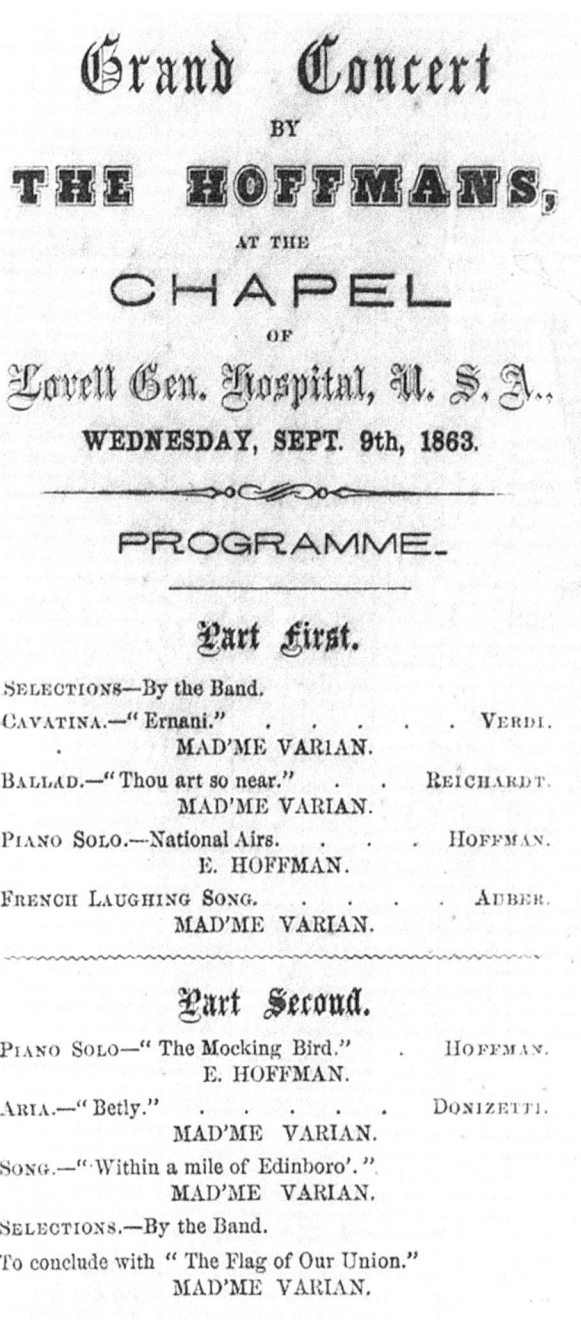

Like many others, the Hoffmans performed at the hospital to raise funds for the men (author's collection).

at Portsmouth Grove would be well fed for the holidays, although some meat may not have been properly stored to maintain absolute freshness. A Thanksgiving meal usually consisted of "boiled turkey, potatoes, mush, gravy, and a piece of pie and one apple and a half for supper."[14] During the holidays, ladies who volunteered to serve the meals usually bestowed small presents upon the soldiers. The day before Thanksgiving in 1864, several men from the hospital guards raised money to buy a barrel of hard cider. The captain found out and told the men to keep their money as he would get it for them. Perhaps figuring he would be confronted with more drunkards than he cared to imagine, he told the men he was unable to find any. George Peck, commenting in his diary about the captain's inability to procure the party liquor, provided this condensed assessment: "So he said."[15]

December was an important month for the young women of Aquidneck Island who organized the annual Young Ladies' Fair to benefit the Auxiliary of the U.S. Sanitary Commission. The two-day event raised an average of $800 annually. Though the timing of the fundraising event seemed to conflict with the Christmas food drive for Portsmouth Grove's hospital, it did not. The Governor of Rhode Island assured all concerned that all necessary supplies for the Christmas dinner would be in place.[16] And so they were. The food was abundant and the meals sumptuous, with only a few exceptions.

An article in the *Fall River Herald* written 62 years after the war reminisced about Sunday steamboat excursions in the summer from Providence, Newport, New Bedford, and Fall River, giving passengers an opportunity to visit Union and Confederate patients at the hospital. They traveled on one of two steamers: the *Perry* or the *City of Newport*. The excursion was usually planned as a round trip from Newport to Providence but also touched "at Portsmouth Grove each way."[17] A one-way fare from Newport to Portsmouth Grove cost 25 cents.[18] Many ladies came laden with baked goods and flower bouquets. When they arrived at the hospital, they immediately set about their work taking care of the Confederate soldiers and the Union men. The ladies were said to comb prisoners' hair and a few gave them money. Others simply came to gawk, and as some correspondents noted, some curious friendships were fashioned between local females and the prisoners. Although the ladies were permitted to chat with the Confederates, some stories they told were reported as tall tales likely invented to impress the womenfolk.

Union men were offended by the show of attention given their enemy and there were more than a few citizens who claimed Confederate prisoners were wearing donated clothes intended for Union soldiers or receiving other preferential treatment. The accusations were probably factual as the accounts were too numerous to discount. One correspondent noted in the *Bristol Phenix*: "Much complaint has been made that articles sent down, designed for the soldiers have not been distributed with the care and discrimination they should have been." Placing the blame squarely on an anonymous hospital administrator — thinly veiled — he continued, "There has been a screw loose somewhere in this respect as well as some others; and we think, if the testimony of hundreds of the men with whom we conversed are to be credited, a certain high official ... is not entirely blameless."[19]

On a more positive note, the hospital was not without humor. A vignette was published locally detailing a brief conversation between a Union and a Confederate patient, convalescing in the same ward. The Confederate, initially extremely ill but now on the road to recovery, was cantankerous as ever, so much so that other patients were annoyed with his demeanor. One day the Union invalid, an adopted citizen from Germany, tried to strike up a conversation with the Confederate. The exchange went thusly:

> "Go to hell," said the Confederate.
> "Do vat?" the Yankee asked.
> The Confederate repeated his sentiment: "Go to hell."
> The German was not at all exasperated.
> "Ah!" said he, "mine friend, you ish too kind, I cannot go to dat place."
> "Why not?" asked the puzzled Confederate.
> "It is now full. It is very crowded der. [General] Sigel he fill it up mit dead rebels. Even the tuyfel [devil] has to sleep out o' doors."[20]

Standing nearby, the medical staff overheard the conversation and were unable to contain their laughter. For the American of German descent, it was an admirable attempt at North/South diplomacy. Though failing to make a friend, his impromptu comeback brightened the day for the medical staff.[21]

Unlike the ill-tempered Confederate, sometime after the heat of battle, men realize they and their enemy are much the same. William Moran of Fall River reminisced years later about a visit he paid to the hospital as a child accompanied by an elder family member. Upon meeting a Confederate army captain, William was briskly picked up by the man. With tears in his eyes, the soldier said, "My little lad, I left in Georgia another such lad as you, and my fondest wish on earth is that I may see him once again." The incident left a lasting impression, though at the time, William could not comprehend the true meaning of the moment.[22]

Chapter 10

New Arrivals: Unanticipated Problems

These are the times that try men's souls.
—Thomas Paine,
The American Crisis, 1776

By the first of September 1862, 2,400 patients were receiving care at the Grove. The hospital was now operating near capacity. Two weeks later, thirty-eight recovered Confederates were to be exchanged at Fort Monroe. Starting their long journey through Providence while under guard, one of the Confederates by the name of William Davis went before Captain Silvie and took the oath of allegiance. All had been prearranged back at Portsmouth Grove, as the necessary paperwork was prepared for the occasion. Imagine the look of condemnation on the faces of his former fellow countrymen when they realized what had happened. William Davis, a reincarnated Union man, was immediately discharged and became a free man.[1]

An important personnel change took place in early September 1862. Dr. Lewis A. Edwards assumed command from Dr. D.J. McKibben. Standing over six feet tall, Dr. Edwards, a regular army major, possessed impeccable credentials for his new assignment. Having graduated from Princeton and the University of Pennsylvania where he received his M.D., he first served with distinction in the military during the Mexican War. Afterward, Dr. Edwards would enhance his physician skills at Santa Fe, New Mexico; Fort Washington, Maryland; and Fort Towson, Arkansas. Before being reassigned to Portsmouth Grove, he was attached to the Bureau of Refugees, Freedmen and Abandoned Lands, and also served as the attending surgeon for officers' families in Washington, D.C.[2] During his tenure at Portsmouth Grove Hospital, he lived up to the advance billing and was highly respected by his staff and wards alike.[3] His initial staff included Assistant Surgeons H. Lawrence Sheldon, U.S.A., and George M. Sternberg, U.S.A., along with physicians Benoni Carpenter, U.S.A., Algernon Coolidge, U.S.A., Philip McNaughten, James E. Marsh, H.B. Livermore, A.M. Paine, Thaddeus Phelps, H.B. Knowles, and Edmund Seyffarth.[4] Dr. Seyffarth served under government contract as an acting assistant surgeon from September 12, 1862, until August 17, 1865, being paid the tidy sum of $100 a month for his services. Born in Germany and schooled at a prestigious university in Vienna, Dr. Seyffarth spent four years learning his profession there. After leaving Germany and Austria and serving as a surgeon on a Russian man-of-war, he found his way to America; specifically Rindge, New Hampshire, and then Lawrence, Massachusetts.[5]

Other physicians appearing frequently in the local press but with no mention in the initial listing by the *Providence Journal* were Dr. William F. Cornick, Dr. Cummings, Dr. James Harris, and Dr. Hentzelman (no first names were found for two of the physicians). They, along with those mentioned previously, comprised only a part of the medical staff by mid–September 1862.[6] More will be said about Dr. Cornick later.

Medical tenure for physicians at the hospital was short-lived. Most of the doctors would spend less than a year at Portsmouth Grove before returning to their respective regiments or private practices. By the end of December 1862, a majority of doctors plying their profession at the hospital were recently hired civilians working under a monthly contract with the government.[7] Whether good, bad, or indifferent, their services would soon be required by men like John M. Lovejoy, who suffered considerably after a long and tedious journey from down south. In a letter to his cousin Cynthia, he tells of his trip as an invalid to Portsmouth Grove after a short stay at the Fairfax Seminary Hospital:

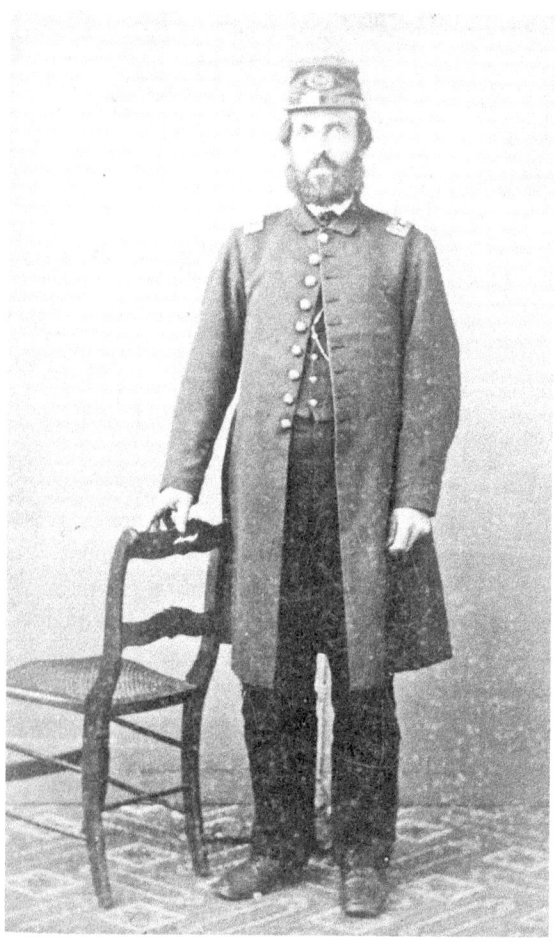

Dr. Lewis A. Edwards, U.S.A., twice served as commander at Portsmouth Grove Hospital. Considered highly capable, he was well respected by patients and staff alike (courtesy Thomas Cottrell).

> We had an awful time coming from Virginia up here. We were ten days on board one of the filthiest transports that flows the ocean. We had to sail from Alexandria down the Potomac to Fort Monroe. There we lay two days waiting for a fair wind ... half on board were sea sick and such a spell of gagging and heaving up Jonah I never saw before nor never wish to again.[8]

Alfred Luther, the Rhode Island lad who lost his right arm fighting at Gaines' Mill, started his journey home in August of 1862. After his capture at a field hospital and spending the next 22 days in a Richmond, Virginia, prison pen struggling for his life, he with other Union men would be exchanged for Confederate prisoners held by the North.[9] An article in the *Providence Evening Press* reported in a news release information obtained from Rhode Island's Adjutant General that Luther had been transported to New York City and was a patient at City Hospital. Soon afterward, he was transferred to Portsmouth Grove. A Rhode Island soldier was now closer to home, only two towns north up Narragansett Bay. Spending less than two months at the hospital, he was discharged on a surgeon certificate.[10] Upon his return to civilian life in late October 1862, his maimed body would serve as testament to the cruelties of the war. Alfred Luther would spend the remaining years of the war living with his parents and reading about his unit fighting in some of the largest battles of the war. Yet, for Alfred Luther, taking a back seat to the theatrics was a godsend. In frightening reality, he knew what the outcome could have been.

Not all injured and sick sent to Portsmouth Grove Hospital came from the battlefields down south. Several black soldiers from the 14th Regiment Rhode Island Heavy Artillery (Colored), training on Dutch Island off the coast of Jamestown in Narragansett Bay, were taken ill and sent to the hospital for recovery. Probably the men were stricken with smallpox, as many had already died of the disease and were buried on the tiny island.[11] Later, the graves were removed to a more established cemetery.

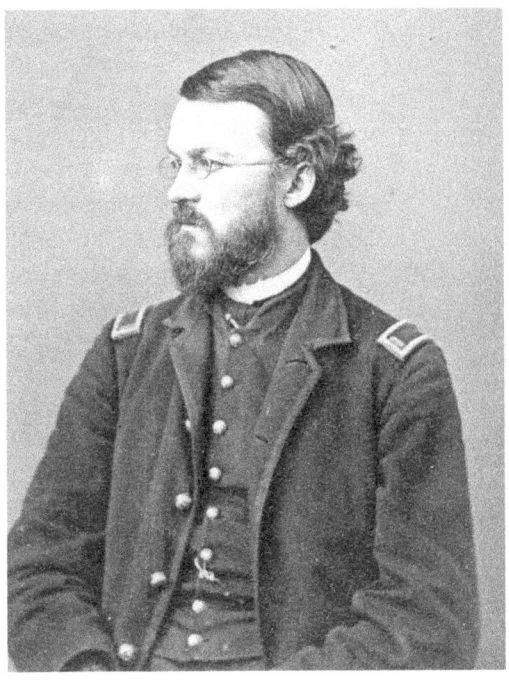

Dr. Edmund Seyffarth served as a contract doctor for nearly the entire time the hospital was open. When this image was taken, Seyffarth was the surgeon in wards 16 and 18 (courtesy Dr. Stephen Altic, D.O.; from his collection).

And then there was 27-year-old Duncan McEachern, born in Glasgow, Scotland, serving with the 13th Regiment Massachusetts Light Artillery, whose feet became frostbitten on the night of December 15, 1862, while performing guard duty at Camp Meigs in Readville, Massachusetts. The frostbite was so severe that all his toes had to be amputated at Pemberton Square Hospital in Boston. He remained there until September 28, 1863, when he was transferred to the Veteran Reserve Corps. From November 1863 until June 1864, he was listed on the rolls of Portsmouth Grove Hospital. Finally, on March 2, 1865, the surgeons issued a Certificate of Disability, and Duncan McEachern was released from the service.[12]

Like most invalids, regardless of mustering state, Rhode Island boys prayed for an early release and homecoming. In a letter from Rhode Island governor William Sprague to Dr. Lloyd Morton and Charlotte F. Dailey dated December 1862, the two-person committee was authorized to visit and inspect various hospitals where Rhode Island soldiers were sick or disabled. Their mission was fourfold:

1. To procure from the Secretary of War an order for the removal of sick and wounded Rhode Island soldiers to the United States Hospital at Portsmouth Grove;

2. To visit the United States Hospitals in and around the city of Washington, and especially that in Alexandria; and, also, the hospitals in Philadelphia, Harrisburg, Baltimore, and wherever else Rhode Island soldiers may be situated, with the particular object of finding out their condition, and make a report of each case to the Department to be presented to the Legislature at its coming Session;
3. The Commission is particularly charged with the transfer to the hospital at Portsmouth Grove, of all wounded and invalid soldiers belonging to Rhode Island regiments from the different hospitals as above directed...;
4. To procure the discharge of every soldier found to be unfitted for further service, and, also, to cause the removal to said hospital of all those cases where health can be better restored within the State....

Leaving Providence on the evening of December 17, and returning on January 24, Dr. Morton and Mrs. Dailey managed to visit four hundred eight Rhode Islanders in sixty-one hospitals and five camps. The entire inspection took only five weeks and four days to complete.

By the first week of January 1863 they had managed to secure the transfer of a large number of Rhode Islanders back to Portsmouth Grove. In a detailed report issued to the General Assembly of the State of Rhode Island on February 2, they determined that of those already sent home, "nearly one hundred will never be fit for duty." Many men suffered from typhoid fever, diarrhea, and rheumatism. In two separate hospitals, three cases of smallpox were also reported. Making note, the committee found many Rhode Island cavalry men were confined to beds as a result of horse injuries. Not surprisingly, they found that nearly all convalescents suffered from exposure and fatigue. The report further noted: "They are discouraged and disheartened by lingering so long in hospitals or the prospect of it."[13]

The report also comprised fifteen pages of soldier's names, hospitals, location, company and regiment, with a remarks column listing their conditions or in some cases duty status (on pass, discharged, and so forth); gunshot wounds, shell wounds and contusions, fractures, amputations, fever, and diarrhea were the status quo. On a smaller scale, but not to diminish the injury or condition, ankle sprains, eye injuries and blindness, heart problems, consumption, and scurvy were also reported. An entry for James Russell, Company F, of the 4th Regiment Rhode Island Volunteers, simply stated: "Never well."

Viewed as an enormous success, the trip seemed to accomplish all its objectives. A convalescent soldier in a Baltimore hospital summarized the feelings of all Rhode Islanders about the commission's visit, speaking in trembling lips, "I am so glad to know that somebody is thinking of us."[14]

This would not be the last occasion of a commission visiting Rhode Island soldiers. Within the first few months of 1863, another commission visited Rhode Island troops in the field and reported "that conditions were generally favorable in spite of delay occasionally in payment of wages due soldiers and difficulty of obtaining supplies promptly after requisition."[15]

Governor William Sprague, a strong advocate of all Union soldiers, not just Rhode Islanders, helped organize hospital visits and inspections. A story published in a local newspaper is worth noting here. A soldier named Hodgkinson, a private in Co. B, 36th

Regiment Massachusetts Volunteer Infantry, was returning home from the war when he boarded a train on his way from New York. Not finding a seat, he was about to sit on his knapsack when a gentleman approached him and urged him to take his seat, saying that he "could not sit comfortably while a soldier was without one." After his offer was turned down, the stranger insisted and the private acquiesced. When an adjoining seat was vacated, the gentleman sat down next to Hodgkinson, and they chatted until arriving in Providence. When the private asked for the gentleman's name, the modest stranger said, "Mr. Sprague." Private Hodgkinson had not only met but had spoken with Governor William Sprague of Rhode Island.[16]

Commissions from several states would also visit the hospital with the intention of returning men back to their home states. After a New York commission visited Portsmouth Grove in February 1863, an order was given to have all New York men ready for a return to their state.[17] Whitman Bosworth, in a letter dated August 7, 1863, said, "A commissioner from New Hampshire has just come through the ward. He is taking the names of all the men from his state and says they shall go to New Hampshire."[18] This would not be the last time New York or New Hampshire representatives would visit the hospital. Connecticut and Maine would carry out similar missions.

Early in January 1863, a few newly assigned hospital guards became ill with smallpox, thought to be of the mild variation. John F. Austin, in a letter to his wife Emily on January 27, 1863, called it "nothing more than chicken pox," trying to ease her fear as he along with all the other patients and staff at the hospital were in the direct line of fire for contracting the disease.[19]

Unique to human beings, smallpox is an infectious disease with two variants: variola major and variola minor. The major form carries an estimated 35 percent death rate, while the minor form, but 1 percent. Most survivors bear facial scars for life after experiencing large spotty eruptions on the face during the disease progression. Weeks after the initial attack, scars usually appear elsewhere on the body where the outbreak first surfaced.[20]

Later during the month, passengers on the steamer *St. Marks* were suspected of carrying the disease and upon confirmation were immediately placed under quarantine in Ward 2.[21] Because many local citizens visited the hospital regularly and convalescents visited stores and families in the area, the town council of Portsmouth took immediate action to protect its citizens from a widespread epidemic. A resolution was adopted on the twenty-second of the month. The first ordinance imposed a $100 penalty for any person from the town who visited the hospital. The second allowed visitations to the hospital under "absolute necessity" only after the chief officer of the hospital granted approval. This required an official pass. The third authorized "the [town]

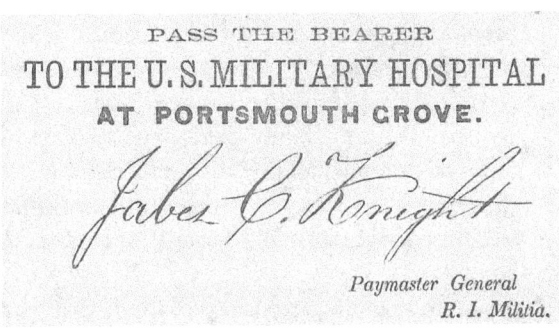

To control the influx of visitors at the hospital especially during the smallpox epidemic, civilians were required to obtain a pass such as this one (author's collection).

council clerk to write the chief surgeon to solicit his cooperation." In consonance, the Newport City Council did the same. Their ordinance set up an invisible "two-way quarantine between the city and the hospital."[22]

When John Austin's wife Emily came to visit him in January, she was greeted with a "No Admittance" sign. Assuming Emily had the required pass, she still needed to see the steward before the privilege was granted to enter the ward. Despite some grumbling, the practice proved effective, as it helped to contain the disease.[23]

Vaccination for smallpox was not a new technique even with the archaic medical knowledge for disease control during the Civil War. Inoculation to thwart the disease had been employed in America since 1721— some say centuries before — but the preventive measure could be dangerous. The vaccine was obtained from a cow or calf infected with cowpox, a close cousin to smallpox. The inoculation method, however, was brutal. With a non-sterilized knife, a deep gash or gashes were made in the person's arm and the liquid obtained from the infected cow or calf was then poured into the wound. Even after the inoculation, the vaccine could prove ineffective, or worse, precipitate more serious complications. Blood poisoning became a real and frightening consequence in many documented cases.[24]

On several occasions from his hospital bed, John Lovejoy wrote his cousin Cynthia, back in New York, about the outbreak and his vaccination: "The Small Pox [is] quite prevalent here. My arm is dreadfully lame from vaccination. It is now the seventh day.... The cases of Small Pox were discovered before they were broke out and was removed from the ward so the danger is all past."[25] Seth Alden also complained of a sore arm after being vaccinated. He writes: "I had a pretty sore arm for a long time, but I have not looked to see where there was any scar left but I presume there is."[26] His arm was not his only problem. Alden was recovering from a leg wound received at Fredericksburg that caused a limp and called for the use of a cane.[27]

The quick and decisive action by Portsmouth town officials and the hospital staff averted a large epidemic. Only thirteen more cases of smallpox were reported.

During the outbreak, twenty-three sick and wounded Rhode Island soldiers arrived in Newport. Presumably no one had smallpox. After being entertained with refreshments like hot coffee, pies, and other like items, they were taken by the steamer *Perry* to the hospital.[28] Imagine their surprise and dismay when advised of the virus. What could have been a calamity became a notable medical achievement. The ordinance, however, did not sit well especially for patients whose relatives came from Newport and were severely restricted from traveling to their homes. "Let the worthy fathers imagine themselves returned from the battle-field weary, sick and wounded and placed in a hospital seven miles from home, and by the foolish notions of a few old fogies, unable to get there — then they would have the same sentiments that we have, and every other patriot." The letter was written to the *Newport Daily News* on February 14 and tersely signed, "Small Pox."[29]

Although the seriousness of the disease was downplayed by patients in letters mailed home, there were a few soldiers who died of the illness. The names, however, are not known. One man was diagnosed with the most serious type: "black smallpox," known to doctors as hemorrhagic smallpox. Decades later, a former ward master still could remember how the deceased appeared: "His body was black as a stovepipe." When the remains were lifted onto a stretcher using a sheet, the ward master witnessed flesh peeling away from the body. The story he tells is not fiction. Black smallpox causes hemorrhaging under the skin and makes it appear charred or black. The skin easily peels away because of all the pus pockets covering the body and is not a pleasing sight.[30]

On March 9, 1863, the ordinances were revoked. Smallpox, however, was not completely wiped out from the island, as could be seen by white warning flags still hanging from homes. In Middletown, a few cases arose simultaneously with the military hospital and the hope was, as one person stated, "that the disease may be arrested within its present limits."[31] But that was not to be. The first death was reported on January 29, 1863, that being the wife of Amos Peckham. Not until the end of May, after a few more isolated cases were reported in Newport, would the disease vanish, at least for the remainder of 1863.[32]

On December 8, 1864, a tent was erected, segregating one soldier suspected of carrying smallpox from the rest of the patients. That night the wind blew down the tent and it took a while before someone would help raise it again.[33] This should come as no surprise as smallpox was a frightening and highly contagious disease. Two weeks later, the disease was confirmed as smallpox. The unlucky carrier was Private John F. Follett, soon to become a corporal in the Hospital Guards—Rhode Island Volunteers. He was fortunate to survive the illness.[34]

On a more uplifting note, in mid–February a New England mother intending to visit her invalid soldier son at Portsmouth Grove regrettably ran out of funds to continue her journey. She had left her hometown with five dollars in her purse thinking the amount sufficient. Several ladies on board the same steamship, *Perry*, hearing of her plight, took up a collection among the passengers to defray her unplanned expenses. The needed funds were obtained and the appreciative woman was able to visit her son and return home without further financial concerns.[35]

Chapter 11

Angels of Mercy

Behold, I send an angel before thee, to keep thee in the way.
— Exodus 23:20

When the hospital was first established, nurses were difficult to find on Aquidneck Island and the surrounding communities on the mainland. Except for military nurses, a few female nurses employed by the U.S. Sanitary Commission, and irregular volunteers, hospital nurses always seemed in short supply. Though ladies were qualified for the profession and even willing to perform their services at Portsmouth Grove, they lacked the daily fare for roundtrip transport from Newport to the Grove. Some local services volunteered to transport the ladies to the hospital at no charge, but how long this service continued is anyone's guess.[1] Trained and experienced nurses would have to be found elsewhere.

One such find, and an exceptional one at that, was Katherine Prescott Wormeley. Katherine Wormeley was born to an aristocratic family in England. After the death of her father, a rear admiral in the British navy and a native of Virginia, Katherine, along with her mother, settled in Newport, Rhode Island, where at the age of thirty-one, she began working for the Ladies' Union Aid Society.[2] The war had just broken out. Under her supervision, she secured a government clothing contract during the winter of 1861–62, which provided employment for soldiers' wives and families.[3] With cloth and buttons supplied by the War Department, the seamstress and her helpers made over 50,000 flannel shirts for the Union soldiers, none of which were returned for imperfections.[4] Katherine was paid 14 cents a shirt, from which she paid the ladies 11 cents. The difference was used to defray her expenses.

When the U.S. Sanitary Commission formed the Hospital Transport Service, Katherine, as a volunteer, boarded the *Daniel Webster*, the first commissioned ship to transport the sick and wounded from the battlefield to safe destinations. Her duties ranged from bathing and feeding incoming patients, to cooking, organizing and replenishing supply closets and pantries. A predominant amount of her tenure was spent in Virginia during the Peninsular Campaign and what was to become a huge learning experience. While there, she wrote about poignant moments captured during the performance of her duties. One incident in particular was brief but left an indelible mark upon her memory. She said, "Last night, shining over blood and agony, I saw a lunar rainbow; and in the afternoon a peculiarly beautiful effect of rainbow and stormy sunset,—it flashed upon my eyes as I passed an operating table, and raised them to avoid seeing anything as I passed."[5] The cruel and personal images of war were difficult to observe, even for an experienced nurse like her.

Katherine was a different breed of woman from the dainty hoop-skirted belles who socialized in the 1860s. Not just intelligent, she possessed foresight, a clear-thinking mind, and other rare gifts that allowed her to excel in a field dominated by males. She had been taught well and learned from the shortcomings of others as she continually confronted "appalling examples of medical and organizational unpreparedness." She also learned during the Peninsula Campaign how to circumvent politics and red tape. In June 1862, she wrote, "I should like to have charge of a hospital *now*; I could make it march, if only I had hold of some of the administrative *power*."[6] Soon she would be granted her wish *and* the opportunity to carry on her admirable work.

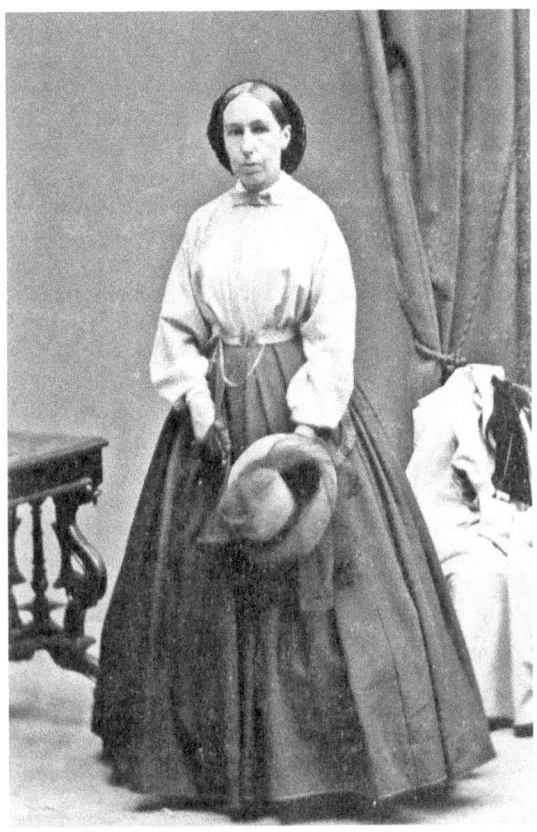

After serving with distinction as a nurse on hospital transports during the Peninsula Campaign, Katherine Prescott Wormeley was named first "Lady Superintendent" of Portsmouth Grove Hospital (courtesy Massachusetts Commandery Military Order of the Loyal Legion and the U.S. Army Military History Institute, Carlisle, Pennsylvania).

Shortly after the Peninsula Campaign, Surgeon General William A. Hammond asked Katherine to accept the lady directorship at Portsmouth Grove. In August 1862, after consulting with her family and friends and despite her poor health, she decided to accept the position.[7] Soon she would be called "Lady Superintendent," a title earned and deserved.[8]

In a letter to Georgeanna Woolsey (nicknamed Georgie) before her arrival at the hospital, she addressed in detail her plans and expectations, while also using Georgeanna as a sounding board:

Miss Wormeley to G

Newport, Sept. 5th, '62

My dear Georgie: I found the new surgeon inclined to one woman for each ward (twenty-eight wards or barracks, of sixty men in each). I hunted him out however. Everything in the domestic management of the hospital being left to me, I shall "gently" avail myself of the courtesy. Now then for your advice my ideas are these. Please give your decided opinion on them. To give five wards, sixty beds to each ward, to the superintendence of five friends—you, your sister, cousin H. Whetten and a lady here whom I esteem and consider efficient. Under these I should put one, two, or three woman nurses, as occasion may require. These five ladies would be responsible for everything connected with their wards, "in general." You know what general supervision means,—cleanliness, beds, linen, due washing thereof, etc, etc, in all of which the women under you should do the actual work whilst you see that they do it. I want to have "the men" intelligently looked after, as only a lady can. I should therefore wish that the ladies should go round with the surgeons "invariably"—to make short notes of each patient's treatment, medicine and diet. Medicines I should want her to make sure were properly and timely given. The special diet lists ordered by the surgeon I should wish to be handed in to me as soon as practicable. I shall put a special diet kitchen at each end of the Barrack St. with a female cook in each, whom I shall attend to myself.

This is in general a sketch of my ideas. What do you say? Will you come? I want to point out to you that no ladies have ever "been allowed" to come into a "U S General Hospital" in this way—much less warmly requested, and thanked, and confided in, as "we are,"—for of course it has nothing personal to myself in it. It is General Hammond's first cordial reception and experiment of ladies in hospital, and is in consequence, as he told me, of the grateful sense he had what we did at White House.

Now as to our own living there—a house is building for us, to be finished by the 12th of this month. It has bedrooms for all the female nurses, a dining room for ditto, an office for me. We shall have to carpet our own rooms, and adorn them as we see fit, the government supplies the common necessities of a bed, etc., for the nurse in general.

I shall want to have you with me at the start. Can you arrange to come?

Write me at once, please. What a vile place you are in; the mails take a week to go.[9]

No evidence has surfaced to date showing that Katherine's plans were negated or changed. Katherine was successful in placing "women in key positions" with supervisory responsibility formerly dominated by males. Further, she was granted the right to disapprove staff positions for doctors "who would not work harmoniously with female nurses and superintendents." Though holding control of the domestic management of the complex, she knew enough to implement changes gradually and wisely until they were accepted in an institution run by males.[10]

Katherine acclimated quickly to her new position and surroundings with self-confidence, tireless energy, and the utmost dedication to her patients, those she respectfully called the "Brave."[11] In family correspondence soon after her arrival, she appeared to be enjoying her new duties and was fairly well established in her "thin board house built for the nursing staff, their rooms 10 × 10, furnished from home with every comfort."[12]

Katherine was also responsible for the diet kitchen, the linen department, and the laundry. Utilizing a steam-operated washing machine, the laundry complex was capable of washing over 4,000 pieces a day. Jane Woolsey describes what she read in Georgeanna's ward notebook one day. The notebook displayed a barracks washing list that consisted of the following items:

120 sheets
60 shirts
70 towels
60 pillowcases
Ditto drawers and socks

In that ward alone, over 1,800 pieces were said to be washed each week.[13]

With twenty-eight separate buildings designed to host sixty-one persons along with attendants, around-the-clock supervision was necessary. Katherine handled the matter by dividing nursing supervision into four separate lots with an assistant superintendent responsible for seven wards each. Understandably, the span of control would increase or decrease based upon patient arrivals and departures.

Nursing assignments, at least in the early stages of the hospital's existence were as follows: one ward master, a woman nurse, and five male nurses to each ward.[14] The numbers would fluctuate depending on patient occupancy. The women nurses were either paid or performed voluntarily, while the male nurses were active-duty service members.

Hospital needs were great, and Katherine Wormeley was continually on a letter-writing campaign to newspapers asking for additional food for her "Brave" men. In one, she requests jellies, preserves, dried fruits and pickles or sauces but "in large quantities, therefore the less expensive kind will suit me best." She also knew how to stir the emotions and lay a guilt trip on potential benefactors. "Thanksgiving Day is approaching ... shall we let these poor fellows, separated from their families, be without some cheerful enjoyment of the day?" she said, concluding with, "I make these requests knowing that your interest equals my own in this matter."[15]

In a letter to a "dear friend" within the U.S. Sanitary Commission, Katherine describes the outcome of the first holiday appeal for the men at the hospital. Rhode Islanders and southeastern Massachusetts residents, she writes "sent me enough for 1,200 men (280 turkeys and geese — 700 mince and pumpkin pies). I had the band of the U.S. Naval Academy — and from first to last, it was a thoroughly successful affair."[16]

No sooner had Thanksgiving passed than Katherine was planning for the Yuletide season. She was looking to serve "roast beef and plum pudding" for dinner. Katherine also wished to have "3 immense Xmas trees" for the men to admire and perk up their spirits. For gifts, she would seek donations of mittens, comforters, and tobacco, as "these would give the greatest delight."[17]

But matters were less than ideal. After confiding to a friend about her happiness helping the invalids, she spoke of a "black spot" that bothered her dearly. The matter had to do with "the cruelty of keeping these men in sheds, in which cattle would suffer." She said there were wallboards "with big

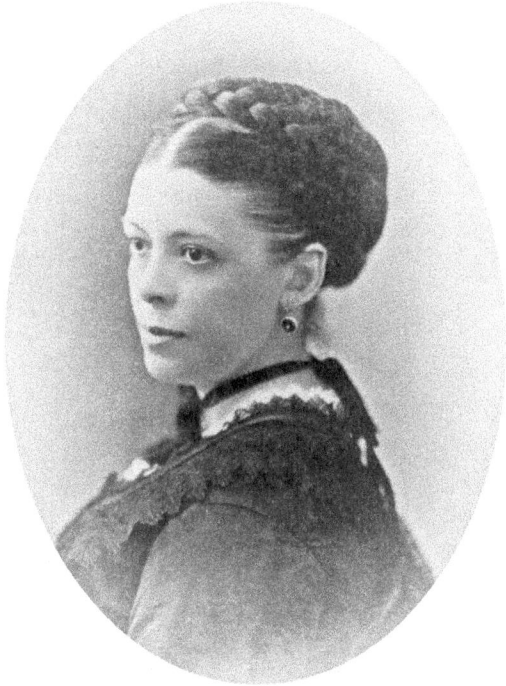

Sarah Chauncey Woolsey and her sisters worked as nurses at Portsmouth Grove Hospital until family concerns about the smallpox epidemic forced them to return home (courtesy Massachusetts Commandery Military Order of the Loyal Legion and the U.S. Army Military History Institute, Carlisle, Pennsylvania).

holes ... and not fitted together [properly]." The inferior construction and low-grade lumber resulted in "beds getting wet" when it rained. "The men cannot keep warm," she said. Sadly, and probably due to government economy, an effort to secure tarpaper prior to shingling of the wards had been disapproved by the quartermaster. As she saw it, "the tarred paper is the real protection against cold." She concluded her thoughts on the subject by saying, "I dread a chilly day. The men are so miserable. What will it be when the cold weather sets in [?]"[18]

Another problem surfaced, and this time it involved her staff. Five months after Katherine's arrival, the first of her aides, Sarah Chauncey Woolsey, was called home by family because of concerns about the smallpox epidemic at the hospital.[19] Initially, the outbreak was reported to be a severe strain, but in most cases proved to be the lesser variant. No matter, Sarah departed for home, but not before leaving a note on scrap paper to Georgeanna, who would double up on Sarah's patients after her departure. The note stated: "Number 41 ought to have soda water and egg beaten in wine every day — Eastman, near the door, be good to him and to D. and C. and M., and read the *Pickwick Papers* to the poor fellow who blew himself up with gunpowder." Her other sisters, previously handpicked by Katherine Wormeley, also departed shortly thereafter.[20]

Katherine's cousin Harriet Whetten would remain at the hospital another year. Invited to become the Lady Superintendent of Carver General Hospital in Washington, D.C., she accepted the position and retained it until the close of the war. Harriet was described by an intimate friend as "a born nurse" who "did more personally for the men" than any of the others.[21]

With her own health failing along with her mother's, along with other unspecified family considerations, Katherine Wormeley resigned her position in September of 1863, about a year after she first arrived.[22] Despite her brief

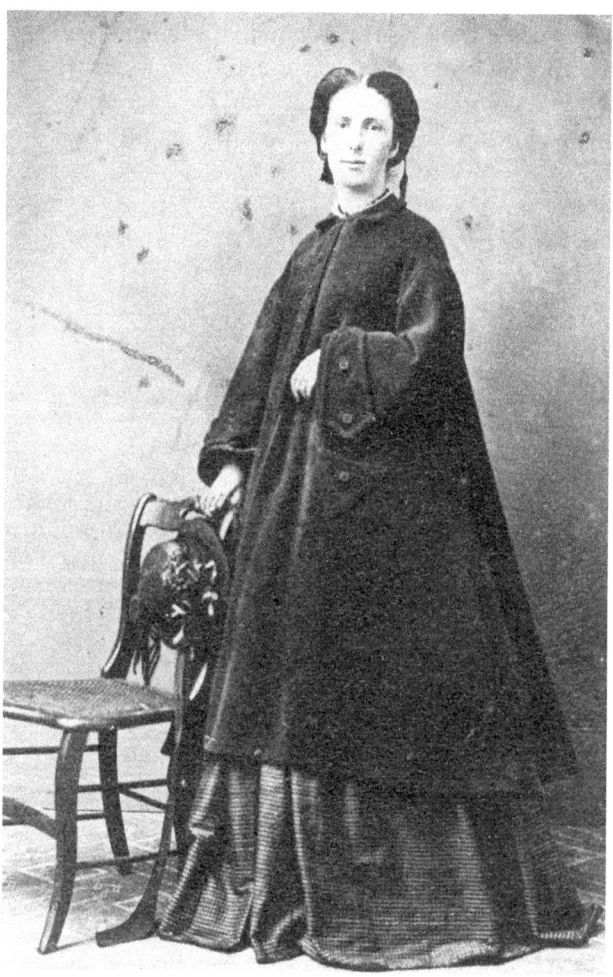

Sixth-generation *Mayflower* descendant Ada A. Brewster, pictured here, and her two sisters served ably as nurses at the hospital (courtesy Dr. Stephen Altic, D.O.; from his collection).

tenure, her effect as Lady Superintendent would resonate for the remaining years of the hospital's existence. Katherine later regained her health and would continue to perform good deeds for the benefit of invalid soldiers. In 1864, as a member of the Boston branch of the New England Women's Auxiliary Association, Katherine Wormeley became the associate manager for Rhode Island and performed charitable work on behalf of all veterans in the state.[23] By the time her work was completed on Aquidneck Island, Katherine Wormeley had collected over $17,000 along with food and supplies for use by the U.S. Sanitary Commission and hospital.[24]

Besides Katherine Wormeley and the Woolsey sisters who nursed with Katherine in the Peninsula Campaign, other nurses are worth mentioning: Agnes Adams Wilbour, her mother Mary Simmons Wilbour, and Sarah C. Dennis. The Wilbour ladies were said to be the first to volunteer their services at the hospital and were already on board before Katherine Wormeley and her staff arrived. About that time, Agnes Wilbour was in charge of hospital linens.[25] Though they were the first nurses at the hospital, many would soon follow.

Also serving as nurses were Ada Brewster of Kingston, Massachusetts, and her sisters Mary and Elizabeth. Elizabeth, affectionately known as Lissie, would go on to become the second Lady Superintendent at the hospital after Katherine Wormeley's departure. The three sisters were descendants of Elder William Brewster, who was a passenger on the *Mayflower* when it sailed into Plymouth harbor in 1620. Period accounts state that Ada and her sisters remained at Portsmouth Grove Hospital until war's end.[26] While there, Ada nursed back to health a young drummer boy hit in the shoulder by either a Minié ball or a shell fragment at Petersburg on July 6, 1864. The injury was said to be more of a contusion then a penetration wound. He was treated with cold water dressings at a field and corps hospital and shortly thereafter was transferred to Portsmouth Grove, where he arrived on the 19th of July. His name was David R. Seville. At the time, Seville served as a private with Company F, 5th Regiment Maryland Volunteer Infantry. From the start, Ada took a liking to this youngster of 16 years, and there is little doubt she affectionately looked after him. He was known as "Ada's boy."[27]

Ada was born May 15, 1842, at her family's home called "Woodside." Early in her life, Miss Brewster became an adventurous soul with a penchant for art. Before the war, Ada perfected her skills at Lowell Institute, where she excelled at brush and pencil sketching.[28] What led her to the nursing profession remains a mystery, but most likely it was her patriotism and a desire to be of service to her fellow man, no different, perhaps, than all the other nurses who served during the Civil War.

Sarah C. Dennis began her career at Portsmouth Grove Hospital as an assistant nurse, later rising through the ranks to oversee 14 of the 28 wards. In a letter to the editor of the *Newport Mercury* in late 1866, a hospital inspector identified only by sex and the initials M.J.J., said she had "yet to see either man or woman to equal in unremitting toil, constant, undivided attention, love and duty, as that shown by Miss Dennis toward those great sufferers." She goes on to talk about an old surgeon who acknowledged Miss Dennis as "a woman who has saved more lives than any two surgeons at this Hospital." She also writes about the day she passed through the ward and found the nurse comforting a dying patient. The patient cried, "O, Miss Dennis, I am going. My dear mother will be here on the noon train, I know you have done all in the power of your kindness to prolong my life until she comes, but it is too late, I must go." Those were his final words. Miss Dennis turned to M.J.J. and said, "Well Mrs. J., the poor boy is gone to rest." She had made every attempt to keep the soldier alive, staying up with him during the night and wetting his lips with brandy. After his death, she heartily regretted the difficult duty of telling the "dear bereaved mother" of the loss of her son.[29]

Miss Dennis, as other nurses, cared for many brave soldiers during her tenure at the hospital. Several cases she managed simultaneously are worth noting. Miss Dennis was responsible for the well-being of three soldiers, described as "Western men," who had had their feet shot away. All were crippled for life.[30] Whether they survived their injuries is unknown, but there is little doubt the poignant memories of these cases would linger for her entire life.

Though little is known about the following individual, she is included here to recognize her laborious efforts while serving as a nurse at the hospital: Mrs. G.M. (only her initials are known). She, along with Jane Woolsey, Miss Harriet Whetten and Sarah Woolsey, was one of Katherine Wormeley's assistant superintendents.[31] Besides the nurses mentioned above, there were several others, such as Annie Boyd, Miss Hazard, a lady remembered only as Mrs. Smith from North Attleboro, Massachusetts, M.A. Atkinson, C.R. Denham, and A.M. Strout of Fall River, Massachusetts. There was also George F. Peterson, a male nurse. These nurses and the others in this chapter are the only names that have surfaced to date.

Most if not all the nurses gave everything they had, not only in time but also the precious little money they earned. Of interest: female nurses who were paid for their services earned a little more than half of what male nurses received and considerably less in benefits.[32] Also, throughout both armies, nurses were expected to purchase various items for patients under their charge from their own meager wages.[33]

When representatives of eight Christian denominations appealed for aid to build a chapel on the premises, the nurses pledged six months' pay to the drive. Contributions were also solicited from

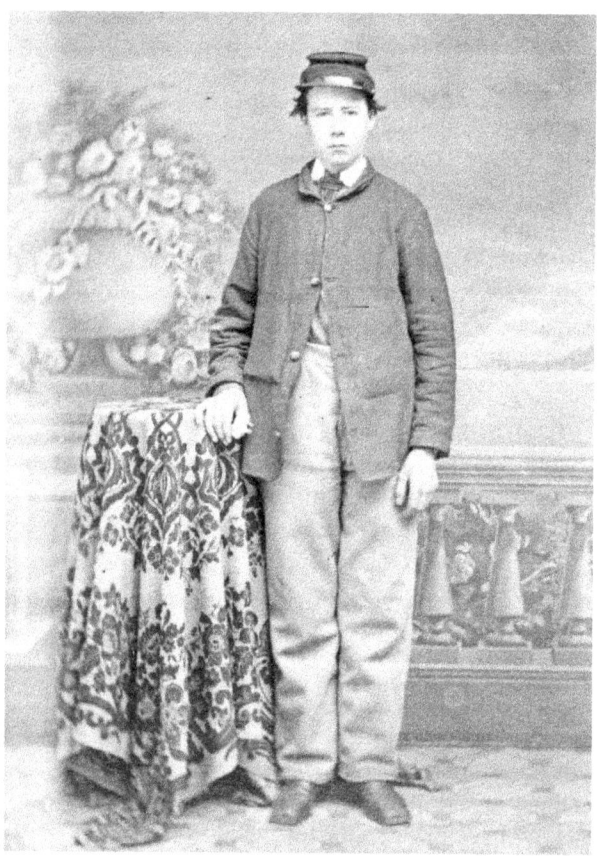

Drummer boy David R. Seville was Nurse Ada Brewster's favorite patient. He was said to be only 15 years old when he came to the hospital (courtesy Dr. Stephen Altic, D.O.; from his collection).

churches and local citizens.³⁴ Mr. R.M. Larned, Agent of the U.S. Sanitary Commission, was tasked with collecting the funds. With over half the money collected, work on the new chapel commenced the following month.³⁵ Nurse Georgeanna Woolsey remembers the initial groundbreaking: "At present it consists of eight holes in the ground and a tolerable fishing pond, but in one fortnight this will be a church and will stand next door to our house, leaving us no excuse for staying at home in the evening."³⁶

Before the chapel was completed, religious services were conducted in the mess hall, a building with a dining area measuring 250 feet long by 30 feet wide.³⁷ Proponents for the immediate construction of a chapel felt that with few activities during the day, patients tended "to gamble and break the rules by running guard and wandering over the surrounding country[side]," claims of which were undisputed by the insurmountable evidence accumulated over the brief three-month period.³⁸

Dedicated on Christmas Day, the new chapel became a godsend to many a soldier.³⁹ The two-story structure included a library and reading room on the first floor that eventually shelved 1,600 books and periodicals dealing with religion, history, biography, travel, and fiction. Books for the shelves were either donated by citizens or purchased from funds obtained through special church collections during Sunday services under the auspices of an organization of clergymen chartered as the Portsmouth Grove Hospital Library Association. The library quickly became a welcome respite for the soldiers. As Stephen Rogers writes: "I shall not have to subscribe for any paper in order to get sufficient reading matter for we have got a fine library with books and papers of almost every description," adding, "I spend much of my time in reading as I have nothing else in particular to busy myself."⁴⁰ Oliver A. Ricker, Company C, 40th Regiment Massachusetts Volunteer Infantry, felt the same. In a letter home he writes: "The library is a good institution to have where the sick and wounded can employ their minds."⁴¹ On the second floor, a five-hundred-seat auditorium was built, complemented with a small melodeon (reed organ) that was primarily used for secular services. In keeping with a religious theme, the worship area was said to be decorated with shields artfully inscribed with Bible verses.⁴²

Serving as the hospital's first chaplain was the Rev. O.S. Prescott, from Trinity Church, an Episcopal parish in the community; but no single parish held a monopoly, as several denominations shared the preaching at the Portsmouth Grove chapel and visiting the men at the hospital. The religious groups included Associated Baptists, Episcopalians, Congregationalists, Methodists, Freewill Baptists, Unitarians, Universalists, and Christian Baptists. The Society of Friends, who worshipped on Quaker Hill near the center of Portsmouth not far from the hospital grounds, was also represented.⁴³ Sunday services were held before noon, along with Bible class at three, and preaching at seven.⁴⁴

The hospital chapel not only served as a place of worship but also as repose for many a soldier. George Peck went to the chapel regularly when he decided "to live nearer to God in future than I have the past years." After attending his first Mass, probably in some time, Peck spoke with the chaplain. "I felt better than for a long time," he said. Not long after, he "partook of the sacrament for the first time in fourteen months." Born again, he noticed "a wakening up of the men" as he became a regular attendee at Sunday services. In his diary there are numerous entries about church attendance, taking communion, and witnessing baptisms of babies (officer's children) and young men who found religion.⁴⁵

To the Churches of Rhode Island.

.... _Church_

....

The Clergymen in the State have sustained a Missionary at the U. S. Hospital at Portsmouth Grove, until the appointment of a permanent chaplain.

There are more than two thousand sick and wounded soldiers in the Hospital, and probably this number will be largely augmented. Many of these, our fellow citizens, are gentlemen of intelligence and piety. The days pass heavily with them for want of useful reading. It is very desirable that a Library, embracing religious, historical and scientific books, should be placed under the care of the Surgeon in charge and the Chaplain, for regular circulation among the patients.

To meet the expenses of the Missionary work already so usefully performed at the Hospital, and to purchase such a Library, it was unanimously voted at a meeting of more than forty of the Clergymen, held in the Lecture Room of the First Baptist Church, Providence, Sept. 22nd inst., that the following gentlemen be a Committee to solicit a contribution from each Church in the State, viz :

REV. DR. JACKSON, REV. BISHOP CLARKE, D. D., REV. LYMAN WHITING, REV. B. F. HAYES, REV. DR. HALL, REV. S. F. UPHAM, REV. C. H. FAY, REV. B. F SUMMERBELL.

THE COMMITTEE VERY RESPECTFULLY REQUEST THAT SUCH A COLLECTION BE TAKEN UP IN EACH OF THE CHURCHES ON SABBATH, THE 12TH OF OCTOBER NEXT.

The collections may be sent to Dea. James H. Read, No. 31 North Main Street, Providence ; or to Dea. Benjamin Marsh, No. 110 Thames Street, Newport.

The Collection from each Church will be duly and publicly acknowledged.

The Ladies have very commendably solicited donations in Books for the Library. Any Books intended for the Hospital may be forwarded to No. 17 South Main Street, Providence ; or to Dr. L. A. Edwards, Surgeon in charge at U. S. Hospital, Portsmouth Grove, R. I.

(Sept. 22, 1862.)

Flyers such as this were distributed to parishioners at area churches to raise funds for the hospital's library. The brief campaign proved highly successful (courtesy Special Collections, Providence Public Library, Providence, Rhode Island).

When Private Moses Whitney went to the chapel one evening, George Peck seemed flabbergasted. Peck couldn't contain himself when he wrote that it was "probably the first time in his life." The next day brought him even more astonishment. "Whitney has been to church again tonight," Peck declared.[46]

Later in the war, when Presbyterian Minister Alexander Proudfit became chaplain, he organized classes for black invalids—illegal in much of the South—and other white illiterates, teaching them to read or improving the skill of those who could. During the Civil War, blacks were not the only illiterates. Civilians from rural farming communities were deficient in reading and writing, and those who became soldiers, North and South, enlisted by signing with their mark ("X"). The mark was always witnessed by an officer who signed next to the mark. But one 36-year-old soldier was determined to learn how to read and write during his stay at the hospital. The patient's name is unknown, but his instructor was identified in writings simply as Ned. Ward master Denham was approached one day by a soldier who asked him to read a letter he had just written. "Why?" Denham asked. The soldier replied that Ned had taught him to read and write, and this was the first letter he ever wrote to his wife, and he wanted to make sure the grammar was acceptable. After reading the letter, Denham looked at the soldier and said, "It is splendid."[47]

Seth Alden attended reading, writing, spelling, grammar, and algebra classes. "I am getting quite a practice now," Alden said to his sister, "but not enough to improve very fast. We have got a very good writing master. He is a good plain writer. He does not put on the flourish that some do." But wanting to concentrate on algebra, he dropped the reading, writing, spelling, and grammar lessons. His decision proved premature. In a letter home, he tells his sister about a book he is reading: "Siners of the Declyration of Indipendance," and adds, "It is not very interesting."[48]

Not limiting his efforts simply to spelling and reading, the Rev. Proudfit taught other subjects of interest to the men, using stationery and second-hand primers furnished by local citizens.[49] For those with higher aptitudes and aspirations, he taught classes in French and Latin.[50]

Apparently the Rev. Proudfit was considerably more adept at teaching than he was at delivering sermons. As Stephen Rogers explains: "I have listened to a sermon today from the chaplain. He is not highly gifted with language but is a very good man."[51] Despite his lack of language skill, his message must have hit home, as Rogers spent nearly a full page of a letter to his parents addressing the chaplain's topic and its meaning.

Then there were the holidays. The first Christmas at Portsmouth Grove Hospital would not be a religious experience or festive occasion for all. There were still many patients suffering from the aftereffects of typhoid fever. Men were dying of the disease and would continue to do so for the duration of the war. One soldier, not identified by name, was feeling blue having had his leg recently amputated. And then there was Johnny. A boy of seventeen, Johnny was a drummer boy in his company before being severely wounded in combat. He now faced the world as a paralyzed veteran, that is, if he survived.[52]

Chapter 12

Late 1862 and 1863

*Hope is a good thing, maybe the best of things,
and no good thing ever dies.*
— *The Shawshank Redemption*, 1994

The arrival was not unexpected, but the time of day was a surprise. The hospital had received a telegram to prepare for a steamer with four hundred and fifty men onboard. Learning that a boatload of patients would soon arrive, the nurses hurriedly cleaned wards, beds, and clothes.[1] On a grey dismal early January morning typical of this time of year on the island, Sarah Woolsey happened to look out the window of her ward to see "a big black steamer off the hospital dock." "The soldiers have come," Sarah exclaimed so all the other nurses would hear. The vessel was the *Daniel Webster* with two hundred and ninety men onboard, not the four hundred and fifty originally anticipated, but still a large number that required immediate care. Many were fresh from the disastrous battle recently fought at Fredericksburg, Virginia.[2] Just as devastating was how the men were treated immediately after the engagement. With no rations, those who did find refuge "lay in rows on muddy blankets soaked with their own blood," their only nourishment being water distributed by volunteers using the few pails and ladles available. According to Clara Barton, who witnessed the unspeakable scene, "500 fainting men hold up their cold, dingy, bloodless hands as I passed, and beg me in Heaven's name for crackers to keep them from starving." Having nothing in the way of food, her only assistance came in the form of compassion, and that did not go very far. Later that night, she returned and subsequently wrote in her diary that the men had yet to be fed. Just as alarming, surgeons required to perform amputations were nowhere in sight. Only after Clara went to Washington to plead her dreadful story was she able to secure the necessary rations and supplies. These soldiers and others like them would eventually be evacuated by rail before being transferred to steamers for passage to northern general hospitals like Portsmouth Grove.[3]

As part of the tally, eighty shot-up and sick men from Rhode Island were on the *Daniel Webster* now docked at the wharf.[4] Of those, Alexander Barker of the 7th Regiment Rhode Island Volunteers nursed a recent amputation to his right arm necessitated because of a severe wound.⁵ During the final stages of the Battle of Fredericksburg, an attack on Marye's Heights proved suicidal. Only one man could be blamed for the carnage: ironically, Rhode Island's adopted favorite son and career soldier, General Ambrose E. Burnside. Unable to convince President Lincoln beforehand of his self-doubts about his ability to command such a large contingent of troops, he reluctantly assumed command of the Army of the Potomac. Before the war was over, General Burnside's name would be associated with a few other battlefield failures that resulted in a tremendous loss of life. Though failing as a military commander, his fortunes changed dramatically after the war when in 1866 he was elected governor of Rhode Island for a three-year term. As a governor his record proved commendable as he garnered significant praise from his constituents.

Private Seth C. Vickery, of Plympton, Massachusetts, now with Company E, 18th Regiment Massachusetts Volunteer Infantry, may have also arrived on the *Daniel Webster*. He had been wounded in the leg by a musket ball three inches above the knee. Prior to military service, Seth was a cobbler and had been married twice, the first time to a 13-year-old when he was 20. The marriage lasted but a short while and was dissolved. The second time, he married Honora (she preferred Ann), a woman three years older than he. A son was born, then three more children in quick succession (two sons and a daughter). On August 9, 1862, Seth enlisted in the army for a three-year term. Now he would spend the next four months recuperating at the hospital.⁶

Unlike previous arrivals, these soldiers were more injured than sick; most patients

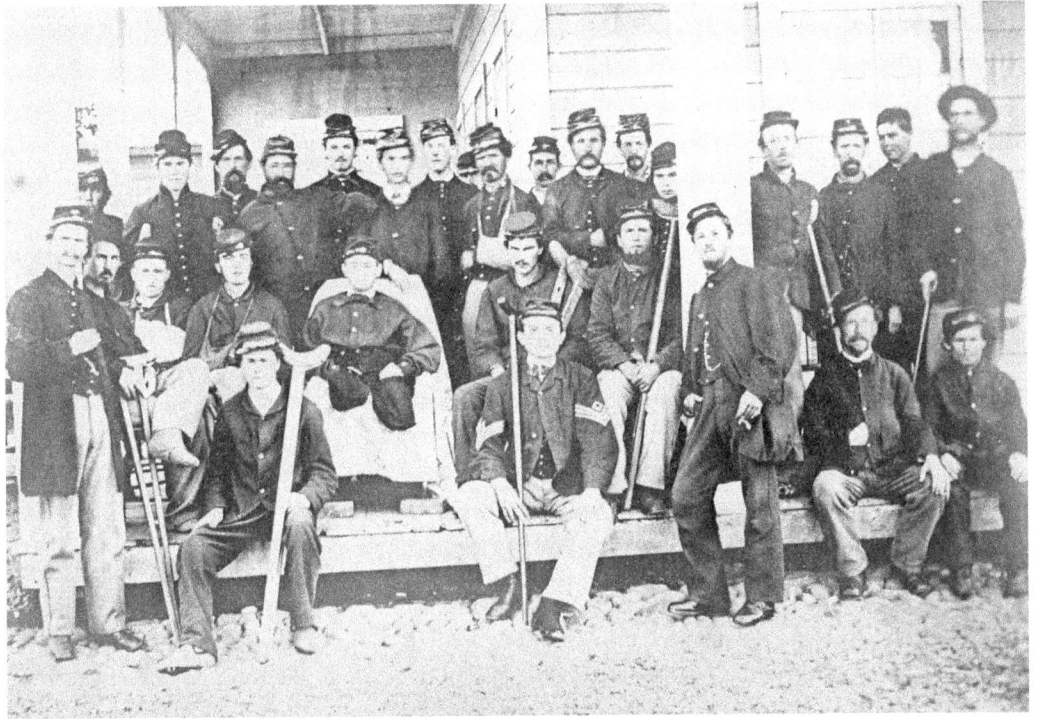

Hospital invalids and crippled soldiers posed for this photograph on the porch of the Administration Building, which also served as officers' quarters on the second floor (courtesy Rhode Island Historical Society, Providence, RI; negative number RHi X3 4885).

arriving at the hospital were suffering from gunshot wounds. With the wounds stabilized in Virginia or en route to Rhode Island, the nurses expected to have an easy time of it. But by 2 P.M. during low tide and no tugboat from Newport in sight, the men had to be brought ashore in shifts by small boats; the new wharf to handle large military transports was still in the planning stage. Luckily "no bad cases" were found on board. Lamenting about the kind of patients she cared for, Nurse Jane wrote home to say, "Georgy and I, who have the medical division, will not profit much. We shall get the sulky old 'chronics' and 'convalescents,' and Sarah and Harriet Whetten will have all the surgical cases; but we shall go to see them all the same, and they shall have all our stores, soft towels, jelly and oranges."[7]

By 7 P.M. the men were landed, placed in wards, and fed a sufficient meal while surgeons continued to perform their normal duties, dressing wounds and prescribing medication. Expressing sympathy for the doctors, Jane said, "They must work all night."[8]

Sometime afterward a nurse whose name is lost to posterity reminisced in a letter to a relative back home about softly washing a boy's face while on duty. Remaining unclear is whether he was a recent arrival or a patient with longer tenure, but it made no matter. Triggering a fond memory, the soldier remarked to the nurse, "Oh! ... that reminds me of home.... That's like my sister; she often did that for me. My eyes—wasn't she a rough one! She'd take off dirt, and skin too, but she'd get the dirt off."[9]

Private Andrew Jacobs, Company G, 21st Regiment Massachusetts Volunteer Infantry, incapacitated by an illness, arrived early in January and could have been onboard the transport as he too fought at Fredericksburg. Jacobs had been transferred from Mt. Pleasant Hospital in Washington, D.C., to Portsmouth Grove Hospital, possibly to be closer to his home in South Hingham, Massachusetts. Andrew Jacobs, like many others, was a brave and dedicated soldier. Prior to his hospital stays, he pleaded with his lieutenant to allow him "to be in one more fight ... to prove that I was not a coward." Jacobs's lieutenant responded, "He had had proof enough that ... he was no coward in the three previous battles." A few weeks after his arrival, while writing from Ward 10, he felt compelled to write that "the hospital here is very pleasantly located.... A steamer runs daily between Providence and Newport stopping here each trip so that visitors from Massachusetts can come here with very little expense."[10]

Oliver Ricker arrived by boat at the hospital near the end of March 1863. Sailing into the bay and landing at the dock at 1 P.M., he and the others onboard were kept waiting until 7 P.M. before being allowed to disembark—a delay that seemed like standard operating procedure for the hospital. During his brief tenure in the army, Ricker performed guard duty in and around Washington, D.C., his regiment operating in a strictly defensive posture. During that time, he knew little but pain and misery, suffering several physical ailments: typhoid fever, occasional diarrhea, cough and colds, a debilitating hip, and occasional back pain. His assortment of problems was noted in his diary on his first full day at the Rhode Island hospital: "Arrived in poor health and a painful hip." Ricker's first hospital visit was the regimental hospital in the field, followed by a stay at Harewood Hospital just two and a half miles outside Washington, D.C. Though he described the hospital as "a very pleasant place and good quarters," he complained that the doctor didn't "do anything for my hip." In most of the subsequent entries, the weather and his poor health and aching hip received top billing.[11]

Seth Alden also enjoyed his new environment but took issue with the protocol:

"They are very strict here. It seems more military. I thought if I get north I should get out of the sound of the fife and drum, but it is not so." Continuing, he said, "They have regular calls and regular guard mounting. We have roll call three times a day ... [and] fall in and march down to our meals, some on crutches and most all the rest with canes."[12] Whitman Bosworth agreed. "I hardly want a job here. They are so strict."[13] How strict was it? Bosworth explains: "It is a guard house offense to pass the front side of the house where the officers are quartered or to pass an officer without saluting."[14] Bosworth may have wished he were back at Hammond General Hospital, where things were a bit easier for him. But at the time he said, "I think that if I were to remain here six months longer, I should be a perfect ignoramus. But as it is I should require at least two terms of schooling before I shall be capable of counting the chickens."[15]

As 1863 dragged on, Portsmouth Grove Hospital was not for want of patients as the flow of sick and wounded continued unabated. Sometimes invalids merely dribbled in, as was the case when fifty-five soldiers arrived in April of 1863 on the steamers *Bay State* and *Perry* from Fort Schuyler Hospital. Under the charge of an assistant Army surgeon, the majority of men proved to be Rhode Islanders.[16] More frequently, soldiers came en masse from battlefields like Gettysburg. Two local boys from Providence, Privates Charles Cargill and Byron D. Snow, were listed as slightly wounded on July 3, the final day of battle at Gettysburg. Each served with Battery A, First Rhode Island Light Artillery. Cargill, previously wounded at Antietam, suffered a leg wound, while Snow nursed an injured back caused by an explosion. How slight their injuries were remains a matter of conjecture, as both spent nearly a year recuperating at the hospital before receiving a disability discharge.[17] So many other invalids arrived from Gettysburg on the same steamer it was said "there were enough to fill all 28 wards."[18] According to John Lovejoy, 817 men arrived on a Monday, one of whom was his friend, George B. Hill, from back home. Hill was nursing a foot injury, the first time he had been injured in eleven battles. "I tell you," John wrote home, "he was a pleased boy to see Allen and I." Allen was John's brother, also a member of the 121st New York Volunteers and a patient at the hospital.[19] John credited Allen for saving his life. Later he wrote, "If it had not been for Allen, no doubt before this, I should have lain beneath the soils of Virginia. We have been a great comfort to each other in hours of sickness."[20] The feeling had to be mutual.

Though John's health continued to improve each day except for an occasional minor relapse, he continued to experience what he described as "a sharp pain in my left side under my ribs." His condition became aggravated when he was put on detail to dry-scrub floors in the ward. "Sometimes after I have been at work ... I have such pains that I can hardly draw in a long breath," he said. Though concerned about his own health, he worried more about his brother's recent illness. Allen had taken ill four days previous with the measles. The prognosis was guarded, but he was expected to make a full recovery. Writing to his cousin, he reported, "The doctor said this morning ... if he did not take new cold ... he has seen the worst part of his sickness."[21]

But Allen's condition did worsen. In a letter to his brother Jonathan, a patient at the U.S. Army General Hospital, Ward B, Armory Square, Washington, D.C., John told his younger brother, "I have not such good news to write. He [Allen] is much worse off than he was when I last wrote to you. He took [a] new cold the 13th that day we scrubbed out the ward and being around on the damp floor, he took a heavy cold which settled on his right lung. And from then till the 18th he was in perfect distress. He raised considerable blood for five days." The only way doctors and nurses could ease Allen's pain was by applying mustard plaster to his sides and placing a canteen of hot water across his chest. Allen did get better, but the recovery would be slow. The spitting up of blood would cease and the pain would gradually lessen. For several more days, Allen remained extremely weak and had to be propped up in bed to take his liquids.[22] John told his cousin in a letter dated June 18 that during Allen's illness, "I have been in the ward almost every moment of the time, the last to bed at night and the first up in the morning."[23] The Lovejoy brothers would soon be joined by other sick and wounded from a battle about to take place in a sleepy small community located in Adams County, Pennsylvania.

After reading the newspapers in mid-June, John Lovejoy wrote to his cousin Cynthia: "The war news is interesting and also exciting. The rebel army is again invading northern soil." A few sentences later, he added, "I hear that some of their cavalry are already in Pennsylvania. Our poor boys now have a hard march ahead of them."[24] On July 27, 1863, commenting on the aftermath of the battle at Gettysburg, Whitman Bosworth wrote to his parents: "The [news]papers state that Lee is in a tight place but as it is not the first time he has been so, he will probably slip out of it." His statement proved prophetic. General Lee and what remained of his battered army did slip away and lived to fight another day, though the consequences of three full days of ferocious fighting, especially the loss of men killed and wounded at Pickett's Charge on July 3, would seriously weaken his chances for final victory over the North. Within the same opening paragraph, Bosworth told his parents, "Could we use up Lee's army and capture Charleston, I think we could then see the light of coming peace."[25]

Whether from Gettysburg or other battlefields, the flow of sick and wounded continued to be a revolving door; there were only so many beds available to satisfy the stampede of invalids now descending upon the hospital. When Oliver Ricker arrived, Private William H. Smith, Company A, 26th New York Infantry, left for Providence to be discharged, while Private James S. Weston, Company E, 18th Regiment Massachusetts Volunteer Infantry departed for his regiment in the field.[26] Many soldiers returned to their units as their conditions improved, while a much smaller percentage would be discharged to return home to family and friends, as they were deemed incapable of serving in any capacity in the army. Some were rushed out the door to make room for the onslaught. For others the door would remain tightly shut. The terminal cases would eventually rest in peace, buried in the "yard" up the embanked road near the top of the hill.

In view of the large and recent influx of patients, collections were taken up at several local churches during Sunday services under the auspices of the Ladies' Union Aid Society. All but one church took up collections and the aggregate sum raised was $1,200, a significant amount to assist the men.[27]

At the chapel, what could have been a calamity turned into a minor annoyance on Sunday night, August 30, 1863. Rising at 6:30 P.M. from a late afternoon nap, Whitman Bosworth went to supper, after which he decided to attend a lecture on missionary ventures in Brazil. Noting that "it was very interesting" and drew "a large crowd," he also said that the event ended "with the floor giving way in the back part of the hall." No one suffered serious injuries and the only real damage was to the men's psyche from the frightening ordeal.[28]

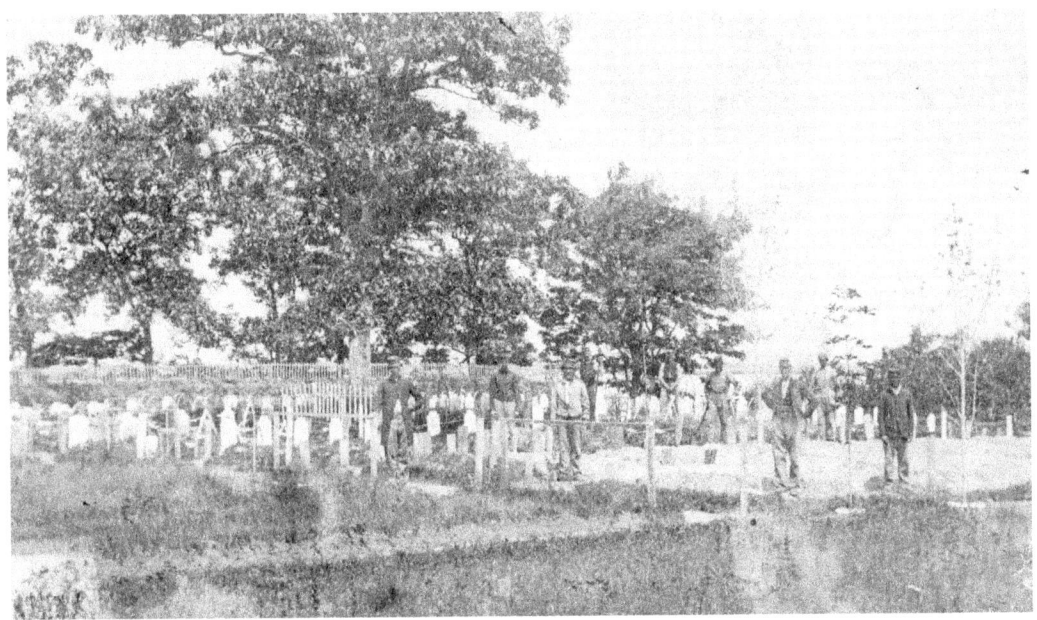

Freshly dug graves are visible in the foreground of this rare image of the hospital's cemetery. Notice African Americans standing to the far right. A few others in the background are holding shovels after completing their onerous assignment. By 1865, 299 bodies would sanctify Portsmouth Grove's soil (courtesy Dr. Stephen Altic, D.O.; from his collection).

Portsmouth Grove was similar to other Union hospitals in treating different types of wounds, but other than through letters and diaries only a few case histories at the hospital are officially recorded: the killing of an inebriated soldier mentioned earlier; post-treatment of a gunshot wound (thigh, penis, and scrotum) caused by a Minié ball; a soldier with a field amputation treated for slow recovery; and a soldier requiring a leg amputation for a serious ankle wound after "stimulating applications" and bromine failed. These cases were unique and would be used as protocols for the future medical knowledge of physicians.

A few words about the Minié ball injury mentioned above. Despite its name, a Minié ball is not a spherical projectile. A Minié ball is a .58 caliber soft-lead bullet with a pointed head designed to decrease wind resistance, thus allowing it to travel faster, and a hollow base that deforms at impact. When fired from a rifled musket, it travels 950 feet per second and is extremely accurate up to 300 yards. What makes it deadly is that when it finds its mark, the bullet tumbles and rips away large amounts of flesh and muscle. Any bone in its path shatters or splinters, and because of the primitive state of surgical knowledge and procedures during the Civil War, amputation was the only means of saving the patient.[29]

Regarding amputations, it can safely be assumed that surgeons at Portsmouth Grove performed a minority of such surgeries, as most patients had arrived with loss of limb from operations performed in field hospitals. Secondary amputations, as they were called, took place forty-eight hours or more after wound infliction and usually resulted in a higher mortality rate from blood poisoning than operations performed immediately in the field.³⁰ Secondary amputations were also performed to clean up, repair, or close wounds that remained open. The fatality rate was said to be 99 percent.³¹ A case in point is taken from the *Medical and Surgical History of the War of the Rebellion (1861–1865)* that relates directly to the hospital:

> Case 1642. Corporal W.A. Armstrong, Co. B. 31st Regiment Maine Volunteer Infantry, aged 23 years, was wounded at Petersburg, July 30, 1864, and was admitted into 2nd division hospital, Ninth Army Corps. Surgeon J. Harris, 7th Rhode Island, noted: "Gunshot fracture of left arm; excision of humerous." On the second day after the resection of the injury the patient was transferred to City Point, and thence to Lovell Hospital, Portsmouth Grove [the name of the hospital was changed from Portsmouth Grove to Lovell in May of 1863]. On August 7th, Surgeon C. O'Leary, U.S.V., reported: "Gunshot fracture of left humerous, upper third. Patient furloughed November 30th and readmitted on January 24th. At this time there was thorough cicatrization of the external wound; formation of false joint by re-absorption of callus; ligmentous union. On January 31st, resection of two inches of the upper third of the bone was performed, by Acting Assistant Surgeon E. Seyffarth, through a longitudinal incision four inches long. Anesthetic: Chloroform and ether. Reaction prompt; considerable loss of venous blood attended the operation, but no arterial hemorrhage. The arm was lightly bandaged, and the bones were brought in contact and secured by an elbow splint. Sutures were entirely dispensed with, as the edges of the wound were easily held in contact by the bandage and adhesive strips, the muscles having been somewhat relieved by a crosscut, about half an inch deep, in order to do away with the 'pockets' formed after pushing both ends of the bone together. During the first six days progress seemed favorable; but on the eighth day there was a severe chill, which was repeated every day or every other day; appetite failed; diarrhea set in, and patient rapidly sank. On the ninth day several abscesses appeared on the inner surface of the arm. These, together with the wound, which had become partially reopened by the extreme tension caused by the swelling of the whole arm, were discharging an ichorous serum mixed with pus, and extremely offensive. The treatment consisted of cold-water applications in the beginning, and afterward of free use of solution of permanganate of potassa, stimulants as freely as could be borne, generous diet, muriated tincture of iron, etc. Death occurred on February 19, 1865. At the 'post-mortem' examination of the shoulder and elbow joint, a small quantity of pus was found in the former, but no metastatic abscesses were discovered."³²

Men fortunate to recover after the stump healed were sent to prosthesis facilities in Central Park, New York, or to Palmer & Co., in Boston, Massachusetts.³³ Patients in Rhode Island with loss of leg must have felt privileged knowing where they would be fitted. In a column that could have been headed "Adding Insult to Injury," soldiers in Washington, D.C., hospitals were transferred to the insane asylum, where "competent surgeons will be in attendance, and where they will be supplied with cork or wooden legs as they may desire."³⁴ In the nineteenth century, insane asylums did more than simply watch over the needs of the mentally disturbed. Partnering with poor farms, they also managed the welfare of indigents.³⁵ Medical enterprises such as prosthesis fittings also sprang up on a space-available basis in these same establishments by doctors and specialists who worked there.

Throughout the war the patient load fluctuated dramatically depending on incoming battlefield casualties and outgoing hospital discharges, but rarely fell below 750. Thirteen months after establishment, the hospital had cared for 6,866 patients while recording only 124 deaths. By that time, 101 soldiers were laid to rest in the cemetery.³⁶

During their recuperation, John and Allen Lovejoy volunteered to become attendants.

Though not officially detailed, John's hope was to remain at Portsmouth Grove Hospital until discharged. He wrote, "I never want to go back into Virginia again for I am perfectly sick of the war."[37] In the same letter he also described the locale: "It is a beautiful place seven miles from Newport. Up the bay towards Providence there are clams and oysters in abundance ... which can be got when the tide is out."[38] Oliver Ricker would also do some clam digging with a few of his friends, later boiling and eating their booty. "They tasted first-rate," he said.[39]

In a subsequent letter, John Lovejoy complained about the weather that "changes regularly every day. One day cold, next warm ... one stormy next pleasant and so on."[40] Private John W. Warner from Hampton, New Hampshire, serving with the 1st Regiment New Hampshire Volunteer Cavalry, would write about thundershowers that "are pretty heavy ones here on the bay."[41] The accounts contradict the testimonial

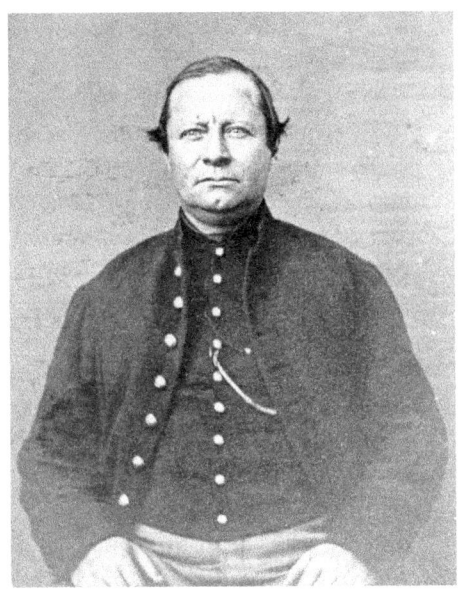

John W. Warner, a New Hampshire soldier, would survive his stay at the hospital and return home (author's collection).

of Dr. William Gibson, professor of surgery at the University of Pennsylvania, a well-traveled gentleman who found the island's climate "the most pleasant and salubrious in the world."[42] Perhaps Dr. Gibson was fortunate to arrive on the island during a glorious summer day. Weather on the island falls somewhere in between: pleasant most seasons of the year with the saving grace of ocean breezes that help moderate temperature extremes, but not always. New England is New England, but Rhode Island is just a tad more moderate due to its southerly position along the coastline.

As if his current illness weren't enough to cope with, on June 18, 1863, John Lovejoy wrote to his cousin Cynthia about another problem: "I have to be bothered with the teeth ache [sic] and when I have the tooth ache, I am as cross as X_____." In his remaining correspondence, Lovejoy makes no further mention about the pain.

John Lovejoy also hoped against hope to be discharged. He wrote to his cousin, "The greater number of the patients that were in this war have been discharged for disability there being only ten remaining besides the nurses, steward and ward master and some of their names are down to be examined for a discharge. If I could have been here at the time I was so sick at Fairfax Seminary, I would have been discharged and at home."[43] The reasons he gave for not seeking a discharge at the time were threefold: first, he did not want to leave his brother Allen alone in a hospital; second, he could not stand up long enough to be examined by the doctor; and third, if he had been discharged, he could not stand straight long enough to ride home. "I was never so weak in my life nor never wish to be again," Lovejoy said.[44] The same day, John penned a second letter to his brother, Jonathan, a member of the 152nd New York Infantry and an invalid recuperating in a Washington hospital. He congratulated him on hearing about his forthcoming discharge and provided some ominous brotherly advice about taking it easy at home, as he had heard of others who were discharged and by not taking care of themselves caused their own deaths.[45]

John Lovejoy was not the only patient looking for a discharge from the service; so, too, were George Peck, Andrew Jacobs, John Austin, and Whitman Bosworth. Each patient suffered from different maladies. Peck nursed a bronchial condition, Jacobs had an undisclosed illness, while Austin experienced a multitude of issues: a lame back, recurring back and side pains, and heart palpitations, also called "soldier's heart" or "stress heart." Heart palpitations were probably a common stress phenomenon for men of the 7th Regiment Rhode Island Volunteers, who saw more combat and served in more battles than any other Rhode Island unit during the war.[46] Like Austin, Whitman Bosworth had a lame leg and a respiratory illness from which he felt faint and dizzy. On occasion his back also ached.[47] These five were a few among those desiring the same resolution: the ever-elusive Certificate of Disability for Discharge. John Austin went as far as employing his wife, Emily, to find medical help on the outside. In a letter to his wife dated February 8, 1863, he told her, "You cannot hurry my discharge," and again three days later, "I have the palpitation of the heart pretty bad; couldn't sleep all night because of the back problem and pain in the side."[48] After a physician took his pulse and examined his stomach, Austin was spoon-fed three drops of an unspecified medication.[49] At least three of the men failed in their attempts for discharge. Andrew Jacobs may have held the rabbit's foot, as his regiment's captain sent a Certificate of Disability on his behalf.[50]

Dr. Green, an assistant surgeon, was ordered to another command and replaced by Dr. Gray, who was put in charge of Oliver Ricker's ward. Ricker described him as "a fine little fellow."[51] Three days later, Dr. Gray, realizing Ricker's incapacities, ordered that the ward master deliver Ricker's rations directly to the ward.[52] On a Saturday afternoon, two weeks to the day after Oliver commenced eating his rations in the ward, Dr. Gray took a bedside statement from him. Ricker writes about the visit, "For what course, I do not know unless it is for an examination for a discharge. I hope that is what it is for, for I want to go home."[53]

As noted earlier in this chapter, the hospital was renamed Lovell in honor of Joseph Lovell, Surgeon General of the United States Army (1818–1836) and organizer of the Army's Medical Department.[54] The hospital was also known by several other names: Wheaton Hospital; Hospital Camp at Portsmouth Grove; U.S.A. General Hospital; U.S. General Army Hospital; Portsmouth Grove Hospital; Lovell U.S.A. Hospital; and Lovell General Hospital, U.S.A. Henceforth the hospital will be referred to under the name Lovell, Portsmouth Grove Hospital, or Portsmouth Grove after the location.

In early spring, rumors swirled that Governor John A. Andrew of Massachusetts, Governor William Sprague of Rhode Island, Secretary of the Treasury Salmon Chase, and General Benjamin Butler would visit the command. As Oliver Ricker told it: "I don't know if they will come."[55] It remains unclear whether Governors Andrew and Sprague actually made it to Portsmouth Grove, but Secretary Chase did appear with several prominent citizens, none of whom were recognized by Ricker. After visiting a few wards, the mess hall, and the chapel at the hospital, they departed by boat at 7 P.M.[56] Two months previous, Brigadier General John Ellis Wool, Commander of the Department of the East, along with his entourage, visited the hospital for a fourth time. As the *New York Times* describes it, "He was received with a salute, and by the Guards drawn up in line at the landing. As the General passed through the wards, many a poor wounded fellow from Antietam, or Fredericksburg, or from some of the Peninsular battles, extended his palm to the old chief, with a glistening eye, and as the General passed on, muttered a 'God bless you.'" After shaking hands, he wished the men well and voiced support for the Union. In the eyes of the men, Brig. General Wool was a curiosity. Approaching his eightieth birthday, he had served in that capacity for over twenty years with more than fifty in the military. No other general in either army could lay such a claim.[57]

After two years of fighting with no end in sight, the war was taking a heavy toll not only on soldiers but those on the home front as well. In Newport, a merchant named Daniel Walker, an Englishman by birth, despondent after losing a son at Antietam who was serving with the 4th Regiment Rhode Island Volunteers and whose remains had recently been brought home for burial, committed suicide at 8 A.M. by slitting his throat with a razor. The ghastly deed was accomplished in the gentlemen's privy and his death did not come easy. After attempting to take his own life, Walker was still able to cause a ruckus that attracted the attention of the neighbors. Shortly after they came to his aid, Walker expired. Later that morning, Coroner John W. Davis wasted little time in conducting an autopsy and summoning a jury for the inquest.[58] Mr. Daniel Walker would become another forgotten victim of the dreadful war.

And still they came. In May 1863 forty-seven sick and wounded arrived in Newport on a commercial New York steamer and were immediately taken to the hospital by the steamer *Perry*. Unlike civilians who secured berths via public conveyance, the convalescents were treated most unfavorably without sleeping arrangements, "packed like sheep or other animals on the floor." One man remarked that "'there were only two of the men that he feared for, last night on the boat,' naming two of the most severely wounded, and who doubtless suffered terribly, lying on the floor of the steamer rather than berths and beds." At the transfer depot in Newport, the invalids were made as comfortable as possible, having the warmth of a fire to take the chill out of the New England spring air. In the meantime, attending surgeons were said to have gained access to a hotel room and secured a warm breakfast while their wards were left without a place to lie down or any nourishment, "not even a cup of coffee to warm their weak and empty stomachs." Soldiers quickly learned to use their ingenuity in these situations. In this instance, several men found a local watering hole to drink away their misery.[59] Whether the Federal government or the city of Newport ever remedied the situation remains unclear. As Mayor Cranston usually addressed such issues, it would be fair to assume corrective action was taken to avoid a replay of the regrettable incident.

Not only did the hospital have its own post office, it may have published its own newspaper. In July, Harry E. Brown, acting as editor, said he was considering publishing a newspaper at the hospital. Such an enterprise was considered "a matter of much interest and curiosity" for the patients and visitors. The plan was to publish biweekly on Thursday but more frequently if interest was shown. Soldiers and nurses were to be solicited for input. The editor said he would discourage articles demeaning to officials at the hospital, articles disloyal to the government, or articles pertaining to religion.[60] To date, no editions of the newspaper have surfaced.

Other hospitals did publish their own news. Satterlee U.S. Army General Hospital in West Philadelphia published the *Hospital Register* as a Saturday edition. The terms were $2.00 per annum in advance or five cents a copy, but single editions were given gratis for every five patients in the wards. By today's standards, the newspaper was less than exciting. The September 26, 1863, four-page edition included poems, literature translated from German, a chaplain's column, a military directory of hospitals in the Philadelphia area, conundrums [question and answer games], and nearly a full page of advertisements. One was for the Sutler's Department at Satterlee, "where soldiers can obtain ice cream, lemonade, mineral water, sarsaparilla," and also "segars [cigars], tobacco, etc." The advertisement concluded with the promise: "Peaches, apples, and all the best fruits of the season at the lowest prices." Knowing the reputation of sutlers, invalids may have seriously debated the last claim.[61]

At Lovell, the situation had improved immensely—so much so that civilians visiting the hospital and departing soldiers returning to the field were complimenting the hospital for the comfort of its facilities and the quality of its convalescent care. Still, accommodations in the area, especially in the town of Portsmouth for overnight visitors, were lacking. Stephen Rogers wrote his parents from Massachusetts that if they arrived after dark they would "have to go some distance outside of the lines in order to get lodging for the night."[62] But day visitors did come, sometimes in droves, as evident by Daniel Austin's assessment that there were a "good many visitors in from the country to see their friends."[63]

In mid–April, Oliver Ricker and the other patients residing in Ward 26 were transferred to Ward 23 so 26 could be whitewashed.[64] The guardhouse barracks was also whitewashed from the second of May through the fourth.[65] Two months later, John Lovejoy

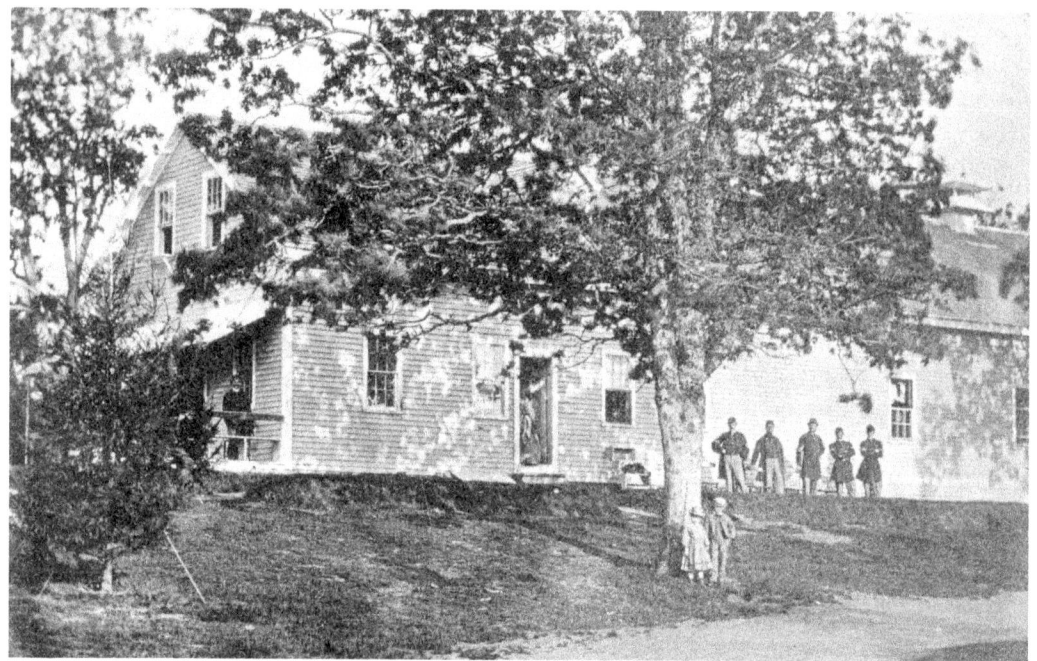

Children standing under a tree in front of a whitewashed ward building while soldiers stand in the background. In a period letter, Dr. Nathaniel Grout Brooks, an assistant surgeon in the 16th Vermont Volunteers, wrote home to say that he was peering out a window when this image was taken (courtesy Lyman John Brooks, descendant of Dr. Nathaniel Grout Brooks).

and other convalescents close to a full recovery were detailed to do the same with their ward, "inside and out." Writing home to his mother, he lamented, "It will be quite a hard job and will keep us very busy."[66] Convalescents also were assigned duties in the kitchen, bakery, mess halls, laundry, carpentry shops, and the stables. Maintaining the grounds also kept them busy and out of trouble.

Patients, at least those who were capable, were expected daily to change linens, make their own beds, and when necessary, clean the floors.[67] The hospital ran a tight ship. As Whitman Bosworth explains, "It is conducted different from any other hospital in these United States. We have to furnish our own underclothes and wash them ourselves. We are not allowed to lie down on the beds through the day except such as are not able to sit up at all."[68] John Lovejoy also added shirts to the list of items men had to procure for themselves. When he was able, he would secure a pass, travel to Providence and buy a few soft flannel shirts, "as the government shirts ... are worse than a hatchel on a person's back." (A hatchel is a comb used to separate flax fibers.[69])

Hygiene played an important role at Lovell, as it did at many general hospitals, and may have played a significant role in saving hundreds of lives, though Portsmouth Grove Hospital may have been more stringent than other similar institutions. Maintaining good hygiene came at a price, however, and it usually meant more housekeeping work for the disgruntled patients. "Our living is not so good as it was in Washington or the Seminary [hospitals]," as Bosworth reckoned.[70]

Three days after Oliver Ricker was transferred to another ward, he was returned to Ward 26. Making note in his diary of the present state of affairs, he said, "There are some very sick men here."[71] Coincidentally, the same phrase would be used by Mrs. Margaret Curtis, a hospital-fund donor to Walt Whitman at Armory Square Hospital in Washington, D.C. No doubt there would be no monopoly on its use throughout all the general hospitals during the war.[72]

As a beautification project, those capable cultivated flower gardens, built stone walls, and placed sod on banks. Adding that special touch, trees were planted.[73] No stone was left unturned to give convalescents proper exercise and to keep the mind active with constructive activities.

But there was more than chores and hard work. Patients amused themselves by playing games of checkers, chess, and cards—usually poker—although gambling for money was unauthorized.[74] How diligently this rule was monitored or obeyed at general hospitals is evident in a letter written by Bugler Heman Packard Kingman to a cousin while convalescing in Eckington Hospital, Washington, D.C.: "Some of the boys amuse themselves by playing cards and I sometimes notice that they have small sums of money lying around."[75] Men experienced a rather boring day if they were non-gamblers or were incapable of performing daily chores like cleaning the ward. Eating, sleeping, lounging outside or in bed, and reading and writing letters were components of their usual routine. Whitman Bosworth had so much free time on his hands, he asked his friend for the name of a lady to write. The friend gave him a name. "I have written her once and received an answer," he said.[76] Bosworth was now corresponding with 12 different people, bragging that "one of my correspondents is a girl in New Jersey."[77]

Oliver Ricker passed some of his time lying in the grass and taking in the sun. When he had had enough, he ventured over to the Quartermaster Department looking for a

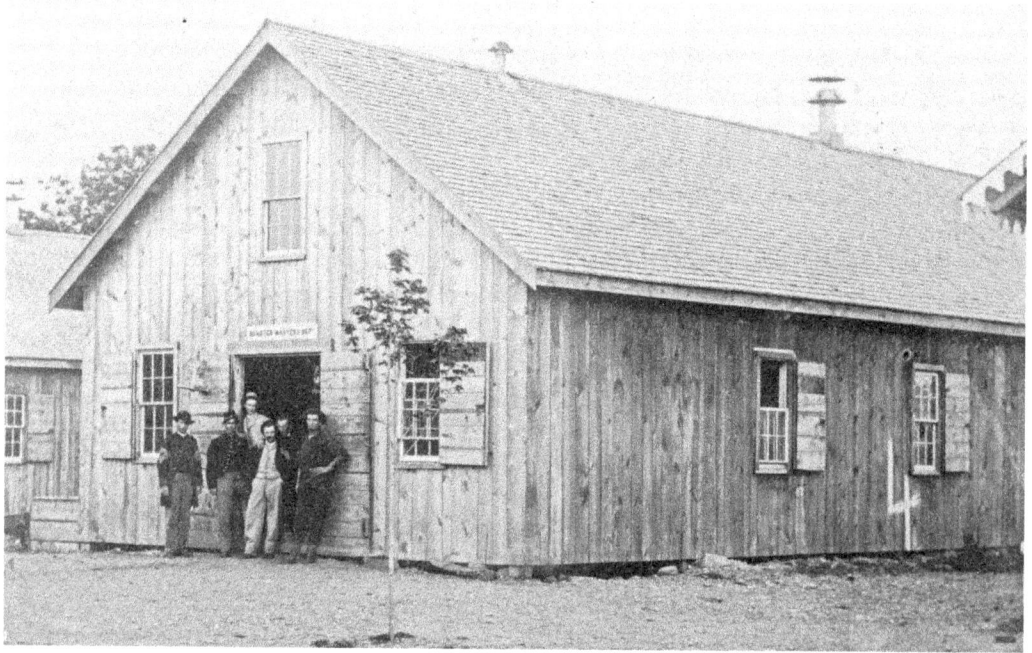

Oliver Ricker attempted to find a new pair of pants at the Quartermaster Department but his efforts proved fruitless. Citizen benefactors helped greatly in this regard by donating used clothing (courtesy Dr. Stephen Altic, D.O.; from his collection).

pair of pants, "but did not find anything to suit." Returning to his ward, he lay down to rest for the remainder of the afternoon.[78]

Many soldiers enjoyed pipe smoking, as evident from photographs that survived the war picturing men at leisure. Chewing tobacco was also enjoyed whenever or wherever the substance could be found.

Not as coveted as letters from home, newspapers were still in great demand. People disembarking from vessels at the wharf with newspapers in their possession were "immediately surrounded by a crowd eager to obtain a copy."[79] Whitman Bosworth's letters are filled with references to newspapers and the comfort they brought along with a temporary respite from boredom. Faithfully he read the *Newport Daily News,* and when a copy could be found, the *New York Herald.* "I have read the newspapers until they are ragged," he said. Newspapers were much in demand, and on numerous occasions Bosworth sent them home to North Ashton, Connecticut, for his parents to read. In exchange, he asked them to mail the *Webster Times* so he could catch up on all the local news and gossip. The *Webster Times* was a weekly publication from a border town in Massachusetts that had a substantial subscription base extending into the northeastern region of Connecticut.[80]

Newspapers during the Civil War, for all their intrinsic value and newsworthy items, were also a vast source of misinformation. Perhaps the patients and staff at Lovell got a huge belly laugh when reading an account in the *Boston Courier* that listed 25,000 sick and wounded at their hospital. An account in a Southern newspaper told of the 104th Rhode Island Regiment — the state's regiments only went as high as 14, and that regiment, the 14th Regiment Rhode Island Heavy Artillery (Colored), was predominantly black.[81]

Over several days, an entrepreneurial soldier in one of the wards set up a stereoscopic exhibition, allowing his fellow patients to view the images for twenty-five cents. Another business enterprise that proved successful was the catching of snakes and bullfrogs. Most likely, they were skinned, fried, and sold as a delicacy. According to George Peck, it was "profitable employment."[82]

One particular day, a soldier in Ward 20 received a gift box of tools. Using a bit of ingenuity, he and his friends fashioned "a nice bagatelle board with glass balls and a cambric [finely woven white linen or cotton] cover"; the board was oblong in design and similar to today's billiards table, and the game was played using a cue stick and balls. The board game proved an immense hit and soon patients from Ward 6 came "to inspect and imitate." They were soon criticizing their neighbors' accomplishment as inferior to what they could manufacture. And build they did. The table they constructed was "seven to eight feet long, covered with scarlet flannel, turned balls and walnut cups," reminiscent of the pool tables that many soldiers enjoy at military bases today. The table and game proved an incredible success, it occupied the men's time for countless hours and contributed to the general health and well-being of the ward.[83]

There were other extracurricular activities in which to partake. John Lovejoy penned a letter to his cousin Cynthia from the hospital reading room in which he explained, "A half dozen [men are] playing checkers and dominoes on the same table on which I write."[84]

There also were simple acts of kindness provided by the staff that helped pass the day. Doughnuts (similar to those baked today) and comic papers were considered "first-rate," and one unidentified nurse at the hospital took a fancy for placing comics underneath the men's pillows for a surprise. She usually followed it up by slipping in a piece of chewing tobacco for good measure.[85] Her thoughtfulness and generosity must have been greatly admired.

But letters received from family and friends seemed to bring the greatest joy. Hiram Keay, a member of Company H, 20th Regiment Maine Volunteer Infantry and a patient in Ward 9, received a letter from his friend, Lydin McKeen, written July 12, 1863, and postmarked five days later from Patten, Maine, a small town in Penobscot County not far from Bangor. The letter provides insight about Hiram's wounds, his profession as a farmer, and feelings about the war from Hiram's friend back home in Maine. Being one of the few letters written to a patient at the hospital still in existence today, it is reprinted in its entirety:

July the 12, 1863

Absent but not forgotten friend, I now take my pen in hand to let you know that we are all well at present and hope these few lines will find you the same. I got a letter from a week ago last Saturday and was very glad to hear from you and glad that you have got better. You said your hand had healed up. I am glad of that. I was afraid you would have to have it cut off perhaps. It will be better than no hand. I should have written the next day after I got your letter but I thought I would wait until we heard from Alden. John wrote that he heard that Alden was sun struck and died but we got a letter from Alden the second day of July and he said that he was well and that he was in the hospital.

They say that Hiram Chesley is wounded in the neck. It came in the days that Edward Cunningham was killed. Oh I should rather be in the hospital than fighting. I should think Mr. Cunningham would feel bad. He wanted his boys to go. I should feel guilty if I coaxed anyone to go. I should think that our folks would feel guilty for teasing you to go.

I think you could have been better off if you had stayed here, but it can't be helped. Mr. Orr says if Sammy was old enough to go he should think that was his duty to go. I don't think it is a duty to have our friends go out there and get shot. What do you think about it?

I don't know whether Mr. Orr has sold any of your potatoes or not. Mrs. Orr told me when they first opened them that she boiled some and they could not eat them. They tasted so bad she said that they could not sell them. They should have to give them to the hogs. He has sold potatoes but I don't know whether they was yours or his.

The last we heard from Martha, she was in Boston but she wasn't a going to stay. She said she was a going back to Salem. She said she had not heard from you since last February and wanted to know where you was.

It has been very cold here this spring. The folks around here haven't got in much of a crop this year. It has been so wet and cold but we have some warm weather and there is a few mosquitoes here.

I can't think of any news to write. I guess I have wrote more news than you can read. Come and see us as soon as you can. Write as soon as you get this and I will try and do better next time. I went to [a] meeting so I could not write. Mr. Orr hain't answered your letter yet. I guess he says he must write.

Wages is good here this summer. James has had a number of chances to work. He has been making shingles.

I can't think of anything more to write. Write as soon as you get this.

Lydin McKeen[86]

Stephen Rogers received a letter from his brother Joe, a fellow soldier serving with the 25th Massachusetts Volunteer Infantry somewhere in the field. He described a portion of the letter to his parents in correspondence home telling of Joe's complaints about "a crust of dry bread and some stuff they *call* coffee ... rather tough fodder for a sick man."[87] Joe may have been in a field hospital at the time.

Allen Lovejoy received a letter from a friend telling him "about one of Daniel Conrad's boys being killed by the kick of a horse." John heard about the incident from Allen, and in a letter sent to his mother and sister Mary, he asked for the particulars and any other local news worthy of his attention. News of any kind from back home, even gossip, was welcomed, whether good, bad, or indifferent.[88]

When making notations in his diary, Oliver Ricker always seemed to include a reference to his wife, Sophia. Either he had received a letter or was anxiously awaiting same. Soldiers like Ricker were not only homesick, but also lovesick. In April 1863, he wrote, "I think of her very often and long for the time to come when I shall be with her again."[89] After Sophia visited him at the hospital, coming from Lawrence, Massachusetts, he simply said, "I was very sorry to have her leave me."[90]

When John Lovejoy ran out of hospital experiences to write about, he turned to the "cause" and easily filled a page or two about his allegiance to the Union and how he would stay the course no matter how long the war lasted. He also dreamed about being home again, noting how he missed "the pleasant hills of Ostego." But more than anything else, he wrote about the day he left Cynthia's house for the last time. In one letter penned during the day on Sunday, August 9, he became rather specific: "I never shall forget that day," he said, "nor the way Aunt talked to me when I was about to leave. I never in my life had to work so hard to keep the tears back as I did then."[91] Similar scenes doubtless played out in thousands of homes as men went off to war. Men seemed inherently naïve about the dangers, but whether through maturity, intuition, or a better grasp of reality, women could foresee the difficult times ahead and the horrors their boys would be subjected to in the not-too-distant future.

John Lovejoy's letter would not be the last he would write that day. In the evening he drafted another letter to Cynthia. This time he thanked her for the photograph she had sent him. "I could not have been more pleased if had had the privilege of seeing you in person," he said. Though neither had seen each other in quite some time, it became increasingly apparent within the multitude of letters traveling back and forth that John and Cynthia were becoming more than simply cousins. Lovejoy's correspondence over the past few months had been strung together using various innuendos. On this occasion, Lovejoy ended his letter by saying, "Your true friend and cousin and well wisher until death," not a profession of love by any means, but by 1860s standards, it was a start.[92] In August 1865, just before his discharge, his letters would open with, "Dearest Cousin C."

Writing and mailing letters was only half of keeping in touch, and the only part under a soldier's direct control. Receiving timely responses was the other half and something that easily became nerve-wracking. When letters went unanswered, some patients became despondent while others tackled the issue head-on. Private Adin B. Thayer, Company B, 16th Regiment Maine Volunteer Infantry had been wounded in the leg at Fredericksburg and sent to Portsmouth Grove for recuperation. He wrote his sister in Waterville, Maine, on January 20, 1863, "I have not received any answer to the last letter I wrote you."[93] Two months later, he wrote again: "I have written to you once or twice and have not received any answer yet, but I thought I would write you a few lines more to let you know that I have not forgotten you. I want you to write all of the news [and] want you to write a good long letter this time."[94]

When no letters arrived from home, Allen Lovejoy admonished his mother, Sally, in a letter written from

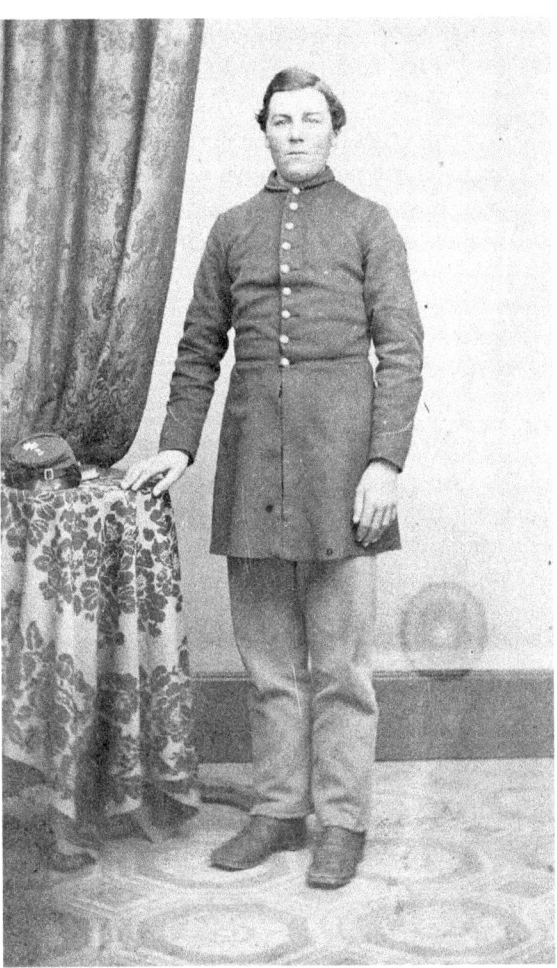

Adin B. Thayer chose to pose formally with his coat buttoned. Captured twice and hospitalized several times, he would die of disease in a Confederate prison. His remains rest for eternity in an unmarked grave at Salisbury National Cemetery (courtesy Gettysburg College Library, Special Collections, Gettysburg, Pennsylvania).

the hospital dated March 23, 1863: "Now mother, don't neglect your boys in that way. Get someone to write for you often." He concluded: "Letters from any of our friends will be gladly received by us."[95] Three months later, he corresponded with his sister Mary at home: "I thank you for being so good to mother as to write her letters for her."[96] In another letter of July 20, Allen expressed his anxiety about money sent home and never acknowledged. "I sent $40 to Almira and she ... never said a word about the money," he wrote. And writing for his brother within the same letter, he says, "John has sent $20 to you some time ago and you have not sent him word, as you should."[97] John Warner experienced a similar scenario regarding lack of letters, but money was not an issue. "It is time for me to hear from Aunt Frances. She has not written but one letter since I was at home," he laments. Summarizing the feeling best for all patients at the hospital, Whitman Bosworth said, "I tell you, time drags heavily without receiving any letters from home or elsewhere."[98]

When letters were not forthcoming from his lady friend back in Bridgeport, Corporal George Phillips, Co. D, 17th Regiment Connecticut Infantry took a different approach. In a letter to his beloved Emma, he said, "I was disappointed until I came to the conclusion that you had not got mine, so I wrote you another, and this is another one still."[99] Whitman Bosworth did the same. Writing from Ward 24, he wrote to his parents and said, "This is the fifteenth letter that I have written you since the 24th of last May and in return I have received three, dated June 2nd and 10th, and July 13th."[100] Phillips and Bosworth learned quickly what others had long since surmised: that mail delivery was unreliable and would continue to be so for the duration of the war. The hospital was not at fault, nor were the steamers that delivered it at the wharf. The bottleneck occurred outside the confines of the hospital. Weather permitting, mail was sorted and delivered several times a day: southern and western at 7:30 P.M. and eastern at 11:30 A.M. and 7:30 P.M.[101]

In a letter dated January 27, 1863, John Austin gave some unsolicited advice to a relative back home through his wife, Emily, when he asked her to "tell Edwin to mend up his heart and find another girl the same way as I did." And adding reassurance, he says, "The next one will be better than the first." And as if that weren't enough, he gave additional advice to the lovelorn: "A redheaded one is always fiery and jealous of you."[102] Different advice was given by Whitman Bosworth via his parents when he heard about his friend Eunice's drinking escapades: "Sarah tells me that *my* [Bosworth's emphasis] Eunice takes to[o] much fire water. Now I want you to tell Eunice that I say she must be a good girl."[103]

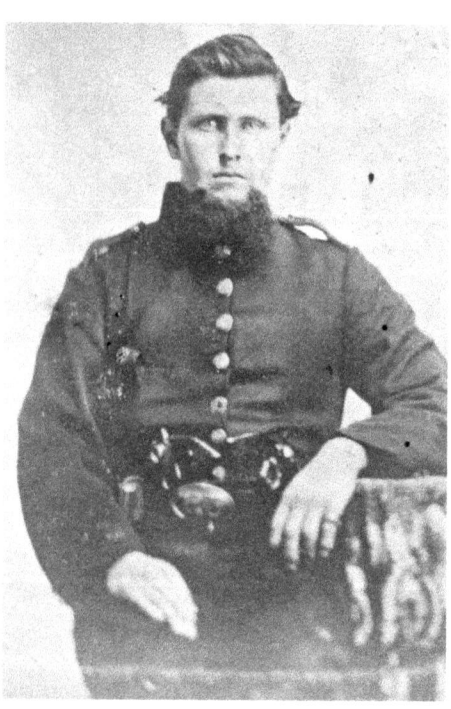

Hailing from Connecticut, George D. Phillips posed with two firearms tucked in his belt. He would desert the hospital to visit his family and a lady friend but would later return (courtesy Connecticut Historical Society, Hartford, CT; collection number MS#90813).

Soldiers also managed to interject political commentary into letters to family and friends. John Warner wrote: "Father has probably seen by the papers before this time how Rhode Island and Connecticut went at the late elections. The copperheads do not stand anymore sight here than in NH [New Hampshire]."[104] No matter how much they despised war and how desirous they were for peace so they could return home to family and friends, soldiers afforded Southern sympathizers little affection. As evident by the presidential election of 1864 and Lincoln's landslide victory over General George B. McClellan, a large majority were Lincoln men. George Peck was elated by the election news: "Ohio is gone Republican by forty thousand majority; Indiana by twenty and Iowa by a large majority."[105] Again on November 11, Peck could hardly contain his exuberance when he wrote, "The election results are not all in yet but far as heard from, McClellan has carried only three states—New Jersey, Delaware and Kentucky."[106]

There were also notations along the way about the conflict. Oliver Ricker concluded a diary entry by throwing in a war bulletin: "The news came tonight of the death of Stonewall Jackson a rebel general. He died of a wound received at the battle of Chancellorsville a few days ago."[107] Considering Jackson's notoriety in the North and his value and larger-than-life stature to the Confederacy, nothing further was added to the commentary that day, or afterward. In a letter written a few weeks prior to his arrival at Portsmouth Grove and days before the Battle of Gettysburg, Whitman Bosworth wrote his parents, "The boys don't seem to like the idea of superseding Hooker by Meade, but it may be all right. I wish Little Mac [General McClellan] had command of the Army of the Potomac."[108] On July 10, 1863, John Lovejoy wrote home to say: "The news from the army is of the very best we could ask for. Vicksburg is ours. It was surrendered the fourth of July."[109]

Letter writing relieved boredom and homesickness, at least to some extent. After deciding to write a letter because he was feeling blue, Stephen Rogers said, "I concluded to try writing and see if I couldn't make the time pass a little more pleasantly." The effort seemed to pay dividends as Rogers stated, "I think I already feel a little better."[110]

Not all correspondence brought joyous news. Such was the case of a letter written by Emma Krinks from her home in Bridgeport, Connecticut, to her beloved soldier, George Phillips. Emma's letter appears not to have survived, but Phillips's response does. He answered Emma's letter by saying, "Now Emma, don't take any notice of William Beardsley. I'll silence him (forget the past). I shall never forgive him or myself for what has already been done. So Emma, let oblivion drown the past. I trust the future will prove brighter for both of us."[111] Did William Beardsley make a pass at Emma while George Phillips was away, or was it another matter entirely?

Before and after letters were written or read, there wasn't a great deal to occupy a convalescent's time. Men would resort to conversation among ward mates. Though soldiers had stories to tell, few had more fascinating tales than William Dennett. At Fort Monroe, he had seen the ironclad *Monitor;* on guard duty he witnessed Professor Thaddeus Lowe's first balloon ride and the subsequent descent back into a valley after being fired upon by the Confederates; he "saw a Negro shot through the thigh while removing guns from a wagon, drawing a gun out by the muzzle"; he toured the White House, Capitol, and Patent Office; and he saw General McClellan, subsequently camping on a hill with others while guarding his well-fortified quarters.[112]

As if the above weren't enough for storytelling, Dennett had a few close encounters to convey. The round that passed through the black man's thigh barely missed Dennett. He also survived a Confederate shelling. "I was hit on the arm by a large piece of hard clay ... thrown out by an exploding 10 in. shell [that hit] about 50 ft. behind me. It made a large hole where it exploded. If I had not laid down when I heard the shell coming, [I would] have been struck with it in the head," he said.[113]

Patients at the hospital were always hard-pressed for cash, and as time went on without pay, the situation became exasperating. Adin B. Thayer wrote his father about the situation and thanked him for the money he sent by saying, "I was glad to get it too."[114] But in a follow-up letter when his funds were near exhausted, he wrote his father, "I have not been paid off yet and I should like to have you send me some money if you can and when I get paid I will send home what I can."[115] John Warner, now convalescing while serving as a hospital steward at Portsmouth Grove, experienced the same small-scale monetary crisis. He, too, wrote home acknowledging the money his father mailed.[116]

On February 23, 1863, Corporal John B. Glenn with the 2nd Battalion Veterans Reserve Corps at Portsmouth Grove, detailed as a clerk at headquarters, wrote home to his sister Callie, "I have not received a cent of my pay yet. I have now 8 months pay due me from the government and not a 'Red' in my pocket." In closing he wrote: "Consequently you need not wonder why I send you this letter with the postage unpaid." Five months earlier, Callie had written asking for money. The request was a twist, as it usually happened the other way around. Glenn's response is understandable: "I could have sent you double what you ask[ed] now when I was at the Regt., but you wrote me that you did not need any and I loaned all I had to a 'chum' of mine who is in the Regt. yet."[117]

Oliver Ricker received a letter from his beloved wife Sophia, and in it he found a small sum of money that he "was very glad to receive."[118] As time went on, Oliver received even more letters from his wife, some containing money, as did the one of April 20, 1863, in which he not only found a picture of Sophia, but also seven dollars and twenty-five cents.[119]

For the typical Civil War soldier, the paymaster always seemed to be on sabbatical and it wasn't uncommon for a soldier to be owed more than a half-year's pay. John Warner states, "We have been expecting the paymaster here every day and I thought of getting a pass after I was paid, but he has not got along yet and no one knows when he will come."[120] In

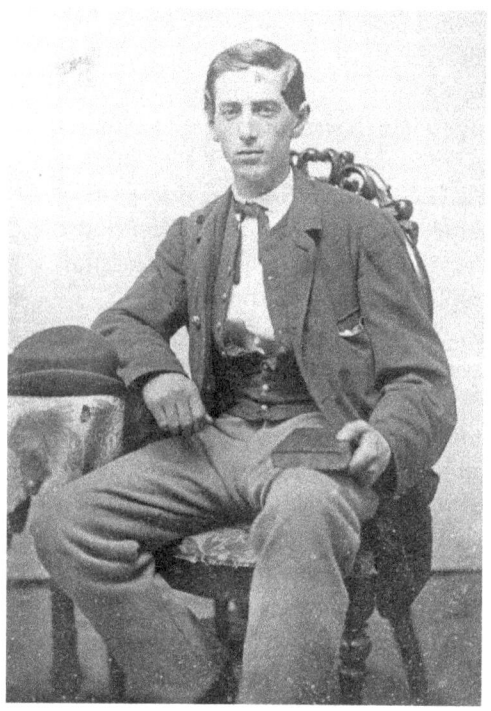

Albert J. Reeve signed the back of this image, titling it "Hospital Steward. Dr. Cornick's clerk at 'Head Quarters.'" Over time, Reeve would be one of several who served in a similar position (courtesy Dr. Stephen Altic, D.O.; from his collection).

another instance, a paymaster did arrive at the hospital supposedly to pay the hospital guards. The men were lined up and marched to the captain's quarters, but were soon advised that they would not be paid. As George Peck wryly explains, "*Our* paymaster was *somebody* else and was coming *sometime*."[121]

Stephen Rogers's father quickly sent five dollars to Stephen after his son requested money to pay his way home while on furlough. Upon receipt, Stephen acknowledged the gift by saying that it was "as good a currency as Uncle Sam ever issued."[122] But in a follow-up letter, Stephen asked for more, acknowledging that he "was ashamed to send home for more money but it has been four months since we were last paid." He surmised it would be another two months before the glorious day. The little money he did have was spent at a hospital in Kentucky before his transfer to Rhode Island. He explained: "I had to spend considerable money ... or go half starved." In the same letter, he expressed that his favorite snack food was apples: "It seems like I could not get along without them."[123] Whitman Bosworth concurred: "There has been a decided improvement in our living here and it makes me feel far more contented and now we can get plenty of apples." Though apples were in abundance, Bosworth complained that there was no other fruit to be had. In another letter to his parents ten days later he reiterated: "I am feeling quite well today—rather better than usual and I hardly know why unless the apples have done one good for I have eaten about a peck since yesterday morning. We have them quite plenty now and quite cheap." Yet again he grumbled, "But we get no other kind of fruit."[124]

Before being reassigned back to his regiment in the field, Rogers wrote his parents that he expected to wait an extra payday before he received his money. "That will make it eight months," he said.[125] Oliver Ricker was slightly less affected. He had only been waiting six months, though he, too, was "in need of it."[126] The situation for all unpaid soldiers at the hospital can only be described as outrageous, although not uncommon, and those mentioned above were only the tip of the iceberg.

To relieve the monetary burden, citizens solicited money for those being discharged while transport officials provided free public transportation for those who remained.[127] The hospital was abuzz after the paymaster arrived on a Tuesday in mid-September 1862. Major Benjamin F. Watson, U.S. Paymaster for Massachusetts, arrived "and paid off a large number" of soldiers, and he agreed to return in a couple of months on another "welcome mission."[128] Probably no one held his breath.

Being paid in the field was difficult enough, but complications multiplied for those confined in hospitals. The problem became so unmanageable that a committee was established to investigate the situation. When President Lincoln was advised of the findings, he expressed his sincere concern and promised to look for an equitable solution.[129] Even though the president and his staff were working on the issue, little progress was made in expediting pay. Surprisingly, about a month later (October 12, 1864), George Peck reported that the "paymaster came this morning and paid off the hospital up to the first of September."[130] Seeing the paymaster two months in a row must have caused a considerable stir among the men.

John Lovejoy's day of jubilation finally arrived. Writing to his mother back home in upstate New York, he said, "Yesterday afternoon I was paid off up to the first of May. I received $100.96 which is my monthly pay from the 1st of Sept. to the 31st of April." Lovejoy obviously meant the 30th of April. In the same letter, he told his mother, "I intend to send you about 75 dollars of it, and I want you to make the best use of it you can." Wisely, Lovejoy would send the money home in increments in case the money was lost or stolen in the mails. "I think I shall send you 20 dollars in this letter, and send ten or twenty in all the letters I write till I have sent 75 or 80 dollars," he said.[131] Using the blank last page of the letter as he sometimes did, John's brother Allen, still suffering from measles in Ward 9, told his mother that he intended "to send Almira about ninety dollars," adding, "I do not need money here, only for postage & I think it will be the safest with her."[132]

On July 29, John Lovejoy wrote home to his mother, telling her, "Since I last wrote, I have been paid 2 months pay ($26.00)." Having, as Lovejoy described it, "considerable money," he bought a newspaper every day and "sometimes two." He could now buy butter to eat with his bread, having had to go without prior to payday. Feeling guilty about his new spending habits, he said to his mother and sister Mary, "Perhaps you will think I am too free with my money, but if you had to live on the food the government furnishes you, you would buy all you ate."

When feeling well enough and possessing a few dollars in their wallets, rehab patients were granted an occasional pass. Most visited Newport or the capital city of Providence, as little entertainment value could be found in Portsmouth, a town of 2,100 rural inhabitants. In Providence, men visited the photographer to have a "likeness" taken for mailings to family and friends. John and Allen Lovejoy, like thousands of other soldiers during the Civil War, were hoping to do just that. Their brother Jonathan had just had his image captured, and John and Allen wanted a pass so they could pose together for a "dagger" [daguerreotype].[133] When the time came, each was granted a pass and headed to Providence, but they may have not traveled together. John wrote home, "I was to the city of Providence last week and had a dozen pictures taken. They cost 12½ cents apiece. They look just like me for all the world."[134] Like the Lovejoy brothers and so many others, Stephen Rogers visited Dexter's Photograph Rooms while in the city "and had several pictures struck off." Rogers decided to wear his overcoat while his pictures were taken and afterwards wrote his parents that he would send one home as soon as they were forwarded to him "on Wednesday or Thursday."[135]

Passes came as a welcome relief for invalids, but furloughs were even more desirable because of their longer duration. On December 9, 1863, the War Department issued General Orders No. 391 that authorized commanders of departments to "grant furloughs to enlisted men in the general hospitals within the limits of their command, upon the approval of the Medical Director or Chief Medical Officer." The orders further directed that "the number allowed to be absent at one time ... be limited to five (5) percent, and the period not to exceed thirty (30) days." There must have been a mild uproar because of the conservative number as the percentage was increased to twenty less than a month later by General Orders No. 2.[136]

Furloughs were granted to patients fairly regularly at the hospital until men abused the privilege. After convalescing at hospitals in Maryland, Virginia, Washington, D.C., and finally Portsmouth Grove, Whitman Bosworth was anxious for his opportunity to travel home on leave. "It is rather unpleasant to be shut up here and deprived of all the luxuries of the season, but so it is, and I don't know how to remedy it. But if they ever give any furloughs, I shall try to get one," he said. Less than a month later, Bosworth wrote home to say, "If anybody can get one, I shall stand a good chance, but I fear that I shall slip up on this for there was an order recently issued to grant no more furloughs on account of so many abusing them over time and deserting."[137] Eventually the order was rescinded.

During the holidays and other times designated by the commanding officer, those able to travel and of "good conduct" were granted furloughs, but only after the orders were forwarded to New York and signed by Maj. General John A. Dix.[138] Holiday furloughs were normally granted after state governors intervened on behalf of their men. George Phillips felt that so many were going home on furlough, he would be one of the few stuck at the hospital. In a letter dated November 24, 1863, he said, "Governor Andrew of Massachusetts is going to get all of his soldiers home for Thanksgiving and that will take so many from the hospital."[139] In a subsequent letter of December 20, he said, "Maine and New Hampshire men are going to have furloughs to go home and talk is that ... I shall have ... a chance to go home for Connecticut soldiers have sent in a petition to Governor William A. Buckingham for a furlough."[140]

Stephen Rogers, coming from Massachusetts and accustomed to snowy weather, longed to be home to take a sleigh ride.[141] On March 26, 1864, many Rhode Island and Connecticut men would get their wish. They were granted fifteen-day furloughs.[142] Stephen Rogers did get his furlough and was, perhaps, part of that group. He longed to tell his sister Ellen about his recent sleigh ride, and as he told his parents in a letter, "I can tell her all there is to tell better with my tongue than with my pen."[143]

When November 1864 rolled around, many men were granted furloughs to vote in the presidential election. On November 2, some four hundred were extended the privilege. The following day, three hundred more went out, and on the seventh, another unspecified number were also furloughed.[144] One of those was Private Benjamin Lincoln, Company G, 4th Regiment of Cavalry, Massachusetts Volunteers, found unfit for duty because of illness. He came to Lovell by way of the hospital at City Point, Virginia, and later through the hospital at Portsmouth, Virginia. After voting in the election, he returned from furlough and was placed on light duty at the hospital because of continued poor health. Benjamin Lincoln eventually returned to his unit in Williamsburg, Virginia, but his illness lingered, perhaps not properly diagnosed from inception. He would survive the war, but shortly after he would die of consumption at his home in Hingham, Massachusetts, on March 29, 1866.[145]

On the seventh, according to George Peck, "the captain gave six men from the Hospital Guards passes to go home but took good care to have none but McClellan men go." This may have been an exaggeration, as the following day (Election Day) Peck was allowed to travel to Bristol "and put in a vote for 'Old Abe,'" returning that evening.[146] What is interesting, if not amazing, is the way Peck said he traveled home. Peck's family resided in a town away from Portsmouth Grove but was separated by Narragansett Bay. As he explains it, his usual method of transport was a rowboat. This seems to be a formidable feat of human endurance to navigate, both in nautical miles and cross-currents, especially in choppy waters. What Peck failed to mention was that some boats with oars were also equipped with sails.[147]

By the twelfth, men furloughed earlier were starting to make their way back to the hospital. Coincidentally, there was an ongoing fear that convalescents granted leave would

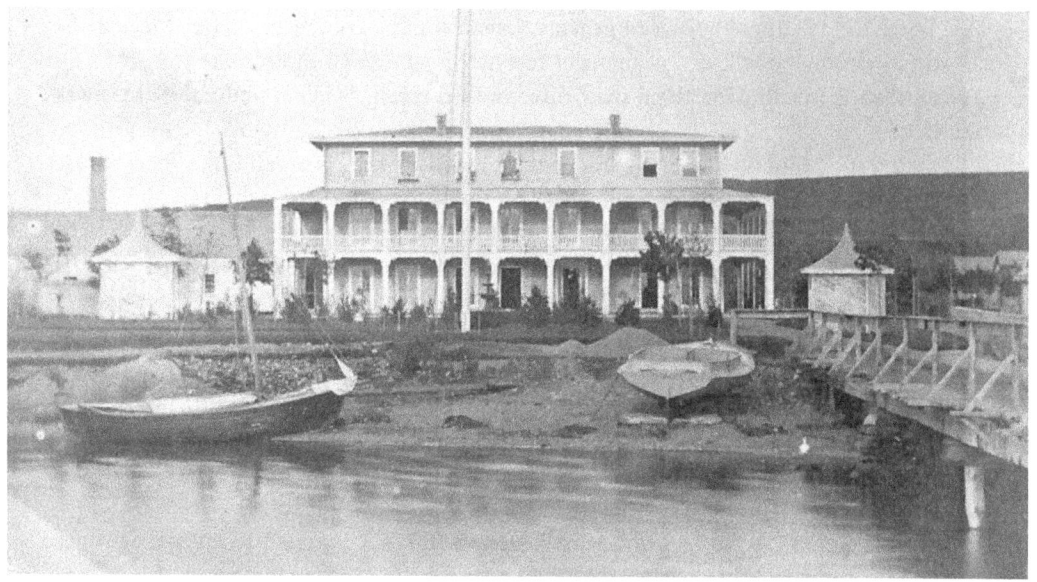

An image of the west side of the hospital administration building that displays a wharf jutting out toward Narragansett Bay (author's collection).

desert. Some did; most returned. Here is what statistics reveal. When comparing desertion rates for the entire Union army hospital system with state desertion rates for units still in the field, general hospitals ranked second, with 33,430 deserters. New York led the pack with 44,913 "skedaddlers."[148] Why did hospitals experience such a serious desertion problem? Running away may have been easier than in the field, where the enemy was thought lurking behind every bush. Also the embarrassment if caught wasn't as difficult to endure, as most friends were still with units in the field. Perhaps the biggest consideration was soldiers in general hospitals were closer to home and the comforts and temptations that the proximity conveyed was simply too hard to resist.

At Portsmouth Grove, Private Edward Jonathan Hoyt would be another to choose desertion. His reason, however, if we can believe his memoirs, is far different from those stated above. Born in Canada, Hoyt learned to hunt and trap alongside Canadian Indians, who called him "Buckskin Joe." But traversing the Northwestern wilderness looking for game with his Indian companions didn't seem to be a big enough adventure. Hoyt decided to migrate to America and join the Union army. After completing a three-month enlistment with a Pennsylvania outfit and seeing action at Bull Run, he reenlisted with the 49th New York Infantry out of Buffalo, New York. He initially served as an infantryman, but his musical talents resulted in his transfer to the regimental band. But serving in the field, regardless of military occupation, proved costly. During the Peninsula Campaign, he contracted typhoid fever, causing him to lament, "I think I will not live long."[149] Unable to shake his fever, he went on sick call and ended up like so many others, working his way through the army hospital system in Virginia, then a military hospital in New York City, before arriving at his ultimate destination: Portsmouth Grove. What he found there appalled him.

Arriving during the early stages of the hospital startup in September of 1862, Hoyt saw the worst in staff and facilities. Describing patient care, he said men were "treated like dogs by one of the most beastly army doctors I ever encountered," giving examples to defend his accusations. While "under the influence of chloroform," the cruel and incompetent doctor tried to straighten a soldier's crooked back "by standing and jumping on him." He also saw the same doctor take a "shirt away from" another soldier "because he had *two* [Hoyt's emphasis]." Further describing the injustices, Hoyt explained how patients "were forced to clean out privies, chop wood, and work on the road to the burying ground when they were not able." The situation continued to escalate, and on November 27 culminated in a riot at the mess hall when the doctor withheld turkey from patients' plates during a Thanksgiving feast. For their transgression, men were placed in the guardhouse or "put on work details in the cold and snow." Hoyt noted, "At least one attempt was made to kill this doctor." He concluded, "I would have shot him myself if I had been given the opportunity." After consulting with his friends

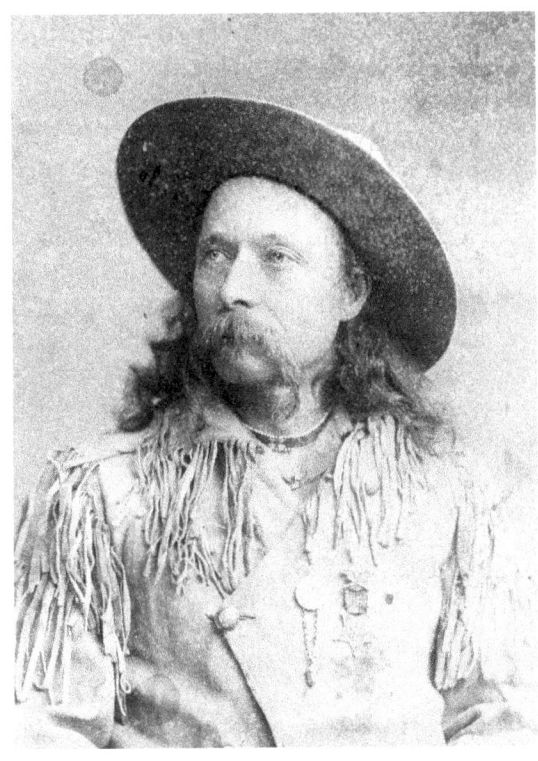

Edward Jonathan Hoyt ("Buckskin Joe") is pictured here while performing at Pawnee Bill's Historical Wild West Exhibition (Vance Hoyt, photographer; courtesy Buckskin Joe Collection, Dickinson Research Center, National Cowboy & Western Heritage Museum, Oklahoma City, Oklahoma).

and fearing that the evil doctor was determined to cause his demise and abscond with all his back pay that had now accumulated to over five months' worth, Hoyt went AWOL.[150]

Men skedaddling from Portsmouth Grove remained a serious issue until the end of the war. Proportionately, and not surprisingly, hospital guards seemed to be the worst offenders, with soldiers deserting nearly every week.

Desertion seemed the easy way out, but many realized it was only a short-term solution that could result in some devastating consequences. Thus, the majority of men took the high road and found ways to avoid the temptation by entertaining themselves during convalescence. With a large hospital population it was easy to find talented musicians. A band was organized to entertain the troops and also perform at local fund-raising events to champion their cause. Buckskin Joe may have been one of them, as he was proficient at playing sixteen instruments. In all likelihood, the number may have been inflated to include the playing of simple instruments such as spoons, washboard, tambourine, mouth harp, triangle, harmonica, cymbals, and drums. That still left considerable room for various string and wind instruments to fulfill a comparatively extensive repertoire. Yet, his musical talents would not satisfy his hunger for returning home and trying to forget what he had witnessed while incapacitated.

Besides playing in the band, there were numerous ways patients could entertain themselves. "Got my ankle hurt today by a bat playing ball," George Peck notes in his diary.[151] Baseball was still in its infancy, but was a recreational activity at the hospital nonetheless.

Peck also wrote about fishing and described one catch "that is a perfect stranger [to] these waters, half eel, half codfish."[152] On another occasion, he "caught a nice mess of scup and tautog."[153] Many men also went clamming, as discussed earlier,[154] in the shellfish-filled waters of New England's nearby North Atlantic. Their efforts served a dual purpose: providing an enjoyable pastime and filling their ever-empty stomachs with added nourishment above and beyond the meager rations usually allowed lower-ranking soldiers.

A few of the winters were extremely cold, and Narragansett Bay froze over at least in the cove areas. Fittingly, the men tried their hand at winter sports, either on the saltwater cove or the freshwater marsh just below the hillside. "Some of the boys are trying to amuse themselves by skating," writes Peck in a diary entry of January 13, 1865.[155]

Birthdays while in the service were not always pleasantly received or a means for celebration, as George Peck points out in a moment of self-pity: "Yesterday [August 14, 1864] was my birthday. Twenty-three years have passed over my head. Years of toil and hard luck."[156] When this was written, Peck had already served three years in the army. The lament was not his last. Ringing in the New Year of 1865 would be difficult for him. "Everything has gone wrong for me today. No pass. And everything I have tried to do has failed," he said.[157] Peck may have had a right to feel melancholy. Before serving with the Hospital Guards—Rhode Island Volunteers, he was a private in the 2nd Regiment Rhode Island Volunteers, hospitalized because of an "inguinal rupture." The side effects would last through his entire enlistment at Lovell. And as if that weren't enough, Peck returned home to Bristol, Rhode Island, to bury his mother who died of an undisclosed illness on March 9, 1864.[158]

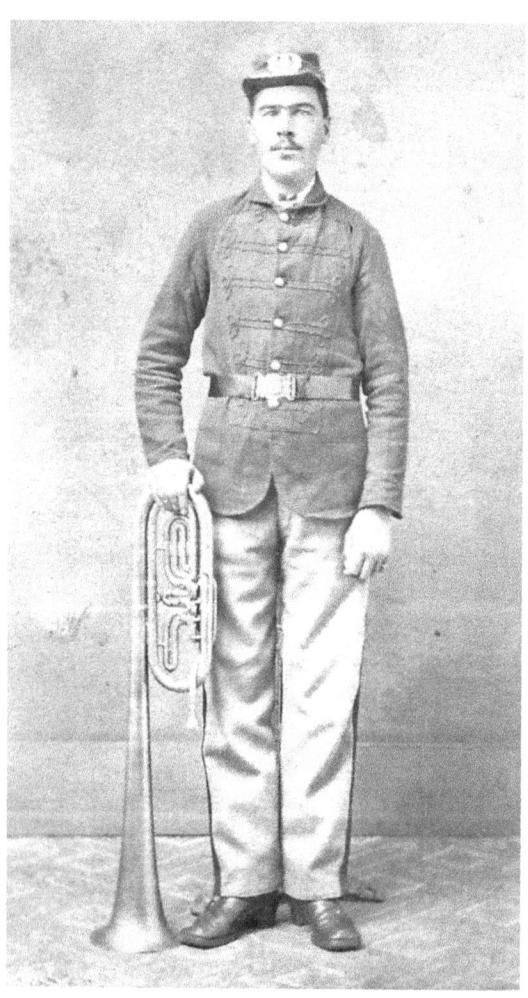

An unidentified musician who performed at the hospital holds his over-the-shoulder horn near his side. This version was said to have been designed by a Providence man (author's collection).

Ne Plus Ultra Opera Troupe!

This Troupe takes pleasure in announcing to the Patients in the Hospital that, through the kindness of the Officers at the Post, they will give

TWO ETHIOPIAN ENTERTAINMENTS!

New Year's Eve and Night, Dec. 31, '63, & Jan. 1, '64.
AT THE USUAL PLACE.

NEW ADDITIONS TO THE TROUPE!!!

FUN! WIT!! AND HUMOR!!!

It is hoped that the Patients will avoid all unnecessary noise and confusion, conducting themselves in as orderly a manner as at the former entertainment.

PROGRAMME.

Part First.

Introductory Overture,	Company
Opening Chorus,	Vocal Corps
Girl in Blue,	Brandimore
Happy be thy Dreams,	Burnes
Off for Charleston,	Dan Taylor
Aunt Dinah's Quilting Party,	Howard
Charcoal Man,	Dan Taylor
Finale,—Chorus,	Company

Part Second.

Quartette—"Come where my love lies dreaming"
  Potter, Raymond, Bishop, and Bowen
Cruelty to Johnny, ... Freeman and Howard

GREAT INTERNATIONAL PRIZE FIGHT.
King vs. Heenan.

Heenan, champion of America,	Dan Taylor
King, champion of England,	Howard
Banjo Solo,	Clark
Music Lesson,	Dan Taylor and Clark
Rattlesnake Jig,	Dan Taylor

Albert Russell will appear in a

VENTRILOQUIAL ENTERTAINMENT,

in which he will illustrate the occult powers of the human voice and its contributary organs.

Part Third.

The whole to conclude with the side splitting Farce entitled

THE TICKET TAKER.

Characters by the Company

Doors open at 6 1/2 o'clock P. M. . . . . Performance to commence at 7 P. M.
Admission TEN CENTS. Tickets to be had of the Ward Masters at the Wards.

Patients and professional entertainers performed in minstrel shows to lift the spirits of patients during the holiday season with proceeds benefiting the invalids (Brown University Library, Providence, Rhode Island).

But matters weren't always bleak for the men. In May of 1863, a combined show of Melville's Great Australian Circus and the R. Sands American Circus came to Newport. The extravaganza concluded with a lifelike steeplechase. Some of Lovell's patients who were lucky enough to obtain passes during the dates were probably in attendance. A year later more entertainment came to town: Van Amburgh and Company's Mammoth Menagerie and Egyptian Caravan, featuring a living giraffe, "the only one on this continent."[159] During the spring and summer months, circuses always seemed to be in vogue.

Minstrel shows were also a popular form of entertainment. The Forrest's Minstrels and Brass Band and Whiting's Minstrels performed several times at Aquidneck Hall with an admission price of 25 cents, an affordable price for soldiers with a pass on a shoestring budget.[160] According to Michael Varhola, in his book *Everyday Life during the Civil War*, minstrel shows consisted of the following areas of entertainment: a sing-along performed by the troop prearranged in a semicircle on the stage; several individual acts; and finally a nonsensical skit combining music and comedy. Overseeing the entire show, and equivalent to today's master of ceremonies, was an interlocutor.[161]

George Phillips was contemplating attending a second minstrel performance at Portsmouth Grove during the Thanksgiving holidays but was hesitant because of the weather: "I am going tonight if it only stops raining long enough."[162] At year's end, George Peck notes in his diary, "The Ne Plus Ultra Opera Troupe gave an entertainment tonight as Ethiopian minstrels."[163] Four shows were scheduled and performed on the hospital grounds: Christmas Eve, Christmas Day, New Year's Eve, and New Year's Day. Supporting performers usually included those from the audience with William Dennett and a few of his wards working overtime as performers. Minstrel acts in the nineteenth century were fashionable and the audience for the shows at Lovell drew citizens from "Providence, Newport and surrounding towns."[164] Participants dressed as Negro caricatures in blackface makeup while performing in dramas and comic variety shows. Amusements like these allowed men a mental boost while providing a safe haven during their humdrum existence as hospitalized soldiers. But judging by today's standards, minstrel shows reeked of racism, with laughs achieved at the unfortunate expense of African Americans. By the early 20th century, such forms of entertainment would gradually meet their rightful demise.

Whitman Bosworth was extended "an invitation to go on a fishing trip and sailing excursion" with his ward doctor. Bosworth accepted though still in poor health with a pain in his side and the passing of blood in his urine. He wrote to his parents: "We crossed the bay [some twelve miles across] in a sailboat and landed at the town of Wickford and then walked into the country about five miles to a factory pond." The real reason for the "expedition," as Bosworth called it, "was to get some small specimens of pouts, flat fish and pickerel for the doctor's aquarium." According to Bosworth, the doctor, knowing he was ill, did all the work, and "I mainly went for the company."[165]

Additional activities evolved at the camp, but on a smaller scale. Men could join arithmetic or algebra classes, a debating club, or a singing group. George Peck participated in all three.[166] Previously, a writing class had been formed.[167]

Charles H. Gowsley from a Pennsylvania regiment seemed to like what he saw at the hospital, stating in a letter, "We have a well conducted hospital here."[168] The opinion was seconded by John Lovejoy in a letter to his sister in which he said it was "first-rate." Lovejoy went on to explain: "This hospital is getting to be a very nice place. It is fixed up very nice [and] outdoors there are nice flowers all over the grounds." Proud of his surroundings, he wished his family could see the hospital complex and how invalids managed their affairs.[169] Lovejoy saw one drawback, telling his cousin Cynthia, "Now I cannot take a walk of over two hundred yards without walking the same ground over again," adding, "I thank God for freedom and liberty but at present I do not enjoy it. For the past four months and a half I have been confined on the bounds of less than eight acres of land [actually twelve] with the exception of once that I had a pass to go to Providence."[170]

Stephen Rogers saw many positives with the hospital, having but one complaint: trying to keep his ward building warm during winter.[171] Seth Alden gazed out the window on a late spring day while writing a letter to his sister and counted twenty sailboats on Narragansett Bay. He thought the place was "quite pretty."[172]

Yet, George Peck would contradict all the charming assessments. Writing on May 6, 1864, he said, "The police party [is] busy planting trees ... they wish to make this mud hole a summer residence."[173] On November 5, 1864, he reconfirmed his earlier opinion: "Policed the whole ground today. Took all day and after we got through, it looked as bad as ever."[174] George Phillips concurred. In a letter to his lady friend, Emma, he said, "I am

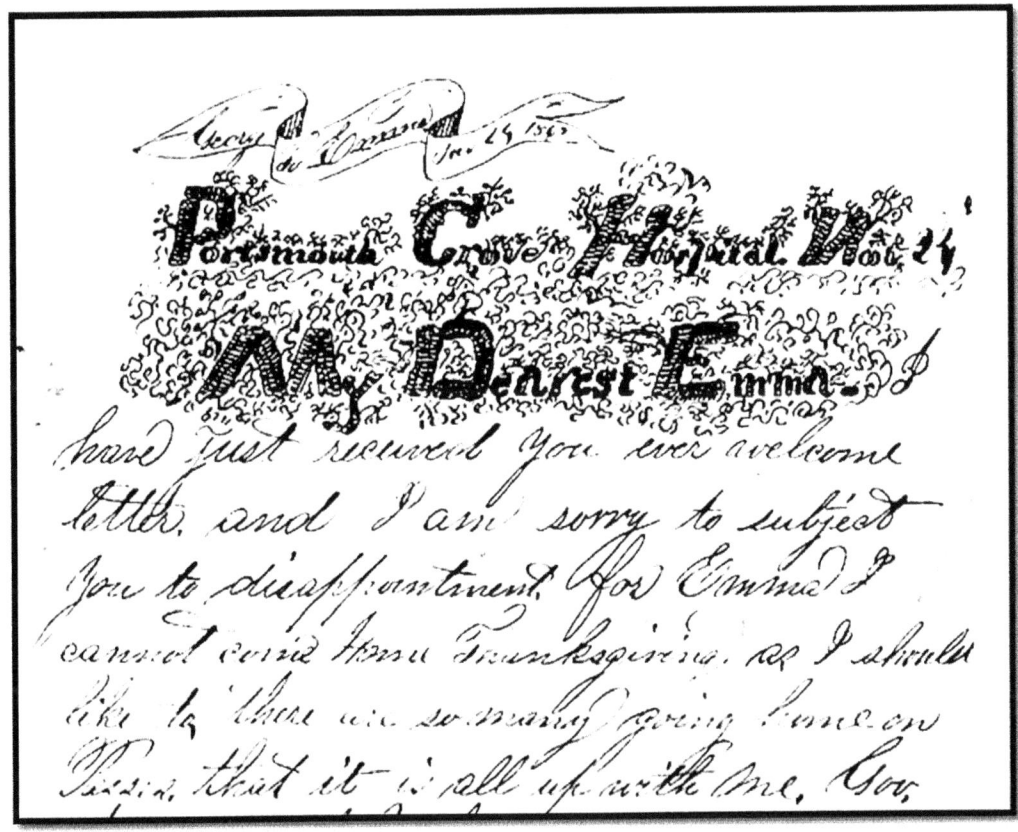

Decorative letterhead sketched by George D. Phillips (courtesy Connecticut Historical Society, Hartford, CT; collection number MS#90813).

glad I am going to leave this place, for I do not like it."[175] Whitman Bosworth also provided a dismal view: "I cannot content myself in this infernal institution and I know of no way to get out of it unless the next examination call[s] myself well and [I] go to the regiment."[176] Neither Phillips nor Bosworth provided reasons for their unflattering opinions.

Evaluating the psychological effect, John Austin offered his opinion, which dealt more with boredom than general maintenance and groundskeeping: "I have got sick of staying here." At the time, he was fairly despondent, which surfaced again in a letter to his wife a month later: "Sometime I get discouraged and that I do not care whether I live or not."[177] With no discharge forthcoming and his back still lame, it's no wonder he felt this way. Stephen Rogers would also experience a tinge of loneliness, as all soldiers feel from time to time. He wrote his parents: "I long to be at home this afternoon. This place seems so dull and not of the world; and it seems more so Sunday than any other days."[178] On another occasion he wrote, "Everything looked so dark and gloomy and I sat down to my potatoes and salt with visions of a little sitting room warm and cozy with a table upon which were warm biscuits, several kinds of pie and a chance to take your own time for eating them."[179] John Lovejoy also experienced and witnessed the same symptoms. He felt that homesickness killed soldiers just like bullets and disease. "It is the worst disease a soldier can have," he said.[180]

Like John Austin and Stephen Rogers, Adin Thayer was jaded by his hospital stay, though he described Portsmouth Grove as "quite a pleasant place."[181] Prior to recuperating from his leg wound at the hospital, he spent time at a U.S. general hospital in Annapolis,

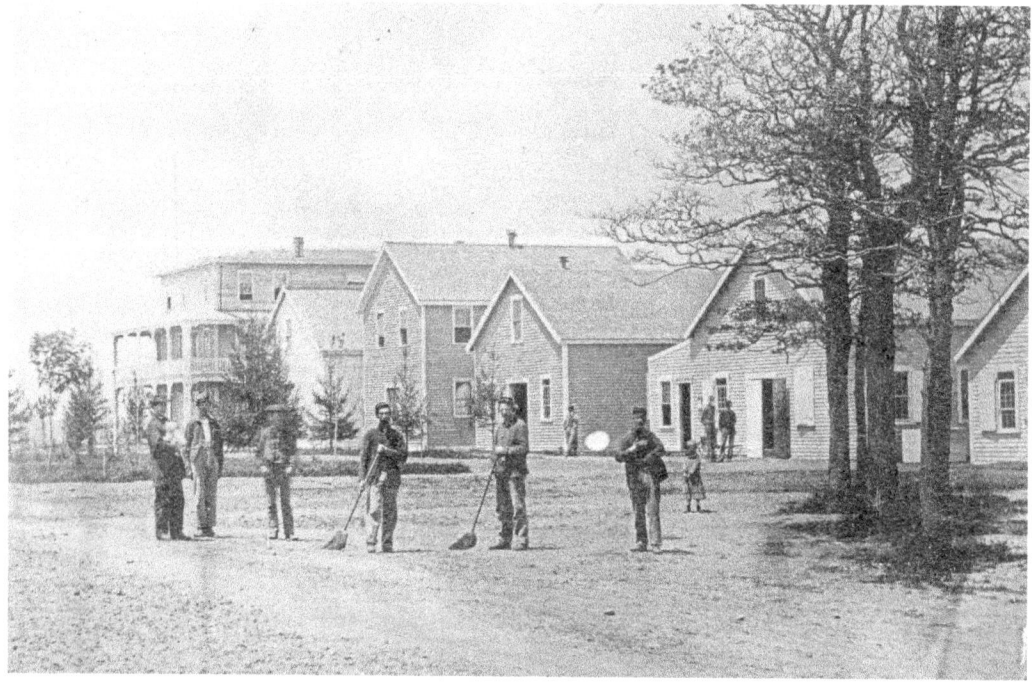

Though policing the grounds was a common occurrence at the hospital, this image was posed for the photographer. Notice two soldiers at each end of the line holding their pet dogs. Standing in the background is a child lucky enough to be photographed that day (author's collection).

Maryland. He may have looked at his release from Portsmouth Grove and return to his unit as a godsend, but that would be short-lived. On July 1, he was captured at Gettysburg and imprisoned at Belle Isle Prison in Richmond, Virginia. His stay lasted ten weeks—ten weeks of misery while facing constant starvation. Thayer lived to fight another day.[182]

George Phillips had arrived at Lovell General Hospital after spending time at Armory Square Hospital for treatment of an undisclosed illness. Unlike Adin Thayer, who was captured by the Confederates after his stay at Portsmouth Grove, Phillips had already been a prisoner of war. Previous to his hospitalizations, he had been wounded and taken prisoner at Chancellorsville on May 2, 1863, before being paroled thirteen days later. Less than a week after setting foot in Rhode Island, Phillips deserted. After spending two weeks AWOL, presumably to visit his lady friend, Emma Krinks, in nearby Bridgeport, Connecticut, or to attend the funeral of his younger brother Alonzo, a private in Co I, Sixth Connecticut Infantry who was killed at Fort Wagner, South Carolina, he returned to the hospital and was immediately placed under house arrest. While recuperating, he was prescribed opium to ease his pain. Eventually, he was granted a disability discharge on June 29, 1865, but not before serving as a coxswain on a mail barge and as a clerk in the quartermaster's department at Fort Wood, Bedloe's Island, in New York harbor.[183]

Soldiers confined to hospitals, especially for long periods, had to find ways to fight boredom. To break the monotony, men volunteered as orderlies or attendants, as did John Warner, William Dennett, and John and Allen Lovejoy. Dennett was appointed an orderly on December 1, 1862. He was immediately put to work "writing in the hospital office" and performing "other light duties."[184] Men like these, well on the road to recovery, were usually moved to Ward 14. Placing such convalescents close to one another, however, proved a problem and an enormous headache for Dr. Edwards. It wasn't long before Ward 14 came to be called "the Rowdy Ward."[185]

Dr. Edwards was at his wits' end with Ward 14 and was convinced the present ward master couldn't keep the men under control or the ward clean. The logical solution was to find a new ward master who could. D.C. Denham, who was already working as a ward master in the hospital, was selected after a brief interview with the commander. The conversation was reported with brevity:

> "Do you think you can get along with these men?" Dr. Edwards asked.
> Denham answered, "I can try."
> "Well," Dr. Edwards said, "that is all anyone can do."

The position was now Denham's and the transfer was affected immediately. After meeting his new wards for the first time, Denham gave them the standard "obey the rules" speech. Years later, when writing about this episode, Denham described the men as "mischievous," "roguish," with some "sulky," and others "quarrelsome."[186] He was probably being pleasant.

On the first night, after tattoo (lights out), the unruliness began. Denham easily heard the noise, not because it was loud, but because his room at the end of the ward had walls that did not extend to the ceiling. Lessening the height of the wall by a few feet in all the wards allowed the ward master to hear a patient who may have had a legitimate need during the night. The wall construction also afforded the ward master a sufficient degree of privacy. Denham came out of his room after hearing the commotion and warned

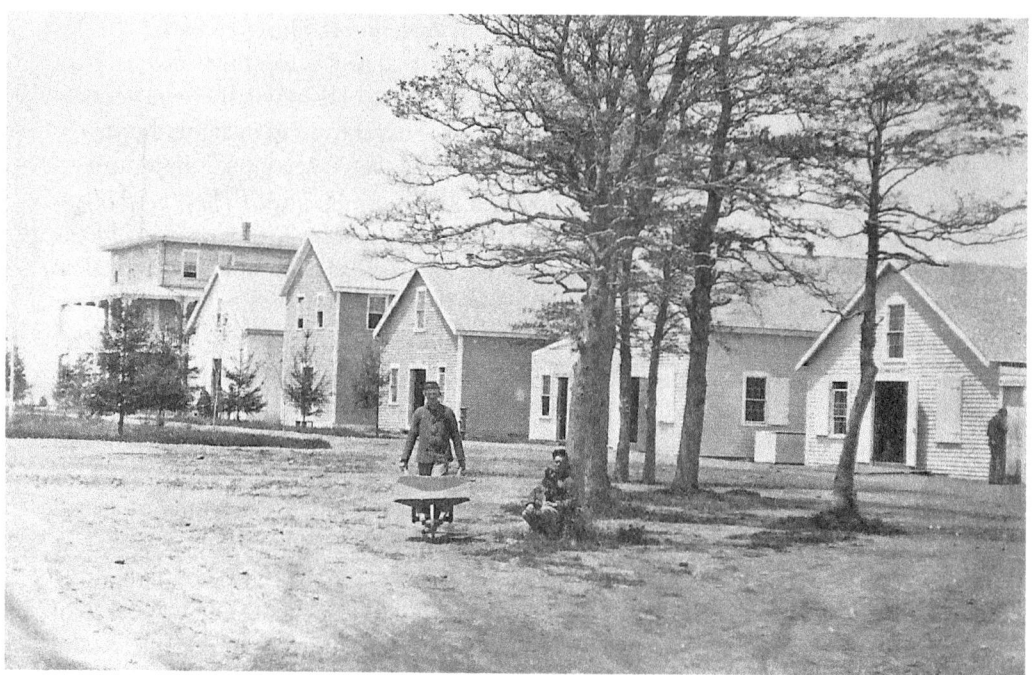

Capturing a view similar to the previous image, the cameraman moved his equipment slightly to afford a full view of the commissary on the far right. The commissary also served as the post office. Left of the building are two other structures: the Kinsley's Express building and the optician's office. Kinsley's Express transported passengers and freight over road, rail, and water between Boston and Newport (author's collection).

the men to go to sleep. By 10:30 the men were still at it, talking, shouting, and carrying on. Denham burst out of his room and issued a second warning. Arriving back in his room, he heard in the distance, "Go to Hell!" then the laughter of several men. Denham chose to ignore the travel advice. Within minutes, he thought he heard a terrier bark and then a big Newfoundland answering the call. Thinking nothing of it, as men were allowed to have dogs as pets although they were not usually allowed in the wards, he tried to get to sleep but was kept awake by a cow mooing, a horse neighing, sheep baaing, hens cackling, and ducks quacking. Soon all kinds of dogs were barking. While tossing and turning, Denham thought he heard the sawing of wood. Seconds later, the barnyard noise started anew. Groggy, Denham stepped out of his room and realized for the first time that the sawing was the work of a ventriloquist and all the animal noises were produced by the patients. "It was perfect," he later admitted. He had a hard time containing his own laughter. As he walked down the center aisle with oil lamps extinguished, the moonlight shining through the window afforded a clear view of the culprits who caused the ruckus. Things quieted down while Denham sent for a guard. Minutes later Sergeant Graves arrived with lanterns and two files of men with loaded muskets. Denham pointed out the delinquents, who continued to profess their innocence but were taken to the guardhouse regardless. Before the night was over seventeen offenders were removed from the ward and placed in confinement. Having to cool their heels for two days resolved most of the disorderly issues, and Denham had regained control of Ward 14.[187]

Eventually, Denham was able to install a substantial degree of order within the ward. Soon he had all the men making their own beds after breakfast and cleaning the floors.

Denham also supported his wards wholeheartedly when he agreed with their issues. Appearing before Dr. Edwards, Denham requested more spittoons for the building. When Dr. Edwards inquired why, Denham explained that his men had much idle time and enjoyed playing cards during the day, which usually kept them out of trouble. With only four spittoons in such a large ward of mobile men, they simply spat on the floor when the urge arose. Dr. Edwards agreed and signed a requisition for not only eight more spittoons but more tables as well. When Ward 14 was inspected by Dr. Remington a month or so later, he remarked, "Well, this is a transformation."[188]

But the day would come when patients would either fully recover and be sent back to their regiments in the field or, if still incapacitated with little hope for a fast recovery, discharged from the service. John Lovejoy would take the first route. His comfort level would change dramatically, however, after his release from the hospital. Prior to his departure, Lovejoy had strong feelings about returning to the war. Writing to his cousin Cynthia, he said, "I was sent here and I must be sent away for I shall never ask to be sent to Dixie. A private is not supposed to know anything. So you see I don't know enough to ask to be sent from a good place to a worse one."[189]

After boarding the New York steamer *Western Metropolis* on the night of August 14, Lovejoy shipped to New York City before boarding the U.S. army transport *Thomas T. Way* for the short ride to Fort Wood, Bedloe's Island, in New York harbor. Arriving on the morning of August 15, he would begin processing back to his regiment in Virginia almost immediately.

The trip did not take very long. "I am again in old Virginia where I was last December," Lovejoy wrote. Arriving at a place called Camp Distribution, he would await transportation back to his unit. Noting his displeasure at what he saw, he wrote, "I have been here long enough to suit me, for this is about the worst place I was ever in."[190] But day by day, Lovejoy's state of affairs would continue to disintegrate. Lovejoy described what he encountered upon rejoining his unit and seeing his friends for the first time in months: the "regiment don't look much as it did when I last saw it." There were but 24 men left in his company.[191] Andrew Jacobs's company would fare no better. "Our regiment is terribly decimated. There are but nine men left in our company," he said.[192] Sergeant Charles Colvin, of Company K, 7th Regiment Rhode Island Volunteers, would see worse. After spending nine months recovering from Yazoo fever at Lovell, he was issued a clean bill of health and returned to his unit in the field. What remained of his hard-fighting regiment in mid–June 1864 was appalling, as evident in the following testament. When Colvin stood in line for his company's rations, he requested them by saying, "Here is Company H." He was the only man alive or healthy enough to secure the provisions.[193]

For some, misfortune would extend hundreds of miles from the battlefield. On October 24, 1863, two hospital guards were lost: Privates Stephen A. Carr and John Taylor drowned after their boat capsized on Narragansett Bay. The circumstances surrounding the mishap and why the tragic event did not receive more in-depth press coverage remain unknown.[194] But what is understood today may shed some light on the mystery. Squalls that materialize out of nowhere, treacherous rip currents, and uncharted rocks near islands could have caused havoc when navigating the passage. Any of these scenarios may have played a part in the soldiers' demise.

By year's end, it was reported that the hospital had been turned into a convalescent camp having only to deal with less severe cases.[195] Such hospitals provided prolonged recovery before designating soldiers for discharge or return to service.[196] Either the account was untrue or someone forgot to inform the appropriate parties down South where to transport the seriously ill and wounded. Over the next year and a half, Lovell General Hospital would continue to see squadrons of battered bodies and desperately ill soldiers.

Chapter 13

1864

Some of the greatest battles will be fought within the silent chambers of your own soul.
— Ezra Taft Benson

At Lovell, the year 1864 rang in with intolerably cold weather. On January 2, temperatures plummeted and ice formed on the saltwater bay. A period account said a thermometer's mercury registered 15 degrees below zero. Stephen Rogers tells his experiences with the cold: "The only trouble is that we do not have fire enough to warm the room such cold blustering weather as it is now."[1] In the guard barracks, coal had run out by reveille — a frequent occurrence — necessitating the foraging of wood after breakfast. A shipment of coal arrived at 10 A.M. but was exhausted by nightfall, forcing the men to cut dead limbs from the surrounding trees until another load of coal arrived. Later in the week the first snowstorm of the season struck. George Peck was elated when he stated the following: "Came off guard this morning just in time to escape the storm, being lucky once in my life."[2]

Winter winds howling and blowing off Narragansett Bay were not only bone-chilling but brutal. Peck describes the sensation: "The wind blew [like a] hurricane" and "the barracks rocked like a cradle."[3]

Coal would not be the only fuel to be exhausted on a semi-regular basis. The men would also have to make do with candles to read or write by after the supply of whale oil was depleted for their lanterns.[4]

With the men confined for discipline reasons, running out of heat during bitter cold weather, and having no worthwhile light to see by, it was no wonder tempers flared. An altercation did break out in the guardhouse, but no one was injured. Perhaps it was too cold for fisticuffs.

The snow that fell on January 2 had to be removed but lay there until the eighth because of the bitter cold. When the cold spell finally snapped, the "boys made a 'snowplough,' and ... cleared around the barracks." Upon completion, the men were served beefsteak for breakfast, an unexpected and well-deserved extravagance.[5] There were some nice unseasonable days in January, like the twenty-eighth, which was "calm and warm, very much like spring," but by mid-February the weather had turned cold again. "Could hardly keep warm at night with a foot of clothes over you," Peck grumbled.[6]

The local newspaper reported officers of the First District in Newport arrested two deserters from the 3rd Regiment Rhode Island Cavalry. Dispositions were not cited. Presumably they were shipped back to their units in the field for court-martial proceedings to face the penalties handed out by the military justice system. In a speech to the Senate a few months later, a Mr. Wilson said there were 40,000 deserters from the army; 10,000 had fled to Canada and the British provinces. According to the same gentleman, within a few months, the provost-marshal system had returned 28,000 deserters to the army.[7]

Among the missing on February 26, 1864, was Sergeant Albert Russell, originally from Providence, Rhode Island. As George Peck described it, "without a doubt he has skedaddled."[8] Russell was not officially recorded as a deserter until March 22, some four weeks later. Private William Bolding, also of Providence, would skedaddle, too, on August 12, 1864, and like James Russell would not be reported as AWOL until two weeks later.[9] Peck had had his fill. Commenting on Bolding and all the others, his diary entry is a simple one-word response: "Deserters."[10]

George Peck was ordered to pack up the belongings of Private John Galligan and Private John Markey on March 24 because "they are supposed to have deserted."[11] Galligan did desert on August 22, 1863. The *Annual Report of the Adjutant General of the State of Rhode Island for the Year 1865* shows that Markey deserted on December 29, 1864, which could mean that he deserted at least once before and was either apprehended or returned of his own volition before deciding on the same course of action again. The date in the report may also be suspect in view of the errors and omissions this document published. A revised edition was printed years later for just that reason.[12]

The desertion problem was not new. In mid–July the following order was issued:

State of Rhode Island and Providence Plantations
Adjutant General's Office
Providence, July 10, 1862
GENERAL ORDERS NO. 33.

All officers and soldiers belonging to the Rhode Island Regiments, on furlough or otherwise, will be required to show a pass or other authority from their commanding officer, to avoid being arrested as deserters.

By order of the Commander-in-Chief
Edward C. Mauran, Adj. Gen.[13]

As the desertion problem worsened, the *Bristol Phenix* reported that the War Department requested assistance from appropriate state authorities to apprehend those without a pass or furlough. Governor William Sprague of Rhode Island, complying with the request, issued an order to all town councils in the state "to arrest such offenders, that they may be returned to their posts or otherwise dealt with."[14] Some returned voluntarily while others were apprehended.

Friends deserting may have been the topic of discussion at the hospital but there were other happenings that got the patients' and staff's attention, some sad and some amusing. On April 8 near the hospital an unfortunate accident took the life of a railroad workman. The exact details of the tragedy went undisclosed.[15] Railroad accidents claiming the lives of railroad workers and civilians alike were a frequent occurrence and published in the local newspapers, usually in somber tones. Most deaths appeared to be the result of the person's own negligence.

Not long after the incident, George Peck would walk into his barracks only to hear the distant singing of black soldiers. "The first thing I heard ... was a Negro melody," he writes in his diary. Pondering the situation, he said, "It takes all sorts to make up an army."[16] Peck may have been surprised when he heard black soldiers singing, but Stephen Rogers's encounter while on pass in Providence was even more dramatic. Paying for stationary and envelopes in a nearby store, he happened to notice a young girl. The storekeeper informed him that she "was a little contraband brought up from the vicinity of Fairfax County Court House." Rogers was dumbfounded at her appearance. "No one would ever have suspected that she had Negro blood in her veins," he said. Further, he noted, "She was almost perfectly white with light curly hair and a very musical voice." Described as cute and talented, she sang several songs for those in attendance, which pleased all around.[17]

African Americans were not the only minority to be found in the hospital and the surrounding community. In a contemporary image included in a presentation album given to Ada Brewster, a nurse at the hospital, handwritten in pencil on the reverse are the words: "Indian. We had 3 in [the] same ward."[18]

By mid–May there would be an influx of new patients. "Twenty came in the Boston train last evening," George Peck wrote in a letter, but providing no details in his diary.[19] In a letter home to his parents dated May 22, 1864, John Warner described the arrival of seven hundred new patients. "We got sixty of them in the ward which I am in, and it has kept me pretty busy since then." Continuing, he wrote, "I expect there will be a few more sent here soon to fill the hospital." The hospital now served an estimated one thousand patients, far fewer than capacity, but still a signifi-

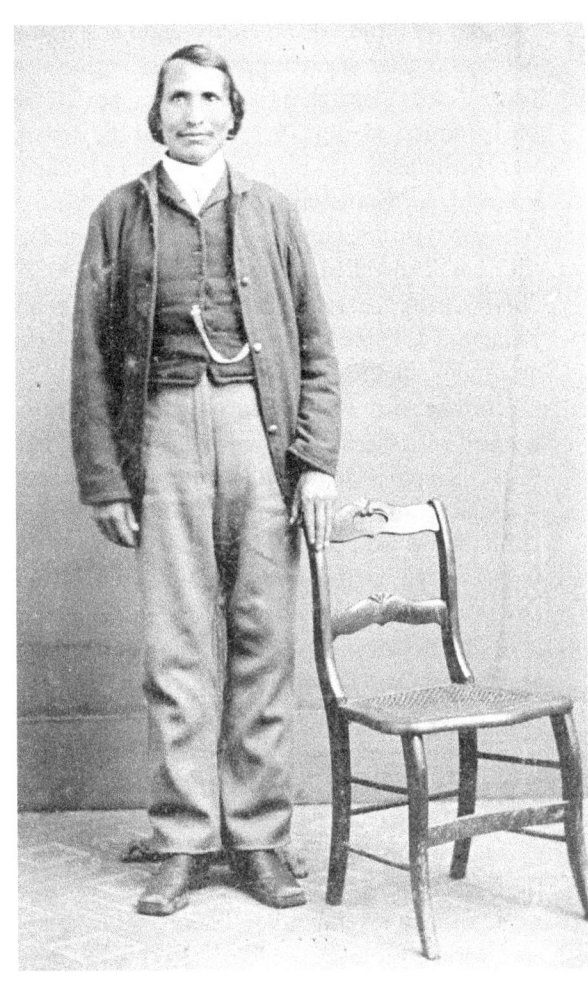

The hospital served several minorities, including three American Indians, all of whom were said to reside in the same ward (courtesy Dr. Stephen Altic, D.O.; from his collection).

cant number. As John Warner and others knew, the figures could change at a moment's notice. Closing his letter, Warner added, "Since the new patients came here, there has been a funeral every day and some days two. It was seldom that there was one before."[20] Death was an everyday occurrence at the hospital, at some times more numerous than others.

With the hospital running smoothly and without major disruptions, Lovell General Hospital became old news for nearly the entire first half of 1864. To find newsworthy items about the hospital was rare except when someone wrote to the newspaper requesting donations of food and clothing from the subscribers. Most local stories about the military concerned the U.S. Naval Academy in Newport and whether the school would be returned to Annapolis, Maryland. National war news was covered extensively but not always accurately; and politics, especially the coming presidential election, composed most of the headlines, accompanied by paid political advertisements.

On a Sunday, June 9, 1864, the situation changed dramatically, as the staff knew it would. Five hundred and eighty-eight sick and wounded arrived on the steamer *Western Metropolis* after departing from Washington.[21] All were victims of the Petersburg Campaign. Initial dispatches erroneously reported that only a few soldiers onboard were seriously injured. George Peck witnessed the debarkation and had his own thoughts: "They were badly used up," he said in his diary.[22] The truth became more frighteningly evident when Mayor Cranston visited the scene. Immediately he put out an urgent request for "contributions of money, old linen, lint, bandages, jellies, and lemons."[23] Weeks earlier, the press had called for food items like "crackers, wines, jellies," and incidentals like "books, games, drawing paper, pencils, fine combs and tobacco, etc."[24] Back in Newport, Benjamin J. Tilley was at it again, hard at work collecting food, clothing and money to accommodate the arrivals.[25]

There were so many invalids on the *Western Metropolis* that the *City of Newport* assisted with the debarkation, which was said to have taken from six to eight hours. Some 80 of the men were so badly wounded they had to be removed by stretchers. The scene was ghastly. After observing the unloading of patients, one reporter predicted, "Many amputations would be necessary." Adding to their misfortune, the soldiers were said to be penniless, having gone without pay for five months.[26] Torn-up soldiers and lack of pay made for a never-ending story at the hospital.

The *Western Metropolis* also carried Confederate prisoners. One had died on passage; another was barely clinging to life "with [a] leg taken off. Many suffered from arm and head wounds." According to Peck, "They were ragged and dirty."[27]

Just as it seemed things couldn't get worse, another 300 sick and wounded were expected a few days hence. In the wards, the scene of melancholy was unrelenting, with much suffering and death. Accounts differed slightly as to the number who died but the average seemed to be between two to three a day. Eventually the funerals would taper off. The staff at Lovell General Hospital was now caring for sixteen hundred and eighty men. Though several hundred more could still be accommodated, no one on the medical staff wished for more.

On the same day the *Western Metropolis* arrived, George Peck wrote in a diary entry: "Two men came here today to enlist, but are not accepted yet. One week here will be about enough for them." And knowing all too well from empirical knowledge, he concludes: "It generally sickens most of the new recruits."[28]

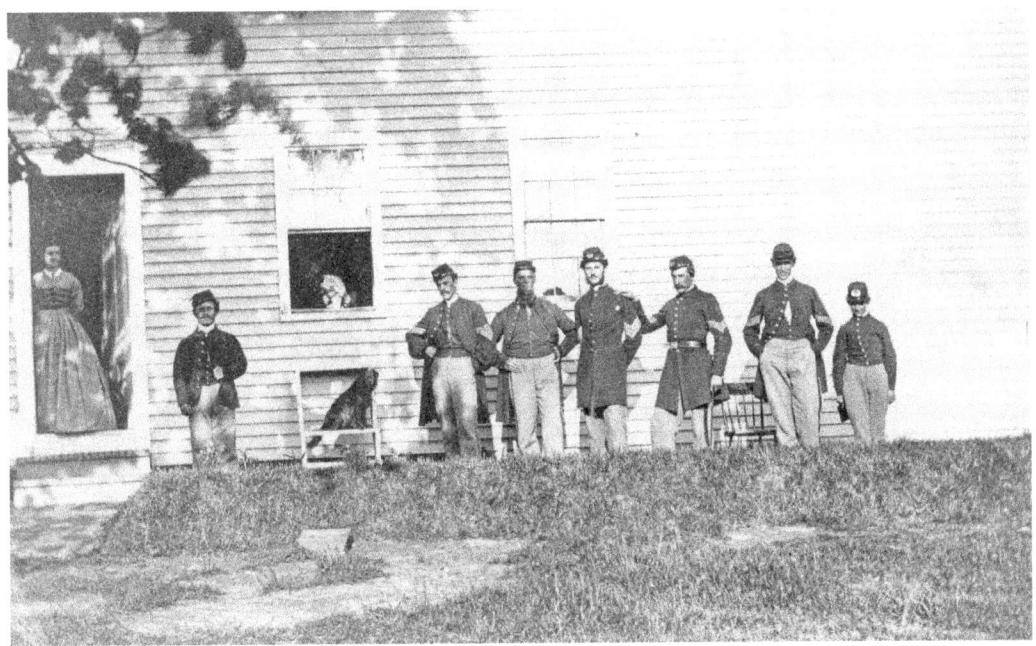

Soldiers came to the hospital as young boys and grown men. Many were born in European and Scandinavian countries. Some were former slaves; a few were American Indians. Some were short in stature, as is a soldier in this image. But in the final analysis, no matter what their physical appearance or pedigree, patriotism was their overriding influence (courtesy Dr. Stephen Altic, D.O.; from his collection).

As predicted, on the following morning more wounded were added to the hospital's caseload, this time 70, not the rumored 300. Arriving on the steamer *Bay State*, the invalids were immediately transported by "special train" along Narragansett Bay to Portsmouth Grove. In the meantime, monetary contributions continued to pour in through Benjamin Tilley's periodical store.[29] Most ranged from $1 to $5 but some were as high as $50 to $100.[30] Rarely, however, were enough provisions purchased to satisfy the soldiers' needs.

To make room for the influx of new arrivals, men were examined by the hospital physicians and swiftly discharged. James Magee, a private in Co. G, 2nd Regiment Rhode Island Volunteers, was discharged on June 17, 1864, in Providence after convalescing at Portsmouth Grove since losing his right leg in the Battle of the Wilderness back on May 5. Originally from Ireland, Magee came to the United States and took up residence in Bristol, Rhode Island. One would suspect the reason for his discharge was for loss of limb, but it actually was because his enlistment had expired. Apparently he was healthy enough to go home.[31]

Later in the month, Corporal John M. Shelow, a 20-year-old corporal from Blair County, Pennsylvania, arrived on the same steamship that carried the first load of sufferers to Portsmouth Grove: the *Western Metropolis*. Shelow had been wounded once before: on June 9, 1862, at Port Republic, Virginia, he suffered a gunshot wound to the knee, a superficial wound from which he quickly recovered. This time, on June 16, 1864, the wound proved more severe and debilitating. While fighting with Company

A, 110th Regiment Pennsylvania Volunteer Infantry, Shelow took a gunshot wound to the face. After the war, Shelow's case was described in the *Medical and Surgical History of the War of the Rebellion (1861–1865)* thusly: "Conoidal ball entered external canthus of left eye, and emerged at outer angle of right eye destroying both." He was now without sight and would have to learn to cope with the disability for the remainder of his life.[32]

As the injured warriors were arriving from the Petersburg Campaign, Assistant Surgeon William F. Cornick, USA, was placed in charge of the hospital as executive officer. Prior to his assignment in Rhode Island, he practiced as a military physician at Fort Monroe, Virginia, and then at the Key West Barracks of the U.S. Army in Florida. At Key West he worked with a multitude of patients suffering from malaria and yellow fever. Like other doctors of the period, at least one of his medical treatments proved highly suspect. According to Andrew McIlwaine Bell, in his book *Mosquito Soldiers*, Dr. Cornick, believing that sweating was a good thing, "submerged his patients in hot bath" laced with several ounces of mustard until the patients nearly fainted, then wrapped them in blankets before placing them in bed. To cure either disease, he prescribed "calomel, castor oil, quinine, and spirits of nitre." Dr. Cornick's tenure at Lovell was short-lived, not because of his skills or treatments, but because his surgeon's assignment was pro tem from the beginning.[33]

For those who managed to survive Dr. Cornick's steamy hot mustard baths and other questionable treatments by well-intentioned but medically-challenged physicians, the holiday recognizing our nation's birth would come as welcome relief. The Fourth of July 1864 would be special for the patients, not because of the celebrations planned for the day, but because they were all treated to ice cream. Pennsylvanians would have even more reason to rejoice. An estimated one hundred soldiers were transferred to their home state.[34] The hospital continued to prune its roster of patients in anticipation of more arrivals.

As expected, two weeks later, the steamer *George Leary* docked with more wounded. One hundred fifty invalids were said to be on-

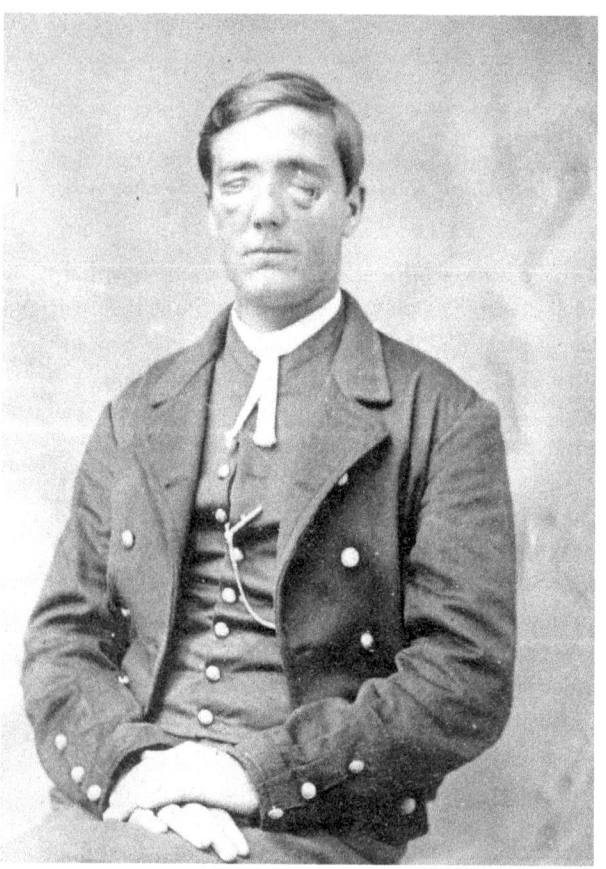

As ghastly as John M. Shelow's wounds appear, there were many others worse off than he (courtesy Dr. Stephen Altic, D.O.; from his collection).

board.³⁵ James Pedley, age thirty-eight, from Syracuse, serving with Company G, 76th New York Infantry, was a likely passenger. He had been seriously wounded near Petersburg on June 13 and was barely clinging to life. His struggle to stay alive ended on July 31, when he succumbed to his wounds. His remains were buried in the yard. After the war ended less than a year later, his body would lie alongside ninety other honored soldiers from New York regiments, the most from any state consecrating the soil of Lovell General Hospital's burial yard.³⁶

At month's end, the transport *Ishland* steamed to the dock with 350 casualties from the Cold Harbor battlefields. Daniel Austin had been wounded in the foot during a skirmish on June 2. Not unlike the others, Daniel Austin had made his way through regimental and field hospitals receiving hasty and poor-quality medical care before arriving at Lovell General Hospital. During his time at Cold Harbor he had witnessed more horrors than most men would face in a lifetime: battlefield deaths; hospital amputations; a soldier with maggots in his wounds; a paralyzed man wounded in his back who would expire next to him; and a man shot through the face who couldn't eat or talk and "smelled bad." Daniel

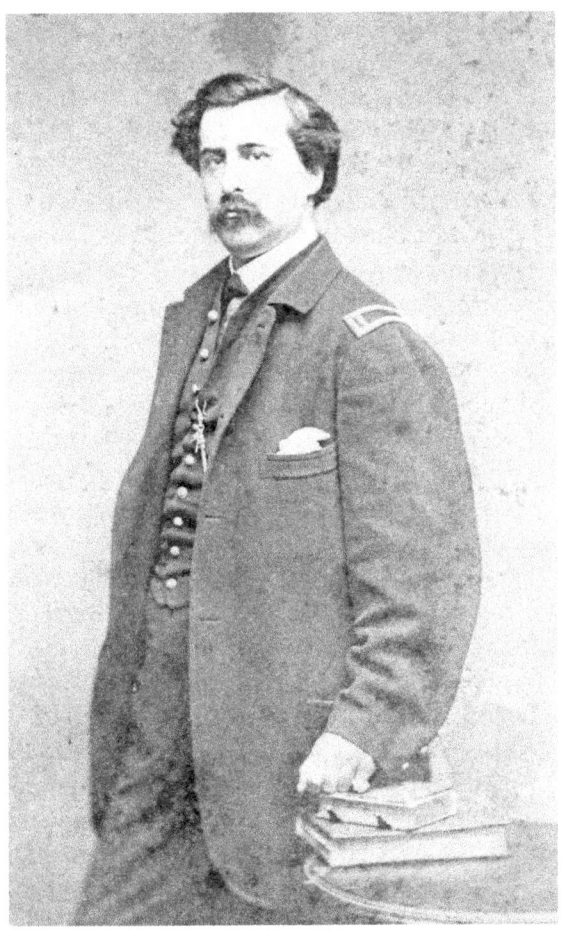

Executive Officer Dr. William F. Cornick, U.S.A., served at the hospital from January 1863 until October 1864. Unlike many of the soldiers under his charge, Dr. Cornick chose to have his image taken at Manchester Brothers Photographers in Providence, Rhode Island (courtesy Dr. Stephen Altic, D.O.; from his collection).

Austin had his own toe amputated because "the bone was fractured so as to render it useless." His experience, however, would be the status quo for most others who served in the war and spent time in military hospitals, whether field or general. Two days later, he watched as gangrene set in his wound. After being treated with nitric acid, he wrote about pus oozing from the wound. He completed the diary entry with this simple statement: "Leg painful." No wonder. A subsequent remark by Daniel Austin tells of a sergeant from Maine who was treated for gangrene and how it "makes him squawk to have it dressed."³⁷

Daniel Austin's trip up New York City's East River to Portsmouth Grove sounded almost like a lark. In two diary entries, he describes "some very pleasant islands" while viewing "plenty of haystacks" and "some men making hay." At 10 P.M. the steamer arrived at the wharf, and just as so many times before, the invalids waited for a ferry to be taken ashore.[38] By now the new wharf had been installed to handle larger steamers, but the *Ishland* arrived at low tide.

Feeling better, on Friday, August 5, Daniel Austin decided to take a walk around the grounds. He visited the "bakery, laundry and dry room" and seemed to be amazed that the washing and baking were accomplished using hot steam.[39]

Five hundred fifty additional sick and wounded arrived at the hospital on a steamer coming up from City Point after the fighting at Petersburg. The invalids were "mostly from Burnside's Corps." According to Daniel, "a few Johnnys [i.e., Confederates, or "Johnny Rebs"] [were] with them."[40]

On an early September day, the U.S. transport steamer *De Molay* arrived with two hundred and fifty sick and wounded soldiers from White House Landing, Virginia, after dropping off seventy patients in New York City, probably those from New York regiments. The debarkation was performed using a schooner, as the two vessels normally called for such duty were unavailable. The men came from the Petersburg battlefields and the casualties were recent.[41]

Less than a month later, the steamer *Baltic* arrived from Fort Monroe carrying four hundred and eighty-seven sick and wounded. For the first time at Portsmouth Grove, a large contingent of black soldiers contributed to the total, one hundred and ninety to be exact. The men had come from City Point, Virginia, and a large number were in bad shape. Two had died on board the *Baltic* immediately after landing and were buried in the cemetery. Several others were in the pangs of death, especially black soldiers who were said to have taken "the greatest proportion of severe wounds." The steamer *Perry* helped with the four-hour debarkation, which had taken longer than usual caused by high winds and rough seas and disparity of deck elevation between the low passenger steamer, *Perry*, and the *Baltic*'s higher configuration.[42] Private Augustus Johnson, Company I, 5th Regiment U.S. Colored was one of the seriously injured after being felled at the Battle of Chaffin's Farm in New Market Heights, Virginia, on September 29, 1864, a fight that favored the Union. After Johnson arrived at Lovell General Hospital, he survived for a short while. Johnson died on October 20. Onboard the same steamer was another wounded African American: First Sergeant Robert A. Pinn, also from the same company and regiment as Johnson. Pinn would remain at Portsmouth Grove for several months before learning he would be awarded the Medal of Honor for his actions at Chaffin's Farm. It was during that engagement, after learning that all the company officers were either killed or wounded, that he assumed command, rallied the men, and gloriously fought off the Confederates. Pinn received the nation's highest military award for valor on April 6, 1865.[43]

Also fighting at Chaffin's Farm on the 29th was a six-foot-tall, brown-haired, blue-eyed lad of 19. Enlisting two years previous in Providence, Perez A. Hopkins was part of the gun crew in Battery F, Rhode Island Light Artillery. Their mission that day was to fire artillery rounds as a way of softening Confederate positions. Then it happened. Hopkins, along with five others, was wounded by a shell or shell fragment that struck the upper part of his right arm. Exactly how it happened remains unclear. An initial report stated he was wounded by a shell fragment fired by the enemy, while another account said his wound was the result of a premature firing of his cannon similar to how Alfred

Luther injured his forearm at Gaines' Mill during the Peninsula Campaign. Whatever the circumstance, an artillery round, whole or part, caused the injury. Because of the severity of the wound, his right forearm was amputated at a field hospital. Hopkins eventually landed in the same hospital as those he fought alongside at Chaffin's Farm. He was now one of the many new faces unceremoniously blending in at Portsmouth Grove.[44]

Thanksgiving was upon the soldiers, and for most it seemed like just another holiday away from home. The citizens of Providence did all they could to rectify the situation, collecting food and produce for the occasion. Three hundred and sixteen turkeys were donated along with five hundred pies and a full complement of vegetables and other fixings. The day of celebration started at 11:30 A.M. with religious services and an address in the chapel by the Rev. Proudfit. Meanwhile, an extra force of men was detailed in the cook room. Shortly after 12 noon, the tables were filled with over two hundred platters of carved turkey along with pies, apples, and other fixings. At 12:30 P.M., after forming outside in two lines — ranks, as the soldiers called them — about a thousand patients marched in unison into the mess hall and took their seats on benches at the long tables. The mess hall was a comfortable setting even in the cold of winter as the building was heated by steam pipes.[45] When all the soldiers were seated, the Rev. Proudfit gave the blessing, after which the hospital band played "The Star Spangled Banner." Only then were the men allowed to dig in, eating from white plates and bowls.[46] When finished, the patients marched back to their wards the same way they had arrived, in a two-row procession. Amazingly, when the uneaten portions were gathered up after the meal, one hundred turkeys and five barrels of apples remained. They would be used the following day for dinner. Provisions were also distributed to those unable to leave the ward because of their infirmity.[47] The day would be a striking success.

In December of 1864, Dr. Edwards, at his own request, after serving from September 1862 through December of 1863 and again from May to December of 1864, was relieved of command. In his stead, Dr. Charles O'Leary assumed command and would remain at the hospital until four months past war's end.[48]

At about the same time Dr. Edwards was leaving Portsmouth Grove, Private Edwin Hill, along with other invalids, boarded a steamer in New Orleans destined for Lovell General Hospital. Hill had been serving with Co. K, 3rd Regiment Rhode Island Heavy Artillery before being taken ill in the swamps of Louisiana. Born in Cheshire, England, Hill now made his permanent residence in Bristol, Rhode Island. Upon his arrival at Lovell, he hoped to recuperate and enjoy the festive season now fast approaching. It was not to be. On December 21, while sailors navigated the treacherous waters off the coast of Cape Hatteras, North Carolina, the ship went down in heavy seas. All onboard were lost. Hill was two weeks shy of his nineteenth birthday.[49]

Back in Newport, the citizens were soliciting donations to prepare a feast for the soldiers' Christmas dinner. The success of the Thanksgiving Day meal was attributed to the fine citizens of Providence, but for this holiday, the citizens of Newport and the neighboring communities of Middletown and Portsmouth did not want to be outdone. The man collecting the donations was Benjamin J. Tilley.[50]

With the holidays arriving at Portsmouth Grove, patients were seen trimming the chapel for the festive occasion. But not all were merry. George Peck relates: "Christmas

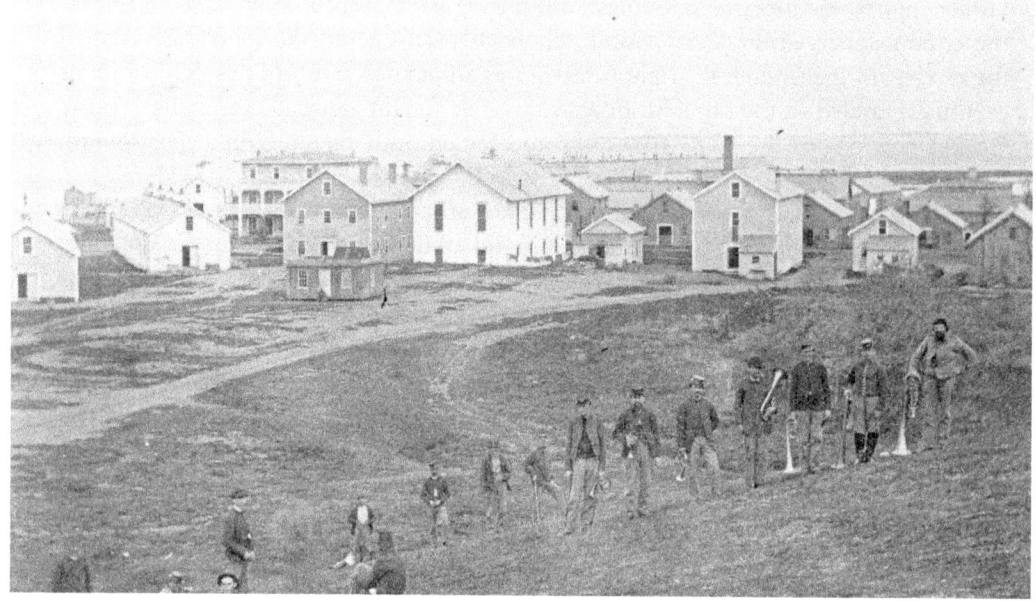

Patients gaze as the hospital band stands for a picture. Note the three-story Administration Building at left center (courtesy Leo F. Kennedy).

eve this evening but rather dull here. One thinks of the time before war when he could enjoy himself but at present our country demands our service and we must bear our trials and let self-denial be a virtue till the war is over." In the same pen stroke, he concludes: "It is rumored the paymaster will be here on Tuesday."[51] But his conjecture may have been nothing more than wishful thinking.

Two days before Christmas, a tank of some unrecorded sort exploded in Ward 5, blowing out windows and destroying a coal stove while disrupting any semblance of serenity in the air that morning. No injuries were reported, but for the patients it must have seemed, at least for the moment, that the war had found Portsmouth Grove and the patients in the hospital.[52]

Christmas Day 1864 was "pleasant and warm" with light winds from the southwest. For dinner, seven hundred patients and staff enjoyed turkey and fixings. Suppertime included pudding, potatoes, and onions along with a regular ration of coffee, bread, and not one, but two apples. Although the dinner was a resounding success, financially the public subscription fell short by three hundred dollars. Unknown to most observers, the deficiency was satisfied by a man of modest means but with a magnanimous heart. His name: Benjamin J. Tilley.[53]

Not all were fortunate enough to partake of the meal and festivities planned for the day. George Peck spent his Christmas performing guard duty.[54]

Two days after the holiday a letter to the editor appeared in the December 26, 1864, edition of the *Newport Daily News* thanking those who had made the day special. The letter was signed simply, "Ward Thirteen (13)." It also extended the following greeting: "We wish you all many a Merry Christmas."[55] In an adjoining column was another reference to Christmas: "A Christmas Present from General Sherman — Capture of Savannah."[56] After nearly four years of fighting, the war was nearing an end. Both the letter and the article may have been read by many soldiers at the hospital, but one man in particular could not have been more proud: Henry Sherman, an Ohio native, had been recuperating at Portsmouth Grove after receiving a wound to the limb. Henry was the nephew of General William Tecumseh Sherman, now a national hero.[57]

Chapter 14

War's End:
Glory, Glory, Halleluiah

I now close my military career and just fade away, an old soldier who tried to do his duty as God gave him the light to see that duty. Good-bye.
— General Douglas MacArthur,
speech to joint session of
Congress, April 19, 1951

On one of the coldest mornings of the year, January 8, 1865, Private John Rapp, Company M, 2nd Regiment Pennsylvania Heavy Artillery, a patient at the hospital, was found lying on the beach not far from the hospital nearly frozen to death after running the guard the night before. Authorities surmised that he had simply got drunk and passed out. A day later after being brought back to the hospital, he died, presumably from exposure.[1] Rapp was one month shy of completing a full year in the army.

Private Timothy Collins, who had precipitated his own undoing on several occasions by falling asleep on watch, was back in the limelight on January 18. While on guard duty, Collins claimed to have shot at a man who ran his beat, calling out, "The man's shot." Knowing Collins and his rap sheet, no one with authority believed his story. All theorized he simply fell asleep, tripped, and dropped his musket, resulting in a misfire. Not wanting to be caught sleeping again and punished for the indiscretion, Collins had, no doubt, concocted the cover story. Playing along with the ruse, Collins was ordered back outside for an hour in the snow to find the intruder, now referred to as "the dead body."[2]

On January 20, a macabre event took place at the hospital. An auction was conducted to sell the effects of dead soldiers.[3] Times were tough and little of anything having material value was wasted. To date, no records have been found to determine who the beneficiaries of the booty were.

A second bizarre incident happened not long after. For reasons unknown, Edmund Cole, co-owner of the hospital grounds currently being leased by the Federal government and still living at Portsmouth Grove, argued with one of the hospital staff. Subsequently, Cole was accused of insulting an officer. On the site was a store called Cole's, "a sort of post exchange" of which Edmund Cole was the proprietor.[4] Edmund Cole apparently had a monopoly; not only did he lease the former resort to the government, but he also acted as Portsmouth Grove's postmaster while owning the so-called post exchange. The post exchange was more likely a permanent sutler's shop. Whether Cole was asked to leave or he did so of his own volition is unclear; but on January 28, 1865, Mr. Cole and his wife Olive moved their personal belongings to Newport.[5]

And if the above were not enough evidence of unusual goings-on, a fire broke out in the stovepipe of Ward 11. The fire was discovered early enough and was quickly contained. Orders were immediately given to extinguish all wood fires at the hospital. At first glance this decision seemed to make perfect sense, as wood fires can be dangerous from sparking and soot buildup; but there was no alternative, as the coal supply had been exhausted until the next delivery. The men had to scrounge wherever they could to find enough dropped coal, perhaps along the railroad tracks, to sustain a fire throughout the night.[6]

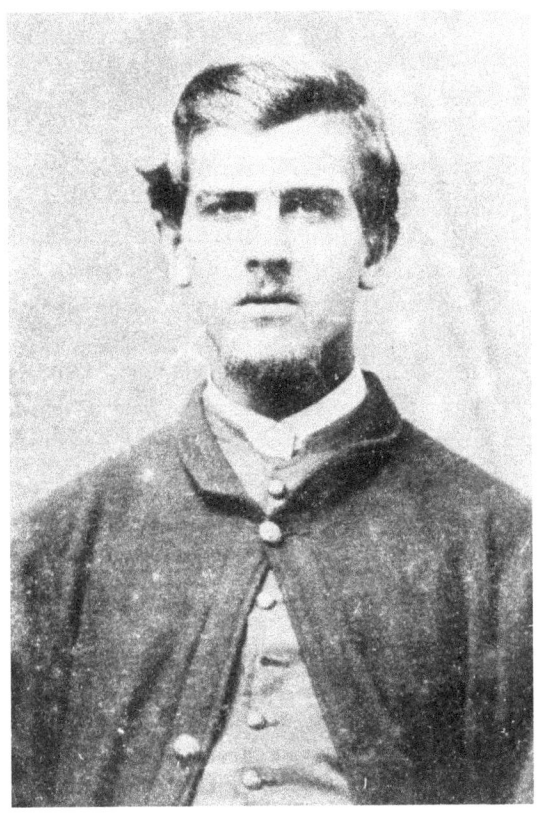

John Rapp met his demise on the shores of Narragansett Bay, dying of exposure after skirting the guard and following up with a night of heavy drinking (courtesy Dr. Stephen Altic, D.O.; from his collection).

Two months earlier, a blaze had started in George Phillips's room. He had left his room momentarily, but after returning, he found it enveloped in flames. According to Phillips, "The wind blew the curtain against a light [presumably either a lantern or candle] but I managed to put it out." Shaken by the experience, he said, "It got the best of me. A little more and I would have had Portsmouth Grove burnt up. What a pity that would have been."[7] In another fire incident that had more comedy than tragedy, a soldier nicknamed Benny lost part of his tent to a fire. George Peck reported: "No insurance but some swearing."[8]

On February 15, 1865, a deserter returned to the hospital. He had been AWOL for more than a year.[9] Maybe he sensed what others who had stayed the course were feeling: that the war was coming to an end. Perhaps he thought this was as good a time as any to expect leniency from military authorities. No one will ever know what caused his change of heart or the penalty he had to serve.

Two months to the day after the deserter turned himself in, news of Abraham Lincoln's assassination hit Portsmouth Grove like heavy artillery. When told of the reprehensible act, Dr. Edwards was said to have turned pale and stated in the simplest terms what almost everyone was feeling: "I can't believe it." Some 10 days earlier, John Wilkes Booth, the assassin, had been seen in Newport while "driven in a carriage to the Aquidneck House where he remained at dinner." Later he was taken to the terminal of a Boston-bound train. Rumors of Booth's travels while in the city ran the gamut, the most interesting being Booth's visiting men of prominence whose allegiance rested with the South.[10]

Later that day, a man bringing supplies from Newport to the hospital made the mistake of being too verbal about his allegiance and the assassination. "Served him right," he said. "Abraham Lincoln ought to have been killed long ago." Shortly after making the remark, the man was brought to Dr. Edwards's office. The immediacy of his removal may have saved him from being lynched, shot, stabbed, or beaten to death by an angry mob of soldiers. According to James L. Swanson, in his book *Blood Crimes: The Chase for Jefferson Davis and the Death Pageant for Lincoln's Corpse*, an estimated two hundred people experienced the wrath of an angry individual or throng for making similar remarks.[11] Following a brief interrogation, one in which the vendor vehemently professed his innocence, Dr. Edwards ordered his release. But many still believed his guilt and eventually the vendor lost a good trade even if it was only to last four more months.[12]

With the war all but over, disability discharges were now the order of business at the hospital. Hugh Finnegan, originally from Ireland, and now a private with Co. G, 7th Regiment Rhode Island Volunteers having transferred from Co. A, 4th Regiment Rhode Island Volunteers, received his on the first of June. Not unexpectedly, it took nearly a year before surgeons would release him from his duties after he was shot in the head by a Minié ball at Petersburg during the siege of Richmond the previous summer. Finnegan sustained a fractured skull and partial removal of the left temporal bone during surgery. This was not the first time he had been wounded. Ten weeks after mustering in on July 7, 1862, Finnegan was injured at the Battle of Antietam. Besides the noticeable disfigurement because of the gunshot wound at Petersburg, he also suffered partial paralysis in his right arm. Yet, in spite of all his injuries, surgeons at the hospital found him qualified to reenlist in the Veteran Reserve Corps.[13]

At his cramped studio, Joshua Appleby Williams, the photographer who took a majority of the images included in this work, would take his final photographs of veteran soldiers. Patrick Baggett, Troop B, 3rd Regiment Rhode Island Cavalry and a native of Woonsocket, Rhode Island, sat patiently with legs crossed and left hand covering the damage done to his right hand and wrist by a Minié ball while he was fighting at Pleasant Hill in Louisiana on April 9, 1864. Four months after being wounded, he was transferred to Lovell General Hospital, where doctors diagnosed alkalosis (abnormally high alkali content in the blood and tissues) along with several ulcerations of the wrist. Baggett's condition improved sufficiently to allow his discharge on January 21, 1865. Dressed in civilian clothes while recuperating from his wounds, Baggett would arrive at Williams's studio to have his likeness taken. Others would follow, but few would match Baggett's singular image. After the exposure was processed, it would prove to be an inimitable photograph that would forever be etched in time. Some 160 years later, Baggett's half-smile and covered hand serve as a fitting reminder of the goodness of man and a veteran's tenacity to fight, maybe even conceal, the physical and psychological scars of war. Baggett, a lad from Ireland with no bona fide profession other than a common laborer, would eventually find his way to Fall River, Massachusetts. There he would find employment and be able to call the industrialized city his home. Baggett left this world prematurely (c. 1890) before reaching his forty-fifth birthday. His exact date of passing is uncertain and is estimated based on failure to pick up his pension claim.[14]

During the first two weeks of June, eight to nine hundred invalids remained on the grounds, but by month's end the number dwindled as many patients were discharged. One of the fortunate, Rufus Messinger, a farmer in civilian life, received his discharge from the hospital on July 10, 1865. A year previous, while serving with Company D, 50th Pennsylvania Infantry, Messinger was wounded at the Crater in Petersburg by a Confederate Minié ball. The round struck him in the middle third of the left thigh and kept him out of action for the duration of the war.[15] Now free of his military burdens, he was ready to head back to the family farm.

By mid–August, having outlived its useful purpose with fewer than twenty-five men on the hospital roll, the staff was ordered to make preparations to disband.[16] Those still incapacitated were transferred to other military hospitals in the region or simply discharged. Jonathan Milton Stewart, Company K, of the Union's 1st Alabama Cavalry, U.S. Volunteers would be part of that final group. He had been shot in each thigh on March 10, 1865, at Monroe Crossroads, North Carolina. On March 15,

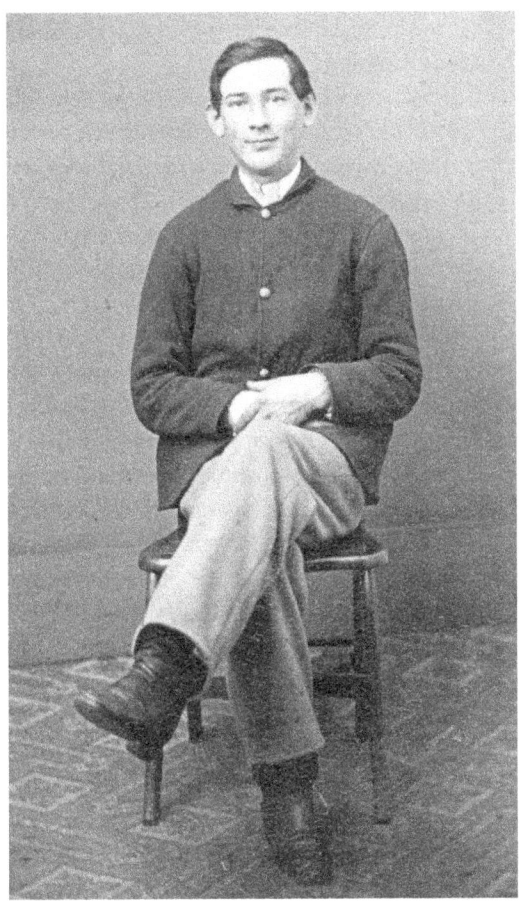

For this image, Patrick Baggett covered his mangled hand. He had been wounded by a Minié ball. Baggett's half-smile stands as a fitting testimonial to the courage and perseverance of the common soldier, both Union and Confederate (initial print courtesy Ron Coddington; duplicate identifying soldier courtesy Dr. Stephen Altic, D.O.).

he was moved up north to Lovell General Hospital, where he arrived on April 21. On July 13, Jonathan would be transferred to a New York City hospital and later discharged on a surgeon's certificate. Anxious to see his bothers, each of whom served in the Confederate army, he arrived home to find but one. To his dismay, Joseph W.S. Stewart had been discharged for health reasons and was shot and killed by "bushwhackers" who thought him a deserter. Jonathan's other brother, Isaac Newton Stewart, survived the ordeal of war. Jonathan and Isaac remained on friendly terms, and family records state that, at least between themselves, they never discussed their allegiances or participation in the war. As for Jonathan's recovery, he remained an invalid and walked with a limp until his dying day.[17]

Lovell General Hospital was officially disestablished on August 25, 1865. Seventy-three Hospital Guards—Rhode Island Volunteers, all combat veterans, mustered out the following day.[18]

There was a bright side to the Peninsula Campaign from which Lovell General Hospital (then known as Portsmouth Grove Hospital) received its first influx of patients. In a letter exchange between General McClellan and General Lee, each "agreed henceforth to treat unarmed surgeons, U.S. Sanitary Commission agents, and other medical relief personnel as neutrals." Further, the U.S. Sanitary Commission would "adopt the principle" to treat the suffering of Union men and Confederates as one and the same. This practice became the foundation of the Geneva Convention of the International Red Cross and is still in effect today.[19]

By the end of the Civil War, more than half a million soldiers had inhaled their last breaths, succumbing to wounds or illness either on the battlefield or in a hospital. Even today, the number of casualties remains staggering. Portsmouth Grove Cemetery would hold only a small number of remains and they would not rest there for long.

During the war years, Union army hospitals cared for over six million patients, treating twice as many sick as wounded.[20] Lovell General Hospital played an important role in this challenge, ranking 12th out of 183 military hospitals for patient bed capacity, surpassed only by those in larger cities or medical care facilities near military installations.[21] Under the command of Dr. Edwards for a majority of the time, Portsmouth Grove boasted 1,464 hospital beds, though several unconfirmed sources placed the number significantly higher (one account listed the peak capacity at 2,400).[22]

The hospital at Portsmouth Grove treated 10,593 patients, with a mortality figure of 308.[23] Despite the dubious startup and the general hardships of the time, patient care was admirable and only rivaled by hospitals in the Philadelphia area that were said to be preferred by soldiers because the food was good, the citizens generous, and the Quaker doctors kindly and efficient. These big-city hospitals received more national press coverage than those in smaller towns and cities. But Lovell General Hospital had one advantage over many big-city hospitals. In 1866, Honorable Erastus Brooks, at the founding of a New York hospital, acknowledged Lovell's low death rate of 3 percent when the national average was 8 percent. He attributed the achievement to proper ventilation, as Lovell General Hospital was "situated on a breezy headland, jutting out into Narragansett Bay."[24] He was remiss, however, if he failed to mention the compassionate and hard-working physicians, nurses, staff, and dedicated citizens who worked diligently at the hospital. Each in his or her own special way contributed immensely to the health and well-being of the patients.

Dr. Lewis A. Edwards would ascend to the rank of brevet colonel, later "the permanent rank of lieutenant colonel,"[25] eventually becoming the medical director of the U.S. Army. He died November 8, 1877, at the age of 54 of what was diagnosed as "progressive softening of the brain"[26] caused by several different factors, but mostly because of brain inflammation. Loss of motor function and an impairment of sensation are immediate and irreversible. Today the degenerative brain disease is called Alzheimer's. His body was laid to rest at Congressional Cemetery in Washington, D.C., next to the remains of 19 United States senators and 71 members of the House of Representatives.[27] Other notables interred at the cemetery are Mathew Brady, famous Civil War photographer; John Philip Sousa, the Marine Corps bandmaster; J. Edgar Hoover, FBI director; and the infamous David Herold, a Lincoln assassination conspirator captured at the Garrett Farm along with John Wilkes Booth in Virginia and later hanged for his treacherous crime.[28]

Dr. William F. Cornick, who served as executive officer at Portsmouth Grove, was reassigned to Key West, Florida, in October 1864, remaining until his resignation a year later. The resignation may have been precipitated because of a promotion denial. In February of 1866, he was hired as a contract surgeon by the U.S. Army and remained at the Key West Barracks, where he was credited with saving the lives of hundreds of patients suffering from yellow fever. The service was difficult. In a report to his superiors, Dr. Cornick gives an idea of the complete isolation he and others faced while there:

> Medical supplies are obtained once a year. About a year's supply is now on hand. Communication with the nearest city is by water or telegraph; the former is very irregular, being liable to interruption from heavy winds. The mails are, therefore, sent once a week, sometimes once a month.... The commissary department is supplied from New Orleans, Louisiana, and the length of time it takes to get the stores from there makes it impossible to have the necessary fresh vegetables. Very many of the stores are always spoiled before they are received at the post.[29]

Whether because of loneliness, hopelessness of the situation, personality disorder, or some other factor, Dr. Cornick experienced frequent bouts of "intemperate habits" during his tenure as a surgeon at the post, and because of this, his contract (paying $125 a month) was terminated in February 1874.

No records have been produced to substantiate his having had a drinking problem earlier, but previous questionable actions while an acting assistant surgeon give hints at such a problem. His behavior was formally questioned by Assistant Surgeon Harvey E. Brown at the Key West Barracks a few months before Dr. Cornick's removal. In January 1874, Dr. Brown drafted a letter to the medical director, Department of the Gulf, explaining his decision to terminate Dr. Cornick's contract:

> I have postponed action in this matter for many weeks in the hope that perhaps the reports which reached me almost daily of Dr. Cornick's habits might be exaggerated, or that his apparent persistent neglect of duty might be unintentional. As an old officer of the Corps as well as a personal friend of many years standing, I felt disposed to give him the benefit of every doubt that might arise. Careful and prolonged observation has however convinced me that any further leniency in his case would be an injustice to the government and perhaps prejudicial to the health of the command. His habits of indulgence in intoxicating drink are firm and persistent, and have affected his mind to such an extent as to render him inefficient and unfit to be trusted with the lives of the soldiers.

Dr. Cornick passed away on July 26, 1906. His remains rest in Emmanuel Episcopal Church Cemetery in Virginia Beach, Virginia, formerly known as Old Princess Anne County.[30]

Little is known about the other surgeons who served at Portsmouth Grove except for Dr. Benoni Carpenter and Dr. Algernon Coolidge. Dr. Carpenter, an 1829 graduate of Brown University, originally from Providence and later a resident of Pawtucket, Rhode Island, also served as a surgeon with the 28th Regiment Massachusetts Volunteer Infantry, the 12th Regiment Rhode Island Volunteers, and the 14th Regiment Rhode Island Heavy Artillery (Colored). He mustered out of service on October 2, 1865. Dr. Coolidge was a great-grandson (maternal side) of President Thomas Jefferson and an 1853 graduate of Harvard Medical School. He and his wife spent their summers in Cotuit, a quaint village in Barnstable, Massachusetts, on Cape Cod. There, Dr. and Mrs. Coolidge were instrumental in organizing, then bequeathing, substantial donations for the building and formation of what now is the Cotuit Library. Dr. Coolidge died in 1912 at the age of 81.[31]

African American Medal of Honor recipient Robert A. Pinn would return to Massillon, Ohio, to work as a contractor and teamster. After attending Oberlin College, he became principal of Cairo High School in South Carolina. He later returned to Massillon, married Emily J. Manzilla, and became a lawyer. Robert and Emily had one child, Gracie. Pinn died on January 5, 1911, at the age of 67. In his honor, the shooting range at the University of Akron, used by the ROTC and the school's NCAA rifle team, was renamed in 1998 and is now known as the Robert A. Pinn Shooting Range.[32]

After the war, a Confederate soldier released from Lovell General Hospital never returned to Southern soil, or so the story goes. A citizen from Newport, James Masterson, reminisced that he personally knew the man. Initially, the pardoned Confederate lived in Newport but later settled in Jamestown, just across the bay.[33] Perhaps the Confederate veteran admired the climate and the area. On the other hand, he may have latched onto one of Newport's attractive socialites, fallen in love, and lived happily ever after.

Another Confederate prisoner described by a newspaper correspondent as "a pitiable case" because of an appalling wound to his jaw (see Chapter 5), most likely is the same unfortunate soldier mentioned here. Peyton S. Rhyne, an illiterate private with Co. H, 37th North Carolina Infantry (Gaston Blues), was shot through the jaw, tongue, and left check at Hanover Courthouse on May 27, 1862. Soon after his capture, he was placed along with 60 to 70 other prisoners on one of two army hospital transports destined for Portsmouth Grove. In spite of ghastly wounds, Rhyne managed to survive on the sweltering deck of a jam-packed steamer and, later, confinement at the makeshift hospital prison that was no more than a group of tents cordoned off from the rest of the hospital population. After nearly three months, he was exchanged and sent south where he continued to be treated at Confederate hospitals. Grotesquely disfigured for life, his facial abnormality made the simple acts of eating and speaking abominably difficult. Adding to his woes, Rhyne lost one of two brothers, Alfred, in a battle at Ox Hill, Virginia. All was not bleak; he married Elvira A. Shumaker and fathered four children. Later, in 1901, he applied for and was granted a small Confederate disability pension. When one of his sons asked him about his injury, Rhyne told him that he credited his survival to the maggot infestation in his jaw that ate away the dead skin while lying on the ground for several days (see Chapter 2 about the spontaneous recovery for gangrene). Continuing to work as a farmer near Gastonia, North Carolina, Rhyne managed to outlive a number of his comrades before passing away in 1908 at the age of 71. Today, many of his descendants still reside in the area.[34]

Duncan McEachern, who lost his toes to frostbite before ever seeing the enemy except as a convalescent prisoner at Lovell General Hospital, joined family members who previously migrated to Grassdale-Digby, district of Victoria, Australia. For the remaining 22 years of his life, he remained a loner. After obtaining a disability pension, he received notice in 1893 that the pension would be revoked because he was no longer a citizen of the United States. After fighting the revocation, he succeeded in having the pension reinstated. Though he was no longer a citizen of the United States, he was entitled to a pension because of his service-connected disability, a fact he brought to the attention of the

Pension Office. Duncan received $12 a month until November 26, 1913, when he died. His remains rest at Hotspur Cemetery in Victoria.[35]

For many, pensions or increases in existing pensions did not come easily. Samuel Wilson II, not mentioned earlier, was a patient at Portsmouth Grove from September 1, 1862, until his discharge in Providence on December 8, 1862. He had served as a private in Company B, 91st Pennsylvania Infantry. Wilson sustained several injuries and illnesses while in the service, including saber cuts inflicted by a fellow soldier after he refused to run after a prisoner who attempted to avoid custody, a left hip injury from a fall, intermittent fever and debility, chronic bronchitis, ascites (serious fluid buildup in the abdominal cavity), and nephritis (kidney inflammation). Wilson was finally granted an increase in his pension for the left hip injury, but only after fighting for it over several years. The pension review board concluded its findings by stating, "The claimant is shown to be an object of charity, and in the opinion of your committee entitled to relief asked for."[36]

A gentleman named William R. Cooper had been wounded in his side on May 3, 1863, and spent over a year at Portsmouth Grove on two separate occasions before returning to his unit in the field. He remained with Co. E, 25th Pennsylvania Infantry until his term of enlistment had expired, at which time he was discharged in Philadelphia on January 6, 1865. He is mentioned here because he, as so many others who ended up in general hospitals in the North, was erroneously listed as a deserter. Cooper's military records were later cleared after his wife Hannah lobbied to have the charges removed. Many soldiers during the war who never deserted also had the unwarranted blemish on their military records. They were victims of erroneous assumptions by company commanders or poor record-keeping by clerks interested in an expedient reconciliation of the numbers. From May 1885 on, Cooper spent his remaining years living at the National Home for Disabled Volunteer Soldiers. His pension totaled $4.00 per month. Upon his death, Hannah applied for and was successful in obtaining a widow's pension.[37]

Hugh Finnegan was one of the luckier veterans, at least as far as pensions go. He filed for his shortly after discharge. With his noticeable disfigurement and partial right arm paralysis from a gunshot wound to the head while fighting at Petersburg, he was listed as two-thirds disabled and granted a pension on Certificate No. 54,802. Finnegan found some work after the war as a common laborer at a print works in the town where he resided and probably remained a mill worker for the remainder of his life. At the time of his death in 1895, Finnegan was receiving a $16 a month pension. Today, several of his descendants live and work on Aquidneck Island.[38]

Isaiah Stauffacher, another soldier not previously mentioned, also had ties to Portsmouth Grove. Like many soldiers during the war, Stauffacher was born in a foreign land (Switzerland). When he mustered into the service at the age of 19 for a three-year enlistment in Co. B, 31st Regiment Wisconsin Volunteers, he left behind eight brothers and sisters and his family's farm of 300 acres. Stauffacher took part in several campaigns during the war, but from the middle of June 1864 until his discharge on July 15, 1865, he spent considerable time in and out of hospitals, the last of which was Lovell. After the war he returned to Wisconsin. Today several of his descendants live on Aquidneck Island.[39]

The road to freedom for Edward Jonathan Hoyt ("Buckskin Joe") after deserting the hospital became a long and arduous journey. Running some two miles north along the railroad track that passed along the hospital's eastern perimeter, he swam across Narragansett Bay under the less-than-watchful eye of a bridge attendant standing above. Staying in shanties and safe-houses during most of his journey, and an occasional hotel in larger cities until his funds were depleted, he constantly felt the presence of military agents searching for deserters. Over the next several weeks he traversed the rugged New England countryside of Massachusetts, New Hampshire, and Vermont. Eventually he reached Canada and the safe confines of his family home, but not before confronting a military agent at the border. A standoff resulted that ended in Hoyt's escape. He had been gone for over four years, and his younger brother did not recognize him, though his mother did. "She threw her arms around me and wept. A loving mother always knows her own child," Hoyt reminisced.[40]

As many men did during the Civil War, Hoyt reenlisted as a substitute, and was paid handsomely after joining the ranks of the 98th Pennsylvania Infantry. Though deserting from the hospital, he was not a quitter, and his bravery in skirmishes was never in doubt either before or after his departure from Portsmouth Grove.

After the war, the rest of his life was nothing less than a wild and exciting ride filled with one adventure after another. His credits include: hunter and trapper; scout; frontiersman; musician; circus performer (tumbler and aerialist); silk smuggler; Indian fighter; silver and gold prospector; and showman for Pawnee Bill's Historical Wild West Exhibition before starting his own ensemble, aptly named Buckskin Joe's Wild West Show. Hoyt even served as a Deputy U.S. Marshal. Along the way, he managed to take a wife, Belle, and have three daughters; at one time or another, all performed in the family business as musicians. Interestingly, a Confederate soldier with whom Hoyt exchanged shots during the Civil War became his close friend after they met again on more friendly terms while prospecting for silver. His name was William Palmer, better known in the late nineteenth century under the daunting nickname, "Butcher-knife Bill."

Buckskin Joe died in 1918 at the age of 78. His legacy of unpredictable and daring exploits continues to entertain readers of Wild West adventures to this day.[41]

On May 14, 1863, Oliver Ricker would get his wish to be discharged because of chronic hip and back ailments. Sent to Providence, he would muster out of the service on May 20. Before returning home to Lawrence, Massachusetts, to see his wife Sophia, he went to Boston and visited with his family. They were "all well and glad to see me," he said. "I now consider myself a free man once more and glad I am for it," he continued.[42] Not long afterward, he and his brother went shopping for clothing in the city, buying a coat, pants, vest, and hat, which cost him $20.37. He was now able to cast off his military attire. A happy man, Oliver Ricker had $86.42 of back pay to play with.[43]

Another lucky soldier was William Dennett. On January 16, 1863, he would be discharged on a surgeon's Certificate of Disability noting his condition as "neuralgia and general nervous derangement." He, too, would visit his brother in the Boston area (Charlestown) before returning home to Saco, Maine, and his beloved Olive.[44]

John Austin's condition eventually improved. He was discharged from the hospital and not long afterward commissioned a second lieutenant on September 9, 1863, as part of the Fifth Brigade.[45] He survived the war and returned home to his wife, Emily, in Ashland, a hamlet in the town of Scituate, Rhode Island. As a souvenir of the war, John brought home the round that struck him in the head, saying, "I am going to keep it to remember them [the Confederates] by."[46]

Twice married, Private Seth C. Vickery was discharged from Lovell General Hospital on a surgeon's Certificate of Disability on March 14, 1863. He would marry a third time to Wareham, Massachusetts, resident Emma Frances Badger on October 6, 1880. She was nineteen; he was fifty-four. There is evidence that that marriage did not last, as four years later, almost to the day, Emma remarried. Seth continued working as a cobbler and was now the recipient of a $12-a-month pension. He passed away at the age of 77 on December 8, 1893, in the town where he was born. The death record listed Seth as married. Was it an erroneous entry, or did he make it to number four?[47]

George Peck, a member of the Hospital Guards—Rhode Island Volunteers and local resident from Bristol, Rhode Island, whose diary added immensely to understanding the inner workings of the hospital, would marry Hattie P. Coggeshall and raise a family. The couple was blessed with a son, Alfred, and a daughter, Gertrude (they had another daughter, Ella, but she died at an early age). For a short time, George worked as a machinist at the National India Rubber Company, as did most of the town. While engaged at the plant, he learned the boot-making trade, which he pursued for the next twenty years. In 1888, he served as Bristol's town treasurer and for a number of years ran for reelection unopposed under both party tickets. As a member and later commander of the Babbitt Post No. 15, Department of Rhode Island, Grand Army of the Republic (GAR), Peck was instrumental in the fund-raising and erection of the town's Civil War monument, an exquisite work of art that continues to be a head-turner to this day. Casual observers who walk or ride down Hope Street would have a difficult time not noticing the enormous boulder and bronze sculptures of the Soldiers' and Sailors' Monument, situated on the southwest corner near the Burnside Memorial Building. As a citizen, Peck also served as a director for several banks within the state as well as a trustee at his church and the town library. He died on September 8, 1914, in his 74th year, due to complications from several diseases. Peck's remains are interred in Bristol's North Burial Ground adjacent to Colt State Park along with another former Lovell General Hospital patient, George W. Simmons, a sergeant from Co. E, 12th Regiment Rhode Island Volunteers.[48] After Simmons was severely wounded in the left thigh at Fredericksburg, he was sent to Portsmouth Grove Hospital to recover. He did get better, but not enough to remain in the service, and on March 5, 1863, he was discharged on a Surgeon's Certificate. After the war Simmons became an undertaker and a politician, serving as a state senator. Hailing from a small community, Peck and Simmons were well acquainted, as both men were members of the Bristol Train of Artillery. Honorable George W. Simmons died on May 6, 1905.[49]

In the neighboring community of Warren, Alfred Luther, the soldier who lost his arm at Gaines' Mill and became a prisoner of war, settled in as a farmer with support from his family and an $8-a-month government pension he was granted, retroactive to October 25, 1862.[50] In late May 1864, he was fitted with an artificial right arm, but found it discomforting and not much of an aid. Eventually he stopped wearing the device.[51] If Alfred felt odd walking around Warren with loss of limb, he must have felt mutual camaraderie with John Butterworth from the same community, who also lost an arm. Butterworth serving with Battery F, First Rhode Island Light Artillery at Whitehall, North Carolina, was wounded in action on December 16, 1862. His arm was amputated shortly thereafter.[52]

In the 1880s, Alfred Luther became a member of the Richard F. Tobin, Post 24,

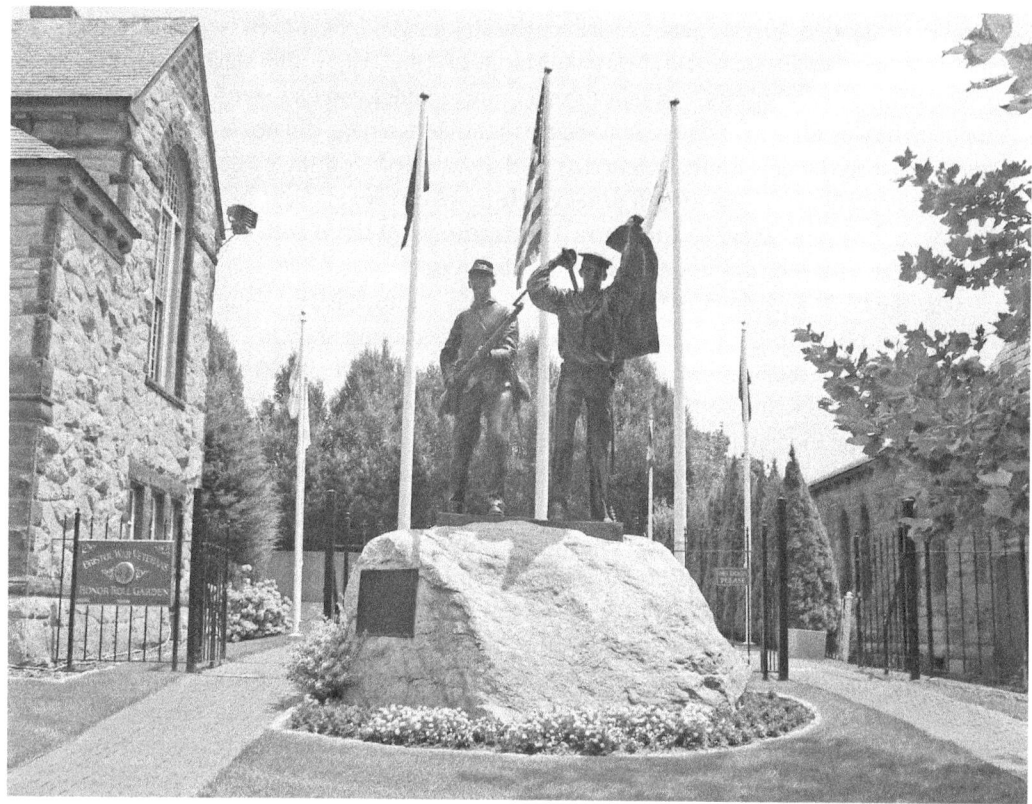

The Soldiers' and Sailors' Monument in Bristol, Rhode Island, was the brainchild of Commander George H. Peck of the Department of Rhode Island, GAR, Babbitt Post No. 15 (photograph by the author).

Department of Rhode Island, GAR and probably took part in their civic and patriotic activities.[53] By 1891, Alfred's pension had increased to $30 a month. With failing health, he was declared legally blind, each eye badly diseased and one with optic nerve damage. Doctors also diagnosed deafness caused by artillery fire during the war, along with severe bowel problems and bleeding hemorrhoids that were attributed to exposure and the intake of poor water and food during his prison confinement. Occasionally, Alfred suffered relapses of malaria, also contracted while serving his country. His physical condition continued to deteriorate until he could no longer care for himself.[54] In early October of 1899, Alfred fell gravely ill at the home of his nephew, Lewis M. Luther. After suffering for 10 days, most of which he spent in a coma, he succumbed to apoplexy. Alfred was 67 years old. His remains lie in Warren's South Burial Ground.[55]

Whitman W. Bosworth enlisted as a corporal on April 20, 1861, but was promoted to sergeant before his capture at Ball's Bluff, Virginia, and imprisonment at Richmond. After an exchange and having survived the terrifying ordeal, he processed through the army hospital system, eventually arriving at Portsmouth Grove. Soldiers' veteran records show he was discharged on August 6, 1864. Returning to his residence in Webster, Massachusetts, he resumed his trade as a house painter. On January 9, 1867, Whitman married Elizabeth and raised a family. They had four children, but sketchy accounts indicate some may not have lived into adulthood. Elizabeth predeceased her husband. Whitman died in 1912 at the age of 72 and is interred at the North Ashford Cemetery, Eastford, Connecticut, a small rural community near the Massachusetts border where he was born and spent most of his youth.[56]

John Lovejoy spent more time in a hospital after his discharge from Portsmouth Grove, but this time for a wound and not an illness. He had been shot in the left ankle by a Minié ball during a skirmish on August 22, 1864, near Charlestown, West Virginia.[57] Lovejoy was taken to the U.S. Army General Hospital, McKim's Mansion in Baltimore, Maryland, for recovery. The wound was minor, with only a slight fracture of the left ankle bone, though it did become inflamed during his trip to the hospital and later caused him substantial pain. In mid-September, Lovejoy was transferred to the U.S. Army Hospital in Chestnut Hill in Philadelphia, Pennsylvania. By the end of September, the exit wound was still drawing pus and doctors had to apply flaxseed poultice to the infected area. Upon recovery, Lovejoy was assigned to the Veteran Reserve Corps and found himself at Headquarters, Co. C, 2nd Regiment now stationed in Columbus, Indiana. After receiving a clean bill of health from the doctors, Lovejoy was transferred back to his regiment in the field. On Sunday evening, Christmas Day, he found himself performing picket duty in Petersburg, Virginia. While taking part in occasional skirmishes, his regiment made their way to Burkes Junction, Virginia. By mid–April, news had arrived of President Abraham Lincoln's assassination and the imminent end of the war.[58]

John Lovejoy managed to survive the conflict, along with his brother Allen, who "spent much of his military life in a hospital or on detached leave in Indiana."[59] Both men would eventually attain the rank of corporal.[60]

A year-and-a-half earlier, Lovejoy said to his cousin Cynthia, "I receive regularly one letter a week from Jonathan. The last news I had from him, he was well with the exception of a boil on his neck, under the ear. I am thankful that his health is as good as it is and I hope it will continue so, for I know how to sympathize with a sick soldier. It is no desirable job to be sick in the army. I hope I may have the privilege of meeting him once again on Ostego soil."[61] It was not meant to be. Jonathan, who had enlisted in the 152nd, would die a short time after arriving home from a military hospital.[62] Still in the army as of July 2, 1865, John Lovejoy found himself wearing his military uniform and "yet a soldier." The good news was that he and his regiment had arrived in Albany, New York, awaiting orders to muster out of the service. In a letter to his "Dearest Cousin 'C,'" he said, "I will send you a relic of the war in this letter one which I prize. A stan[dard] from the flag which I have fought under since we last met." When describing the regimental flag, he said "[it] is all in rags, torn by bullets and by constant exposure to the weather."[63]

In the beginning, John Lovejoy's opening salutation of letters written to his cousin Cynthia back home in upstate New York said unpretentiously, "Dear Cousin," but a short while after arriving at Portsmouth Grove it had changed to "My Dear Cousin Cynthia." In his final letter home from his home state to Cynthia he closed with, "Your affectionate cousin and true friend ever. Yours truly, John M. to Cynthia Allen."[64] After writing copious letters to her during his entire term of enlistment, he finally mustered the courage to tell her how he felt, though no known letters exist to confirm this assumption. It was a love solidified over time and distance through the mail that had perhaps flickered before Lovejoy went off to war.[65]

John M. Lovejoy and Cynthia A. Allen became Mr. and Mrs. Lovejoy soon after the war. Upon arrival of their firstborn, a boy, John and Cynthia named him Upton in tribute to John's highly respected regimental commander Emory Upton.[66] A deeply religious man, John was a staunch Republican and Abraham Lincoln supporter in the 1864 presidential election. After the war, he became an avid GAR member, a secretary and treasurer of the

> "Lovell" General Hospital, U. S. A.,
> PORTSMOUTH GROVE, R. I.
> Dec. 31st 1864
>
> Sir:
>
> I would respectfully inform you that the following named men of your command are at present patients in this Hospital, admitted by proper authority. They will return to their Regiment as soon as they are "fit for field service." Should any of the within named die, be discharged, transferred to Veteran Reserve Corps, &c., you will be immediately notified.
>
> In obedience to Par. 1236, Revised Army Regulations, 1863, you will please forward their Descriptive Lists.
>
> Corpl. James L. Watson
>
> I have the honor to be,
> Your Ob't Servant.
> Chas. O'Leary
> Surgeon U. S. V., in charge.
>
> To the Commanding Officer
> Co. K 142 Reg't N. Y. Vols.

Without a hospital commander's letter such as this, soldiers could be carried indefinitely on regimental rolls as deserters (State of Rhode Island and Providence Plantations, Office of the Secretary of State, Archives Division, Providence, Rhode Island).

121st Regimental Association, and a veterans' advocate.[67] Before his death, John had been ill for several years; his most recent sickness lasted 10 days. He was 57 years old when he passed away in his hometown of Roseboom, New York, on May 24, 1900. John's wife Cynthia would follow eight years later and be laid at her husband's side. John's newspaper obituary concluded with the fitting remark, "We believe that God whom he so faithfully served has crowned him victor and that he is *mustered* in the Grand Army above, where all is peace."[68]

Allen Lovejoy survived his brother John. The two had been inseparable throughout the war while serving under the same regiment and later while recovering together in two military hospitals (Fairfax Seminary and Portsmouth Grove), but bad blood developed between their mother and Allen's wife. Allen subsequently moved to Gloversville, away from his original homestead. Little is known about the cause of the dispute and the remainder of Allen's life is shrouded in mystery.[69]

Blind for the balance of his earthly existence, veteran John M. Shelow returned to his home in Tyrone, Pennsylvania, but not after spending June through August of 1864 at Lovell General Hospital and at Satterlee General Hospital in Philadelphia until war's end. The *Medical and Surgical History of the War of the Rebellion (1861–1865)* states that Shelow was fitted with artificial eyes. Several years after the war, he married Jane Benton, who proved to be "a faithful helpmate." They had no children. A deeply religious man, he continued as a patriot, joining other veterans from the community as a member of the Colonel D.M. Jones Post No. 172 Grand Army of the Republic. Considering his severe disability, Shelow managed to outlive the majority of his fellow wards from Portsmouth Grove. He died in 1920, four months shy of his 76th birthday, after a bout with shingles and other undisclosed illnesses. Survived by his wife, a sister, and a brother, he is buried in Grandview Cemetery, Tyrone, Pennsylvania.[70]

On August 18, 1864, at the Battle of Weldon Railroad, Adin B. Thayer, the soldier who would survive several hospital stays for a wound and different illnesses, would be captured a second time and sent to Salisbury Prison in North Carolina. During that same year, General Ulysses S. Grant stopped all prisoner exchanges. For Thayer, the policy proved disastrous. While imprisoned and with no hope of exchange, he became ill and before long succumbed to the ravages of chronic diarrhea on January 23, 1865, joining the ill-fated ranks of 44,558 Union soldiers who lost their lives to diarrhea or dysentery during the war.[71]

When Salisbury Prison inmates doubled from 5,000 to 10,000 in a short period, the Confederates had to contend with ever-increasing numbers of deaths each day, so much so that burial details could not keep up with the identifications. During 1864 and early 1865 in an abandoned cornfield, 18 trenches were dug, spanning some 240 feet, where an estimated 11,700 Union soldiers were laid to rest, one atop another, most without coffins. Even though the number of burials is disputed to this day, no person can argue that the estimate of nameless burials is appalling. Today, visitors can walk the grounds of Salisbury National Cemetery near the former site of the prison and view the burial trenches and the three stone monuments erected there — two from Pennsylvania and the other from Adin Thayer's home state of Maine. Salisbury Prison has the regrettable distinction of having one of the highest prison death rates during the war, and an even more appalling statistic: 99 percent (not a misprint) of the burials are anonymous.[72] Adin B. Thayer's remains lie in one of the 18 trenches, unidentified, as are most of the other forgotten souls.

On a more joyous note, the beloved "Lady Superintendent" of Lovell, Katherine Prescott Wormeley, recovered from her illness and continued her benevolent and tireless work with the U.S. Sanitary Commission. She would live a full life, passing away on August 4, 1908, in Jackson, New Hampshire, caused by complications from a fall on the front steps of her home at the age of 78. Her remains were cremated and later interred next to her husband in Island Cemetery, Newport, Rhode Island.

By war's end, the Connecticut Woolsey family had contributed a mother, seven sisters and one brother to the cause. All the ladies were nurses, while the lone brother, Charles, served in the regular army.[73] After years of service, the ladies found themselves in an all-too-familiar position: subservient females in a male-dominated society. As Georgeanna Woolsey describes her situation, she was "a woman with experience and management skills without a place to use them."[74] Her statement was not unfounded. After her stint at Portsmouth Grove, she gained valuable nursing experience at Gettysburg soon after the tumultuous battle. Georgeanna's sister, Jane, may have done better. Jane gave teaching a try, educating freed slaves at the Lincoln Industrial School in Richmond, and later worked at the Hampton Normal and Agricultural Institute teaching sewing and housework classes.[75] In 1872, she became the resident directress at New York Presbyterian Hospital but resigned her position because of ill health in 1876. Never fully recovered, she lived the next fifteen years with her sister Abby before passing away on July 9, 1891.[76]

Nurse Sarah C. Dennis became Mrs. Thomas H.B. Taylor. On October 27, 1866, a new addition would arrive, Frank S. Taylor. Remembered as popular and kindhearted, Sarah would be congratulated on this special occasion by friends who were fortunate to receive her benevolent care.[77] Upon the establishment of Newport Hospital in 1873 as a twelve-bed cottage hospital, Mrs. Taylor served as a matron.[78]

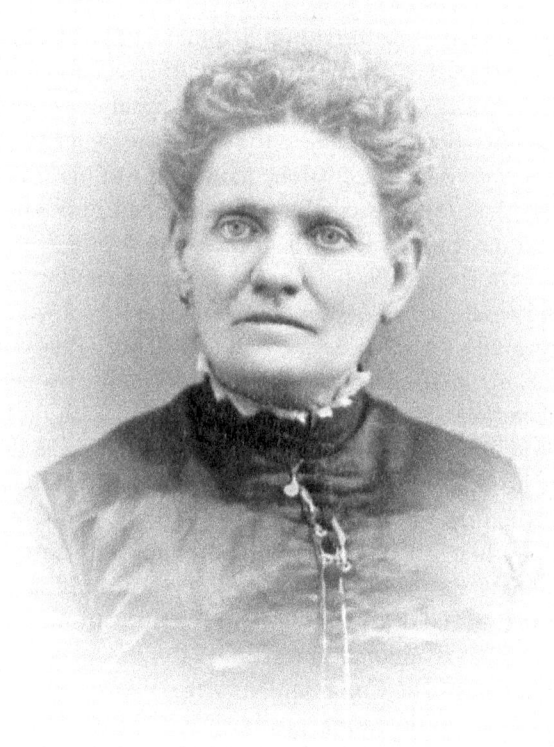

Sarah C. (Dennis) Taylor was a hardworking and well respected nurse at the hospital (courtesy Massachusetts Commandery Military Order of the Loyal Legion and the U.S. Army Military History Institute, Carlisle, Pennsylvania).

While at Portsmouth Grove, Nurse Agnes Wilbour met Private George H. Richardson, an accomplished carpenter by trade, from nearby Fairhaven, Massachusetts, assigned to Company F (later reorganized as Company B), 2nd Regiment Rhode Island Volunteers. He was a patient at the hospital, having arrived from the field on July 9, 1863, suffering from sunstroke. They would fall in love, marry, and raise a family of three children. During Mrs. Richardson's travels in Newport, she was said to be a popular figure. Respectfully addressed as Mrs. Richardson in public, she was affectionately called "Little Ma" by her immediate family. According to family history, George, a poet by avocation, managed to stay at the hospital until mustering out on July 7, 1865, perhaps because of his value as a craftsman, but nobody knows for certain. George is also credited for building the second story library, if not the entire second floor, of the Newport Historical Society. The husband and wife lived on Whitfield Street, less than a block from the institution. George died at the age of 78. Mrs. Richardson passed

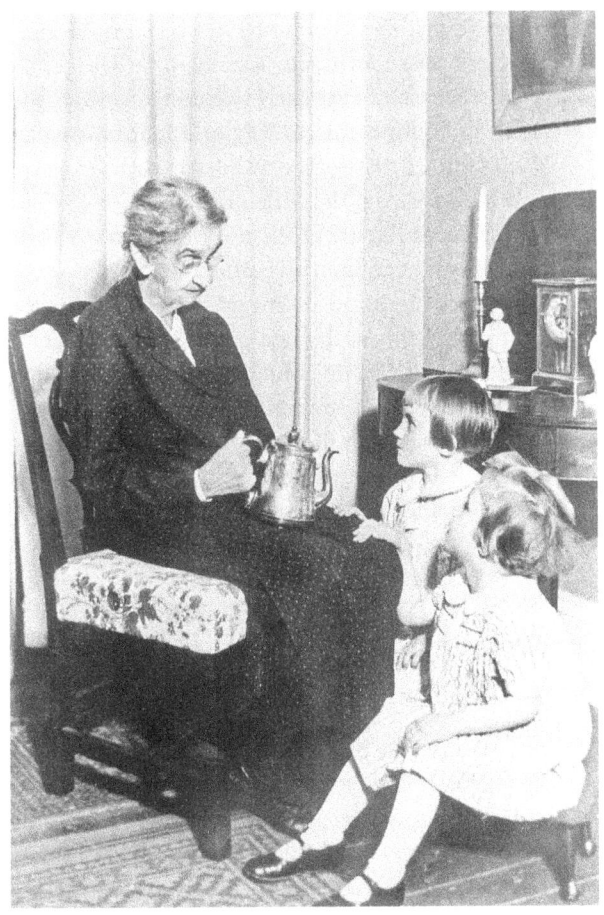

Agnes Wilbour Richardson, pictured here with her great-granddaughters. The teapot Mrs. Richardson is holding was presented to her by patients while she served as a nurse at the hospital. She was also given a watch (courtesy Ed Regan, descendant of Mrs. Richardson).

away in 1933 at the ripe old age of 94. Prior to her passing, she was purported to be the last surviving nurse from the hospital and one of the few nurses still alive who had served during the war. Today her descendants are scattered throughout the land, but some still reside on Aquidneck Island.[79]

Sixth-generation *Mayflower* descendant and adventuress Ada Brewster, who also served as a nurse at the hospital, blazed the trail as kind of a female Buckskin Joe. An accomplished artist, Ada traveled the country drawing and painting the people and locations of a quickly expanding America. Between war's end and 1867 she taught her craft at Baker University in Baldwin City, Kansas, and during the mid–1870s, she spent time working for the U.S. Mint in Carson City, Nevada, where, it was said, "she weighed the first trade dollar coined by the Federal government."[80] The remainder of her life was spent as a teacher, portrait artist, and illustrator living in San Francisco, California; New York City; Nantucket, Massachusetts; Tallulah Falls, Georgia; and St. Petersburg, Florida, before returning to her home in Kingston, Massachusetts.[81] Her love for hospitals and the care they gave continued, as evident by her membership in the Brockton Hospital Ladies' Aid Association in the early twentieth century; she contributed cookbook recipes to them for hospital fund-raisers.[82] Prior to her passing in 1929, she was one of a handful of surviving nurses that served at Portsmouth Grove.

Maud Howe, the little girl who with a friend stumbled upon what she believed to be a scene of torture at the hospital, was the youngest of four daughters and fifth of six children of the influential Samuel Gridley Howe family. Her father established the Perkins School for the Blind in Watertown, Massachusetts, and her mother, Julia Ward Howe, wrote the highly acclaimed poem "The Battle Hymn of the Republic" that later replaced the lyrics of the tune "John Brown's Body." Homeschooled and introduced early to Newport society, Miss Howe married English artist John Elliott in 1887. For a time, they lived in Italy. During her lifetime she wrote prolifically; her last book was published when she was 90. It is from this book, *This Was My Newport* (1944), that the torture account was extracted. In 1917 Mrs. Elliott and two of her sisters were awarded the first Pulitzer Prize for a biography: *The Life of Julia Ward Howe* (1916). She died in Newport in 1948, just shy of her 94th birthday.

As for Portsmouth Grove Hospital's first commanding officer, Dr. Francis L. Wheaton, whether he ever set foot in Newport again after his retirement from the military is a subject of conjecture. If he did, it must have been incognito. In and around Providence, however, he was known as a prominent citizen. An unsubstantiated account states Dr. Wheaton spent his post-military years at Brown University, but if he did, his legacy is invisible. Neither the John Hay Library at Brown University nor the Rhode Island Historical Society has an image or details about his life after the war. One hundred fifty years later, after assessing his brief command at Portsmouth Grove, it is difficult to ascertain whether he deserved the condemnation he received from Aquidneck Islanders. The entire military hospital scene during the early years of the war was chaotic, and Portsmouth Grove Hospital's disorganized establishment was not much different from other hospital startups at the time.[83] To place the entire blame on one man's shoulders is, perhaps, unreasonable and unjust. Even those present at the time found it "difficult to determine [to] how much credit such stories are entitled."[84] One such story, printed some 36 years later and taken from a conversation of August 1862, asserts that a Robert Coggeshall met Dr. Wheaton and didn't like him from the start. Mr. Coggeshall found Dr. Wheaton to be a "brute, and ... not fit to be here." As an indirect slap in the face, Mr. Coggeshall said, "He thinks the liquor or brandy he drinks, if given to the weak soldiers would be better all around and many others think the same."[85]

Interesting to note, during Dr. Wheaton's brief tenure at Portsmouth Grove, many of his subordinates from Yorktown and later from the hospital came to his aid, several writing letters explaining his circumstances using words like "difficult," "trying," and even "peculiar." All three seemed appropriate. Dr. Wheaton passed away at the age of 92 on December 26, 1895, at his residence in Providence. His death was attributed to hardening of the arteries and old age.[86] Was he a victim or a villain? We may never know. But in a belated letter written two months after Dr. Wheaton's departure from Portsmouth Grove, the writer may have hit a vital nerve when he said, "It is easier to see the flaws and defects in a machine of such large proportions, than to run the machine ourselves."[87]

14. War's End 151

Benjamin J. Tilley's health failed shortly after the war. His childhood malady, along with frequent visits to the hospital, negatively affected his health. Suffering for more than six months with illness, he died on July 31, 1866, at the age of 45. In his obituary, the *Newport Mercury* described him as "a man of modest and unassuming demeanor, always as gentle as a child, of sterling good sense and apparently freer from vice than almost any person whom we know." His funeral was held at the Zion Episcopal Church (now Jane Pickens Theater at Washington Square in Newport), and his remains were conveyed for burial by the Masons, the Sons of Temperance, his family and friends, and a large crowd of mourners.[88] His wife, Mary G., would live another 45 years before passing away in 1911. Their remains lie side-by-side at Island Cemetery in Newport, the same grounds where Katherine Wormeley rests. The people of Aquidneck Island, and the soldiers Benjamin befriended as they convalesced, not only lost a fellow citizen, but more importantly an island treasure.

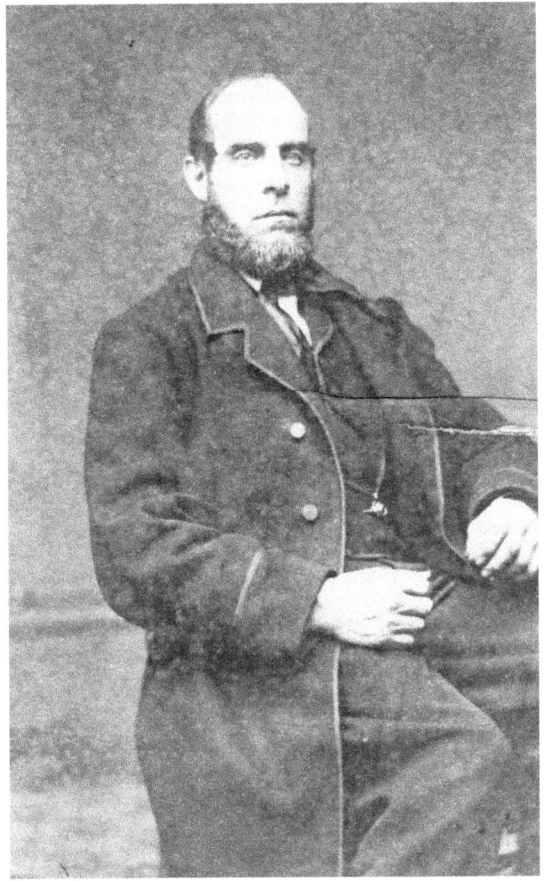

Benjamin J. Tilley: a soldier's friend to the end. Less than a year after his charitable work ended in August of 1865, Tilley passed away, his death accelerated perhaps by a childhood illness and his unrelenting dedication to patients at the hospital (courtesy Dr. Stephen Altic, D.O.; from his collection).

After a stint as commander of the U.S. General Hospital in Cleveland, Ohio, Dr. George Miller Sternberg would go on to serve as surgeon general of the U.S. Army. During his nine-year tenure, he helped establish the Army Medical School. Dr. Sternberg was also credited with discovering the microorganism that caused pneumonia, and he later contributed to the diagnosis and treatment of the illness. Dr. Sternberg was cited for developing ambulance services and many battlefield treatments that are still in existence today. He was also an early pioneer in bacteriology and a one-time president of the American Medical Association. Retiring as a brigadier general after serving in three wars, Dr. Sternberg received an honorary LL.D. from the University of Michigan (1894) and Brown University in Providence, Rhode Island (1897). After achieving a distinguished civilian medical career, he died at the age of 77. His remains and those of his wife, Martha, rest together at Arlington National Cemetery.[89]

Lovell's fifty-eight buildings, furnishings and medical supplies were put to auction.[90] The government made it known that the buildings would not be "sacrificed." If fair prices were not obtained, officials said the structures would remain as is, "to be used, if necessary, for the assembling of cholera patients."[91] The auction was a success, perhaps not as resounding as the government intended, but still raising about $22,000 for the U.S. Treasury.[92] John N.A. Griswold, Esq., purchased the engine and works with the intention of shipping them south. One structure remained on the premises for a while and was later used as a pest house for smallpox victims; others were transported up Narragansett Bay by barge to the coal mines at the northern end of the island. A pig farmer was a beneficiary of another building.[93]

On July 29, 1865, Edmund and Olive M. Cole sold the former hospital grounds to Governor William Sprague of Rhode Island through the agency of Doyle and Dike of Newport. The selling price was $25,000 with a deposit of $11,000 and a mortgage for the balance. The property was then conveyed to Byron Sprague, a relative and real estate investor, who held it for many years.[94]

In late 1865, with a growing family, Herbert Ashley of Portsmouth wanted a larger house. After the hospital closed, Mr. Ashley went to the auction four miles from his home and successfully procured either lumber from a torn-down structure or an intact building—reports are contradictory about his purchase. If it was a small building, it could have been carted away along dirt roads or moved up river by oxen after the bay froze. The Brownell/Ashley/Grant House, originally constructed c. 1750, was the recipient of the acquisition. Today, the late–1860s renovation encompasses a kitchen designed with an early American flair. Because the addition was built directly on stones, insect infestation was inevitable. Over the past decade, the wide floorboards had to be replaced. Some boards were salvaged and used to replace a sagging section of floor in an upstairs bedroom; remaining lumber was salvaged and kept in the adjacent barn in case future repairs are necessary. The ceiling posts and beams were also replaced because of structural weakness. The addition measures roughly 13 feet long by 14 ½

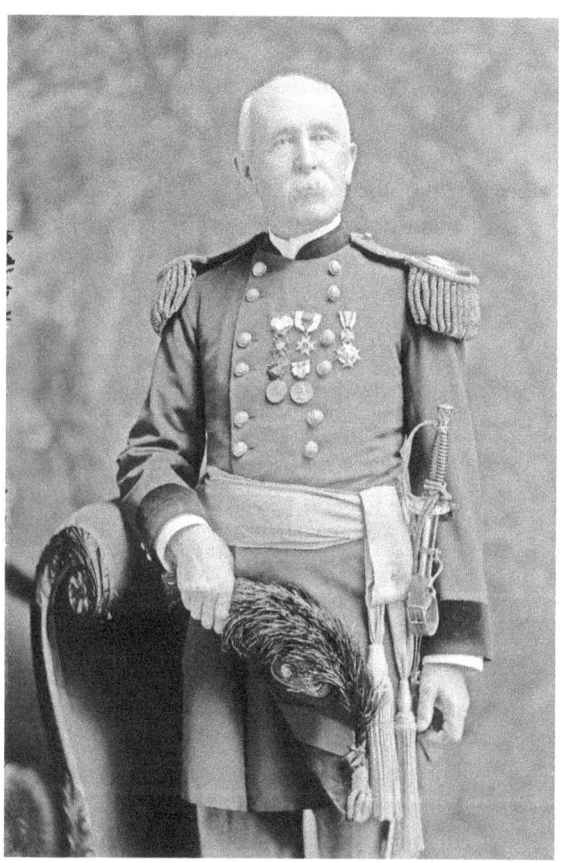

As a young lieutenant, Dr. George Miller Sternberg came to Portsmouth Grove Hospital suffering from typhoid fever. Upon his recovery, he served as a highly capable surgeon. Years after the war, he was extended the honorary title "Father of American Bacteriology." Dr. Sternberg retired from active duty as a brigadier general after serving as the 18th U.S. Army Surgeon General (Arlington National Cemetery).

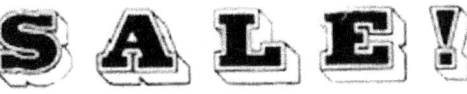

GOVERNMENT SALE!

LARGE SALE OF MEDICAL AND HOSPITAL PROPERTY.

In accordance with instructions from the U. S. Medical Purveyor, there will be sold at the "LOVELL" U. S. General Hospital, Portsmouth Grove, R. I., on

Thursday, Sept. 28th, 1865,
AT 9 O'CLOCK A. M.,

The following named articles of Medical and Hospital property, viz:

All the Bedsteads, Bedding, Hospital Clothing, Furniture, Books, Instruments, Medicines and appliances of whatever character, now remaining at said Hospital.

1,900 Iron Bedsteads, 2,000 Linen Sheets, 6,000 Cotton Sheets, 5,000 Pillow Cases, 5,800 Blankets, 2,300 Counterpanes, 2,600 Bed Sacks, 1,600 Pillows---hair, 100 Mattresses---Hair, 2,000 Cotton Drawers and Shirts, 3,000 Towels, 100 Quilts, Dressing Gowns, Socks, etc., a large and complete supply of standard Drugs and Medicines, a large supply of excellent Surgical Instruments, Dressings and appliances.

Also, a large lot of Furniture, Cooking Utensils, Crockery, Lamps, Fixtures, etc.

☞ Sale unconditional and without reserve. Terms Cash, in Government Funds.

The Sale will be continued from day to day, until all is sold.

W. F. EDGAR, Surgeon U. S. A.
WM. MASON, Auctioneer.

PORTSMOUTH GROVE, R. I., September 20, 1865.

Knowles, Anthony & Co., Printers, No. 5 Washington Buildings, Providence.

Since there was no reason to maintain the grounds after the war, an auction was held to sell the hospital buildings and furnishings (courtesy Portsmouth Historical Society, Portsmouth, Rhode Island).

feet wide by 12½ feet high, and is the only known structure with written provenance that can be traced directly to the hospital.[95] The house is also reputed to have a spirit. The present owners have not seen the apparition and neither subscribe to nor deny the spectral existence. Could a Civil War soldier from the hospital at Portsmouth Grove be lurking within?

Less than a half mile east of the Ashley House is another structure said to have been moved by barge from Portsmouth Grove after the hospital closed its doors. The austere design and construction fit perfectly with the image of a Civil War–era hospital building. When the building is compared to more contemporary designs, its beauty rests in its absolute simplicity. Unfortunately, no written documents have surfaced to support the family legacy that this building was part of the original Portsmouth Grove complex. The well-maintained structure is currently a private residence.[96]

Having served its useful purpose, the Portsmouth Grove Post Office was subsequently disbanded. Today, envelopes postmarked from defunct post offices like Portsmouth Grove sell at auction and are considered highly desirable items by postal history collectors.

Even the steamer *Perry* that carried passengers up and down Narragansett Bay for decades and helped to unload patients from government steamers—the vessel pictured in a J.P. Newell's lithograph of Lovell General Hospital—would take its last passenger excursion along Narragansett Bay. As reported: "A name for reliability ... has been sold to parties in New York, and ... taken thither."[97]

Soon all that remained was the cemetery. That, too, would disappear three years after the war. Of the 308 reported burials, 9 were removed by family and friends, leaving 299 remains (292 identified as military, 4 unknowns most likely military, and 3 civilians).[98] With good intentions, the federal government requested that the state maintain the cemetery. Gov. James Smith was to ask the next session of the General Assembly to pass the necessary legislation to authorize funds to maintain the grounds, yet nothing happened. Knowing that several hospital cemeteries were scattered throughout the northeast and making little progress with state officials, the federal government decided to consolidate several hospital cemeteries at a single location. Previous accounts in the mid-twentieth century erroneously listed Arlington National Cemetery as the new burial site, all because of the failed memory of an elderly citizen who visited Portsmouth Grove as a child shortly after the war. Starting in May 1868, soldiers were exhumed and reburied at the Cypress Hills National Cemetery, Section 1B, in Brooklyn, New York, in a three-acre section that came to be known as the "Union Grounds." (For a list of burials see Appendix B; for a map of the site see Appendix C.) Originally, this location was a private cemetery; the government purchased it to rebury Civil War soldiers who died at various military hospitals in the North. By September 1870, 3,170 Union and 461 Confederate soldiers would be at rest on the premises.[99] Today, there is no permanent administrative staff at the site; however, locating gravesites that are listed in Appendix B, Roll of Honor, is relatively easy.

Should you visit the pastoral setting of Cypress Hills National Cemetery, walk to plot 3300 and pay your respects to Private David Miller, Company I, 102nd Pennsylvania Infantry who endeared himself to several wartime correspondents before passing away at the age of 61 on July 17, 1862, only a few weeks after his arrival at Portsmouth Grove. Also visit nearby plot 3333 and behold the grave of Private John Robinson, Company F,

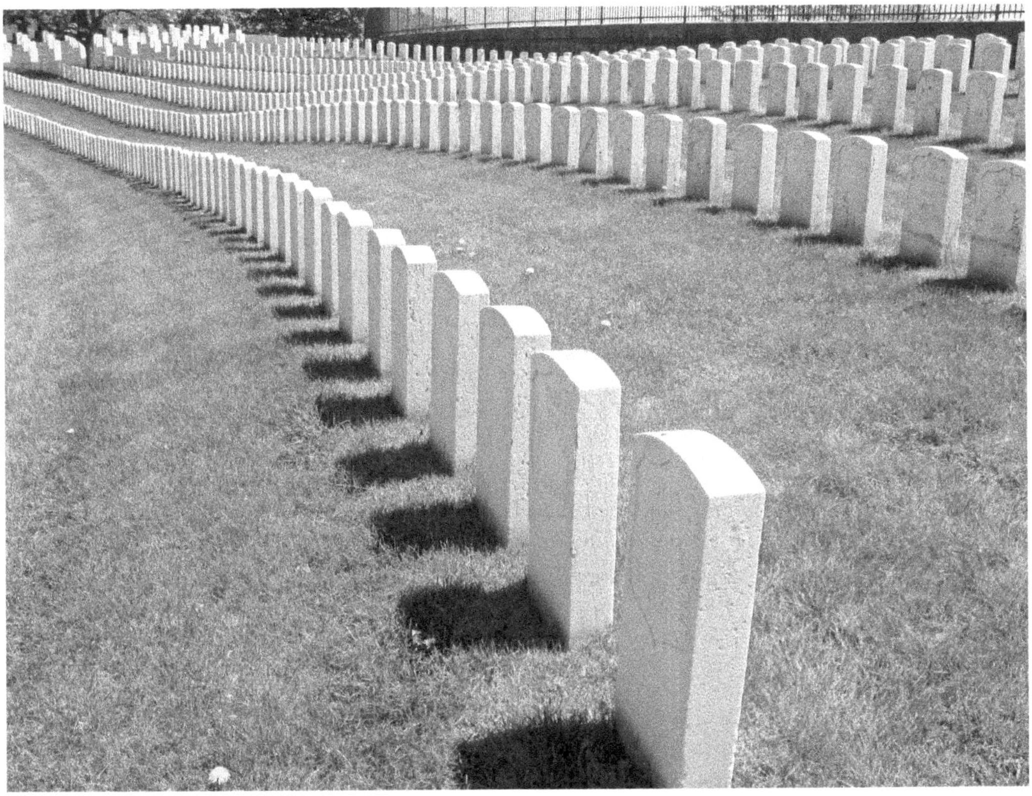

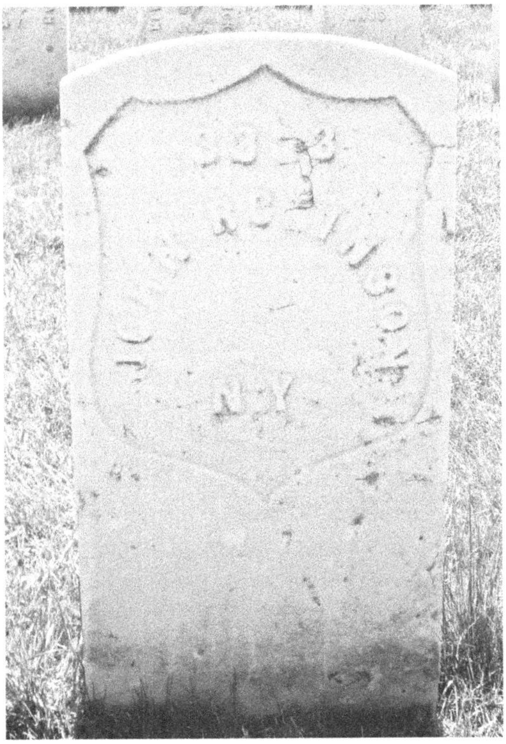

Top: Cypress Hills National Cemetery, Union Grounds, Section 1B serves as the final resting place for nearly 300 soldiers and a few civilians originally interred at Portsmouth Grove's Burial Yard (courtesy Ken Garthee). *Bottom:* A soldier rests in peace: the gravesite of Private John Robinson. Inscribed by a close friend on a wooden marker at the hospital's original burial yard were the words, "He never turned his back on the enemy or on a friend" (courtesy Ken Garthee).

88th New York Infantry, the man who was among the first to die at the hospital. A friend inscribed on his initial wooden grave marker, "He never turned his back on an enemy or on a friend"—understandably, but still unfortunately, national cemeteries will not allow additional inscriptions on grave markers. Resting in plot 3497 are the remains of Private James Doran, Company K, 8th Michigan Volunteer Infantry. Three months after enlistment, he was wounded at the Wilderness in Virginia and died on

October 21, 1864, at Lovell General Hospital from disease contracted while in the field. Doran was barely 20 years old and only eight months into his enlistment before meeting his Maker. Not to be forgotten is Corporal William A. Armstrong, Company B, 31st Regiment Maine Volunteer Infantry who appeared on the road to recovery but succumbed to infection not long after a secondary amputation was performed on what remained of his arm. Corporal Armstrong now rests in peace at plot 3519.

Today Cypress Hills Cemetery, which includes the national cemetery and the Union Grounds, encompasses roughly eighteen acres on the boundary of Kings and Queens Counties. Over the years the cemetery has accommodated the remains of soldiers who fought in the American Revolution, the Spanish-American War, Korea, Vietnam, and other national conflicts. Twenty-four Medal of Honor recipients consecrate the Brooklyn soil — a meticulously maintained cemetery in a surprisingly bucolic setting within the city. The hallowed ground of Cypress Hills National Cemetery is a glorious place and affords an ideal setting for visitors to pay their respects to American servicemen.[100]

And what about the nine remains claimed by family and friends? To date, two gravesites have been found: those of Private Samuel S. Whiting and Corporal Walter H. Sawtell. Whiting, as noted in a previous chapter, is buried at First Cemetery, in East Greenwich, Rhode Island. Sawtell, who fought with the 25th Regiment Massachusetts Volunteer Infantry, survived but ten weeks after arriving at Portsmouth Grove. He succumbed to wounds received at Drewry's Bluff, Virginia, and his remains lie at Woodside Cemetery in Westminster, Massachusetts.

Those buried at Portsmouth Grove accounted for only the unfortunates who died on the premises. There were others on furlough from the hospital who passed away, such as Private William B. Heath, who was taken ill in the field and sent to Portsmouth Grove in July 1862. Heath's father came to the hospital in September and took his son home to Delaware County, Indiana, only to see him die within a week.[101] How many more on furlough would meet a similar fate? Ten? Twenty? Fifty? The answer may never be known.

At first, battlefield deaths were recorded as "killed" or "died of wounds." It wasn't long before the War Department realized that more needed to be done for families of the deceased to assist with identifying remains. Clearly marked burial sites with memorial tablets was the first solution, followed by regulations that required the preparation of a detailed Record of Death and Interment card "for every soldier who dies in the military hospital, or in the field, where his body can be recognized."[102] Because of the sheer number of battlefield deaths, the regulation was difficult to implement in the field, but in general hospitals the regulation was followed to the letter. Three copies of the form were required: copy 1 was kept at the hospital or by the attending surgeon; copy 2 was sent to the adjutant general in Washington, D.C.; and copy 3 went to the sexton or quartermaster.[103] At Portsmouth Grove, a comprehensive register of interments was kept; however, the listing includes a multitude of surname spelling errors and some with incorrect regiment and battery information. Appendix B is included as a corrected version.

The Rev. George W. Chevers, who conducted the ceremonies at the initial burials during a chaotic time at Portsmouth Grove, by his own estimate presided over half the burials at the hospital cemetery for the next two and a half years. The Rev. Chevers would not live long after the hospital officially closed, passing away at the age of 59 on October

31, 1867. His remains lie next to his wife, Sarah, in a family plot at Rhode Island Historical Cemetery No. 9, adjacent to St. Paul's Episcopal Church in Portsmouth.[104]

A month after the soldiers' remains were moved from Portsmouth Grove Cemetery to Cypress Hills National Cemetery, the following letter arrived at the desk of a state official in Providence. The letter was directed to either the Governor's Office or the Secretary of State:

Oshkosh, Wisconsin, June 23/68

Mr. George H. Stewart
Dear Sir

I wrote a letter sometime ago directing it to the USCM. I have had no response from it. I now address you & though I have no claim whatsoever upon you yet, I believe that as friend & brother in Christ, you will readily give the information I seek. I lost a son in the Army & he was buried at Portsmouth Grove, RI. The government as I notice has lately been moving some of the bodies of the soldiers to Cypress Hill Cemetery, LI [Long Island]. If you will be kind enough to inform me whether they have moved all or intend to move all & break up the cemetery there, I will be truly obliged to you. My sons name was Luther M. Loper.

Yours with respect
Isaac Loper[105]

The subject letter is currently in the possession of the Office of the Secretary of State, A. Ralph Mollis State Archives Division. On the middle right edge of the paper is written "ans [answered] June 30th, 1868, GS." Though the letter elicited a prompt response, no copy of the return correspondence is on file. We can only conclude that Mr. Loper was advised that his late son's remains were sent to Cypress Hills National Cemetery for reinterment and was peaceably laid to rest at plot number 3564. Though Wisconsin was the home state of Sergeant Loper, the deceased veteran enlisted and served out of state with Co. G, 115th New York Infantry. The practice of hailing from one state and serving in another was a common occurrence during the war.

Though the hospital library ceased to exist when the hospital closed its doors, the Portsmouth Grove Hospital Library Association took years to disband. Initially, books deemed useable by the library committee "were shipped to the Freedmen of the South," while those in poorer condition were discarded, but it took until September 8, 1884, before the remaining funds left in the association's bank account were distributed. The benefactor of approximately $2,200 was the "C. Fiske Harris Collection or the similar collection belonging to Hon. John R. Bartlett." Both collections were located at the Providence Public Library in Providence, Rhode Island. The funds were earmarked for building and maintaining the said collections.[106]

Fourteen years later, on September 2, 1898, Rt. the Rev. Thomas M. Clark, Bishop of Newport, wrote to the surgeon general in Washington, D.C., suggesting that the hospital formerly sited at Portsmouth Grove be reestablished to lodge the current contingent of military men fighting in the Spanish-American War. Acknowledging that the previous hospital "was well remembered," the secretary, who replied instead of the surgeon general, said, "It seems unlikely, however, that further hospital accommodations will be required so far north. The sick will come from a tropical climate and hospitals in a milder winter climate than that of Rhode Island would appear to be desirable."[107] His argument made

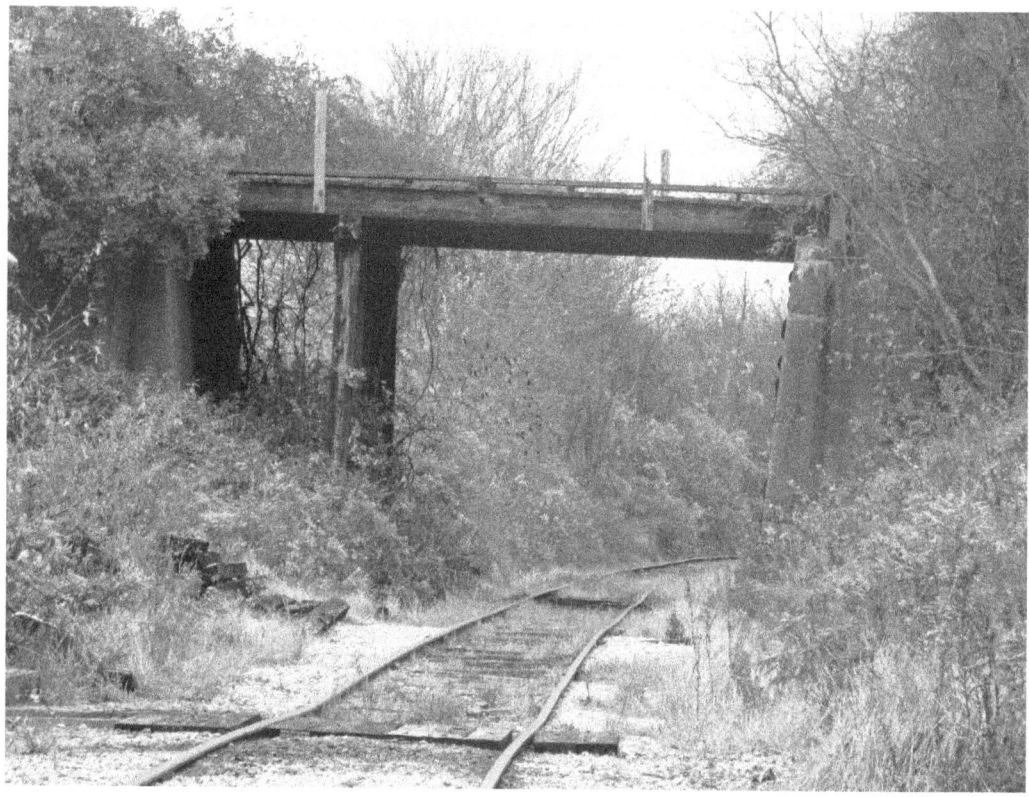

The embanked road that led to the burial yard is now an overgrown pathway that abruptly ends at a fenced area of a defunct military tank farm (courtesy Ken Garthee).

perfect sense, as men requiring hospitalization would come from the Caribbean and the Pacific. The case for reopening the grounds as a hospital was closed.

For nearly a hundred years, the site of Portsmouth Grove's cemetery was thought lost to posterity. A rudimentary pencil sketch of the grounds was published in Dr. Seebert J. Goldowsky's scholarly article in 1959 that was copied from an undated period lithograph titled *U.S. General Hospital, Portsmouth, RI*, and credited to J. Baker and J.M. Taber Jr.[108] The small drawing, reproduced at the bottom of the page within Godowsky's article, depicts a horseshoe entrance, a few graves surrounded by trees, and a grieving widow standing in the center. Part of the mystery was solved in January 2010 after the original plan for the hospital grounds was found at the state archives. The penciled plan, measuring roughly 19" by 27" on heavy Manila paper, depicts the entire hospital complex in rough draft with block diagrams representing the buildings and slightly curved lines representing roads. At the upper east side of the drawing, just off the embanked road leading through the marsh, are the words "Burying Ground."[109] Another revelation surfaced when a photograph of the cemetery came to light. The image, however, sheds no new information about the exact location of the burial ground, though it does provide a glimpse of how it appeared and how large it had become by 1864. Even if the precise location is found, with all the changes to the land by the military over the years, nothing remains that would distinguish its allotted purpose. Perhaps that is the way it should remain.

Today there are seventy-nine national cemeteries scattered throughout the country containing the remains of thousands of Civil War veterans. Unbelievably, 54 percent of the soldiers and sailors buried at these shrines are unknown, a chilling statistic representing just how impersonal America's Civil War was and how heartbreaking it must have been for surviving family members in their attempt to locate their sons and brothers.[110]

At the beginning of the twentieth century, those who visited the former site of the hospital at Portsmouth Grove seemed shocked at what little remained. A Portsmouth resident remembers seeing water hydrants but nothing more. Words like "vanished, disappeared," and "obliterated" were frequently used in articles published about the site, as if the entire complex had been sucked into a gigantic black hole.[111]

The land at Portsmouth Grove subsequently reverted to private ownership. Around 1895–96, part of the complex became a rifle range for the Newport Artillery Company.[112] In 1901, Bradford Coaling Station was constructed to supply coal to steamers and military transports navigating Narragansett Bay, but that, too, was short-lived.[113] After the introduction of diesel fuel engines, the station became antiquated. Before closure, the railroad changed the name of their depot from Portsmouth Grove to Bradford Station. In 1904, the town of Portsmouth also changed the name of the street originally leading to the hospital from Portsmouth Grove Road to Bradford Avenue. Today Bradford Avenue is a private way that leads to a campground before ending abruptly at fenced government property. A quarter of a mile south, Stringham Road, built by the navy, offers the only paved access to where the hospital once stood.

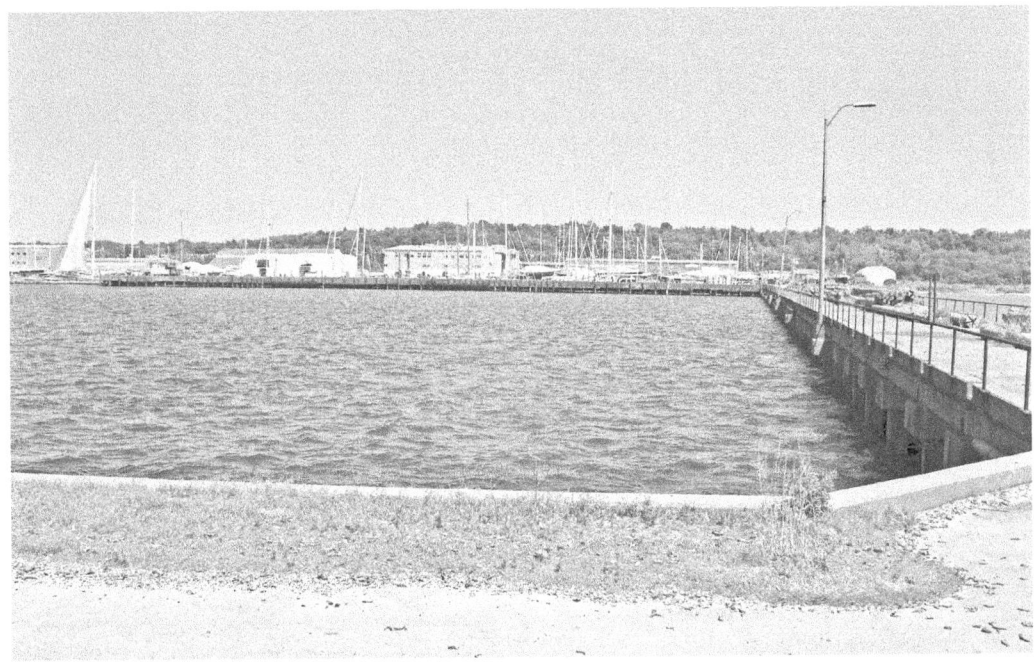

Situated on the grounds of the former hospital at Portsmouth Grove is the Melville Boat and Marina District. Long ago, the word "Grove" was dropped in favor of the town name, Portsmouth, thus losing its period identity. Notice the long wharf enhanced during World War II but now in need of repair (photograph by the author).

During World War II, the navy commenced a mammoth buildup on Aquidneck Island. Over 6,000 acres of shorefront property was acquired. Lovell's former 12 acres was part of that transaction and renamed Melville after Rear Admiral George Melville of the Bureau of Engineering. Melville became a training center for navy patrol torpedo (PT) boats and an anti-submarine net depot.[114] Here, John F. Kennedy, later to become the country's thirty-fifth president, would take his training. Also a navy fuel supply depot was constructed on the eastern ridge but eventually became inactive, as did the PT boat training center. In the early 1960s, construction was started on a nuclear-powered submarine base along with appropriate shore facilities, but the plans barely got off the ground before they were canceled.

Today, the site is home to the Melville Boat and Marina District. When the Newport Dinner Train passes the area and passengers glance out the windows, only a few may know the history, understand the suffering, and appreciate the sacrifice of those from each side of the conflict who spent what seemed like an eternity at Portsmouth Grove Hospital and, like John Lovejoy, have long since mustered to a better place above.

In a letter home while a patient at Portsmouth Grove Hospital, Seth Alden told his sister, "After a man is dead he is soon forgotten."[115] Perhaps the testament herein will contradict his dire assessment so that the legacy of courage and perseverance of the men who died at the hospital, those like Seth Alden fortunate enough to survive the ordeal, and the compassionate men and women who served there will carry on for generations.

Appendix A
Hospital Guards— Rhode Island Volunteers

Name	Rank	Residence	Date of Muster	Remarks
Christopher Blanding	Captain	Providence, RI	Dec. 6, 1862	Mustered out, Aug. 26, 1865
William S. Chace	1st Lieutenant	Providence, RI	Nov. 12, 1862	Mustered out, Aug. 26, 1865
John H. Hammond	2nd Lieutenant	Providence, RI	Dec. 13, 1862	Mustered out, Aug. 26, 1865
James E. Blackmar*	Sergeant	E. Providence, RI	Dec. 6, 1862	Mustered out, Aug. 26, 1865
George W. Weeden	Sergeant	Providence, RI	Dec. 6, 1862	1st Sergeant, Mar. 1, 1863; honorably discharged Nov. 18, 1863, to accept commission in 14th RIHA (Colored)
Horatio N. Slocum	Sergeant	Providence, RI	Dec. 6, 1862	Mustered out, Aug. 26, 1865
Albert Russell	Sergeant	Providence, RI	Dec. 6, 1862	Deserted Mar. 22, 1864
Stephen G. Luther	Sergeant	Providence, RI	Dec. 6, 1862	Mustered out, Aug. 26, 1865
Michael Nolan	Corporal	Newport, RI	Dec. 6, 1862	Deserted Feb. 9, 1863
Samuel H. Redman	Corporal	Providence, RI	Dec. 6, 1862	Deserted Aug. 1, 1863
William P. Dillabar	Corporal	Providence, RI	Dec. 6, 1862	Discharged for disability, Jan. 10, 1863
George H. Peck	Corporal	Bristol, RI	Dec. 6, 1862	Mustered out, Aug. 26, 1865
Stephen F. Fish	Corporal	Providence, RI	Jan. 14, 1863	Promoted to Sergeant; mustered out, Aug. 26, 1865
James H. Williams	Drummer	Providence, RI	Dec. 6, 1862	Mustered out, Aug. 26, 1865
Daniel H. Goff	Fifer	Smithfield, RI	Dec. 6, 1862	Mustered out, Aug. 26, 1865
Aigan, James	Private	Providence, RI	Jan. 19, 1863	Corporal; deserted Dec. 29, 1863
Allen, Antoine	Private	Smithfield, RI	Dec. 6, 1862	Dishonorably discharged, May 3, 1863
Amadon, Jeremiah	Private	Smithfield, RI	Dec. 6, 1862	Mustered out, Aug. 26, 1865
Ballou, James	Private	Smithfield, RI	Dec. 6, 1862	Mustered out, Aug. 26, 1865
Bamfrey, John	Private	Smithfield, RI	Dec. 6, 1862	Corporal; mustered out, Aug. 26, 1865
Bolding, William	Private	Providence, RI	Dec. 6, 1862	Deserted Aug. 27, 1864
Boyce, Peter	Private		Never must'd	Discharged previous to muster
Brown, William	Private	Newport, RI	Dec. 6, 1862	Mustered out, Aug. 26, 1865
Burns, Bernard	Private	Smithfield, RI	Dec. 6, 1862	Mustered out, Aug. 26, 1865
Campbell, Peter	Private	Providence, RI	Jan 14, 1863	Discharged for disability, Jun. 10, 1863
Cargill, William H.	Private		Aug. 10, 1863	Mustered out, Aug. 26, 1865
Carpenter, Curnel A.	Private	Providence, RI	Dec. 6, 1862	Mustered out, Aug. 26, 1865
Carr, Stephen A.	Private	Providence, RI	Dec. 6, 1862	Drowned Oct. 24, 1863

Name	Rank	Residence	Date of Muster	Remarks
Cavanagh, Michael	Private	Providence, RI	Dec. 19, 1862	Deserted Jan. 17, 1863
Chappell, John H.	Private	Johnston, RI	Jun. 6, 1864	Mustered out, Aug. 26, 1865
Coghill, Thomas A.	Private	Providence, RI	Dec. 6, 1862	Discharged for disability, Dec. 10, 1862
Coit, William M.	Private	Bristol, RI	Dec. 6, 1862	Mustered out, Aug. 26, 1865
Cole, Charles W.	Private	Providence, RI	Dec. 6, 1862	Mustered out, Aug. 26, 1865
Collins, Timothy	Private	Smithfield, RI	Dec. 6, 1862	Deserted Aug. 14, 1865
Creed, Francis	Private	Providence, RI	Jun. 8, 1863	Mustered out, Aug. 26, 1865
Crofton, James	Private	Smithfield, RI	Dec. 6, 1862	Mustered out, Aug. 26, 1865
Davis, William	Private	Providence, RI	Dec. 6, 1862	Mustered out, Aug. 26, 1865
Denton, Joseph	Private	Providence, RI	Dec. 6, 1862	Discharged for disability, Oct. 5, 1863
Dill, George	Private	Bristol, RI	Dec. 6, 1862	Discharged for disability, Oct. 5, 1863
Drohan, John E.	Private	Fall River, MA	Dec. 12, 1862	Sergeant Mar. 14, 1864; mustered out, Aug, 26, 1865
Duffy, Thomas	Private	Pawtucket, RI	Dec. 6, 1862	Mustered out, Aug. 26, 1865
Ellis, Joseph M.	Private	Providence, RI	Dec. 27, 1862	Mustered out, Aug. 26, 1865
Farmer, Henry H.	Private	Providence, RI	Dec. 6, 1862	Mustered out, Aug. 26, 1865
Farrell, Edward	Private	Providence, RI	Dec. 6, 1862	Discharged for disability, Mar. 20, 1863
Farrell, Terence	Private	Providence, RI	Dec. 6, 1862	Mustered out, Aug. 26, 1865
Flemming, Michael	Private	E. Greenwich, RI	Dec. 6, 1862	Mustered out, Aug. 26, 1865
Follett, John F.	Private	Barrington, RI	Dec. 6, 1862	Corporal; mustered out, Aug. 26, 1865
Ford, Isaac	Private	Providence, RI	Dec. 6, 1862	Mustered out, Aug. 26, 1865
Galligan, John	Private	Cranston, RI	Jul. 30, 1863	Deserted Apr. 28, 1864
Gallighan, William	Private	Providence, RI	Dec. 6, 1862	Discharged Aug. 22, 1863, on surgeon certificate
Gavin, William	Private	Olneyville, RI	Dec. 6, 1862	Mustered out, Aug. 26, 1865
Gero, Alexander	Private	Maine	Dec. 6, 1862	Deserted Feb. 1, 1864
Gleason, Silas	Private	N. Providence, RI	Dec. 6, 1862	Mustered out, Aug. 26, 1865
Gove, Edward	Private	Cranston, RI	Dec. 6, 1862	Deserted Apr. 16, 1863
Gray, John C.	Private	Providence, RI	Dec. 10, 1862	Mustered out, Aug. 26, 1865
Greene, William	Private	Providence, RI	Dec. 6, 1862	Mustered out, Aug. 26, 1865
Grey, William	Private	Providence, RI	Dec. 6, 1862	Dischared for disability, Mar. 19, 1863
Gwyne, Charles	Private	Canada	May 16, 1863	Deserted Dec. 29, 1863
Haley, Michael	Private	Providence, RI	Dec. 6, 1862	Mustered out, Aug. 26, 1865
Hall, Chandler	Private	Providence, RI	Dec. 27, 1862	Mustered out, Aug. 26, 1865
Harper, Thomas	Private	Smithfield, RI	Dec. 6, 1862	Mustered out, Aug. 26, 1865
Harrigan, William Jr.	Private	Johnston, RI	Dec. 22, 1862	Mustered out, Aug. 26, 1865
Hawes, Marcellus D.	Private	Wrentham, MA	Dec. 6, 1862	Mustered out, Aug. 26, 1865
Heath, George W.	Private	Providence, RI	Dec. 6, 1862	Mustered out, Aug. 26, 1865
Henderson, Alexander	Private	Slatersville, RI	Dec. 6, 1862	Mustered out, Aug. 26, 1865
Hicks, Charles F.	Private	Providence, RI	Dec. 6, 1862	Mustered out, Aug. 26, 1865
Higgins, John	Private	Smithfield, RI	Dec. 6, 1862	Killed by officer of guard Feb. 28, 1863
Irving, William S.	Private	Providence, RI	Dec. 6, 1862	Discharged Dec. 24, 1862, on surgeon certificate
Johnson, Alfred A.	Private	Warwick, RI	Dec. 6, 1862	Corporal; mustered out, Aug. 26, 1865
Kelley, John	Private	S. Kingstown, RI	Jun. 13, 1864	Deserted Jun. 30, 1865
King, Anthony H.	Private	Cranston, RI	Dec. 6, 1862	Mustered out, Aug. 26, 1865
Leonard, James	Private	Cranston, RI	Dec. 6, 1862	Mustered out, Aug. 26, 1865
Locke, Mark	Private	Warwick, RI	Dec. 6, 1862	Mustered out, Aug. 26, 1865
Markey, John	Private	Boston, MA	May 23, 1863	Deserted Dec. 29, 1864
Mattison, Jacob	Private	Bristol, RI	Dec. 6, 1862	Mustered out, Aug. 26, 1865

Appendix A

Name	Rank	Residence	Date of Muster	Remarks
McCaffrey, Patrick	Private	Providence, RI	Dec. 6, 1862	Mustered out, Aug. 26, 1865
McDermot, Michael*	Private	Providence, RI	Jun. 8, 1863	Mustered out, Aug. 26, 1865
McWilliams, James	Private	Slatersville, RI	Dec. 6, 1862	Mustered out, Aug. 26, 1865
Medbury, Theodore H.	Private	Barrington, RI	Dec. 6, 1862	Deserted May 31, 1865
Merchant, Curtis	Private	Providence, RI	Dec. 6, 1862	Discharged March 19, 1863
Mitchell, William J.	Private	Providence, RI	Dec. 6, 1862	Mustered out, Aug. 26, 1865
Munroe, James B.	Private	Providence, RI	Dec. 6, 1862	Corporal; mustered out, Aug. 26, 1865
Newell, Albert F.	Private	Providence, RI	Dec. 6, 1862	Deserted Jan 13, 1863
O'Keefe, David F.	Private	Boston, MA	Dec. 11, 1862	Corporal; mustered out, Aug. 26, 1865
Peck, Charles W.	Private	Providence, RI	Dec. 6, 1862	Mustered out, Aug. 26, 1865
Pierce, John F.	Private	Johnston, RI	Dec. 6, 1862	Mustered out, Aug. 26, 1865
Pierce, William Jr.	Private	Foster, RI	Dec. 6, 1862	Discharged Feb. 9, 1863, on surgeon certificate
Pierce, Wilson D.	Private	Rehoboth, MA	Dec. 6, 1862	Mustered out, Aug. 26, 1865
Pyers, Edward	Private	Providence, RI	Dec. 6, 1862	Mustered out, Aug. 26, 1865
Ray, Thomas	Private	Providence, RI	Dec. 6, 1862	Deserted Dec. 5, 1862
Rohr, Herman	Private	Providence, RI	Jan. 8, 1863	Mustered out, Aug. 26, 1865
Ryder, James	Private	Smithfield, RI	Dec. 6, 1862	Mustered out, Aug. 26, 1865
Smith, John	Private	Portsmouth, RI	May 19, 1863	Mustered out, Aug. 26, 1865
Smith, Nathan A.	Private	Providence, RI	Dec. 17, 1862	Corporal; mustered out, Aug. 26, 1865
Stewart, John	Private	New York, NY	May 12, 1863	Deserted Jun. 30, 1865
Street, Ralph	Private	Greenville, RI	Dec. 6, 1862	Mustered out, Aug. 26, 1865
Sullivan, James	Private	Smithfield, RI	Dec. 16, 1862	Deserted Aug. 25, 1863
Tanner, Charles H.	Private	Providence, RI	Dec. 6, 1862	Died Jan. 9, 1865 of disease
Taylor, John	Private	Smithfield, RI	Dec. 6, 1862	Drowned Oct. 24, 1863
Taylor, John A.	Private	Providence, RI	Dec. 6, 1862	Corporal; mustered out, Aug. 26, 1865
Waldron, Alfred B.	Private	Bristol, RI	Dec. 6, 1862	Corporal; discharged Mar. 19, 1863,
Wathey, John	Private	Providence, RI	May 25, 1863	Corporal; mustered out, Aug. 26, 1865
Watson, Caleb	Private	Smithfield, RI	Dec. 6, 1862	Mustered out, Aug. 26, 1865
White, James P.	Private	Smithfield, RI	Dec. 6, 1862	Mustered out, Aug. 26, 1865
Whiting, Moses G.	Private	Bristol, RI	Dec. 6, 1862	Mustered out, Aug. 26, 1865
Whitmarsh, Thomas B.	Private	Providence, RI	Dec. 6, 1862	Mustered out, Aug. 26, 1865
Wilkinson, John	Private	Providence, RI	Jan. 19, 1863	Mustered out, Aug. 26, 1865
Williams, Esek	Private	Providence, RI	Dec. 6, 1862	Mustered out, Aug. 26, 1865
Yost, Charles E.	Private	Providence, RI	Dec. 6, 1862	Mustered out, Aug. 26, 1865

*Due to illegible handwriting, poor record keeping, or transposing, some surnames are suspect: for instance, Blackmar is probably Blackman and McDermot may be McDermott. There may be other errors.

Source: Annual Report of the Adjutant General of the State of Rhode Island for the Year 1865, Providence, Providence Press Company, Printers to the State.

Appendix B
Roll of Honor

The following soldiers died at Lovell General Hospital, U.S.A., Portsmouth Grove, Rhode Island, and were reinterred at Cypress Hills National Cemetary, Section 1B, Jamaica Avenue, Brooklyn, New York, in May of 1868. The section is known as the Union Plot. Names may differ in the following list from what appears on the headstone. After extensive research, the most plausible spelling was selected.

Name	*Rank*	*Company and Regiment*	*State*	*Death of Death*	*Cypress Hills Plot Number*
Alspach, David S.	Sergeant	A, 50th Infantry	PA	August 14, 1864	3449
Anderson, Stillman	Private	G, 11th Infantry	ME	July 12, 1862	3304
Angle, David	Private	E, 1st Infantry	KY	November 18, 1862	3362
Armstrong, William A.	Corporal	B, 31st Infantry	ME	February 19, 1865	3519
Austin, Albert H.	Private	H, 1st Battery	NY	September 19, 1864	3467
Austin, William	Private	F, 169th, Infantry	NY	July 8, 1865	3568
Bailey, Addison D.	Private	I, 12th Cavalry	NY	May 18, 1865	3536
Balch, Ambros E.	Private	A, 33rd Infantry	NY	July 15, 1862	3294
Barger, Jacob	Private	K, 203rd Infantry	PA	April 27, 1865	3524
Barker, Chauncey C.	Private	G, 7th Infantry	WI	October 6, 1864	3489
Barnes, William H.	Private	G, 56th Infantry	NY	August 12, 1862	3355
Barnhart, Samuel L.	Private	G, 69th Infantry	OH	June 24, 1865	3556
Barr, Samuel	Private	A, 61st Infantry	PA	August 23, 1862	3371
Beadle, Oliver H.	Private	L, 56th Infantry	NY	July 23, 1862	3296
Bean, George P.	Private	K, 9th Infantry	NH	May 15, 2009	3515
Belton, Robert A.	Private	B, 2nd Infantry	MI	August 25, 1864	3458
Berry, Lewis E.	Private	A, 87th Infantry	IN	May 3, 1865	3530
Bishop, George B.	Private	A, 100 Infantry	NY	September 5, 1862	3344
Bliss, Seth	Private	K, 55th Infantry	IL	April 30, 1865	3527
Bowditch, William P.	Private	B, 158th Infantry	NY	October 13, 1864	3483
Bowsir, Milner	Private	G, 47th, Infantry	NY	June 19, 1865	3559
Boyer, Jacob	Private	G, U.S. 22nd Colored	US	November 15, 1864	3512
Boyer, William H.	Private	G, 6th U.S. Colored	US	November 14, 1864	3511
Brabson, William F.	Private	1, 101st Infantry	PA	July 13, 1862	3305
Broadheart, Abel	Private	F, 16th Heavy Artillery	NY	October 19, 1864	3492
Brown, Benjamin F.	Private	G, 57th Infantry	PA	August 5, 1862	3350
Brown, Bradish B.	Private	E, 31st Infantry	ME	August 29, 1864	3459
Brown, F.M.	Private	A, 7th Infantry	ME	July 12, 1862	3292
Brown, James H.	Private	B, 179th Infantry	NY	June 29, 1864	3392
Brown, Joseph	Sergeant	D, 6th Cavallry	OH	June 19, 1864	3406

Appendix B

Name	Rank	Company and Regiment	State	Death of Death	Cypress Hills Plot Number
Brown, William S.	Bugler	6th Battery	ME	July 16, 1864	3421
Buck, Orsborne	Sergeant	B, 8th Cavalry	PA	August 6, 1863	3379
Burgess, Edwin D.	Private	D, 4th Infantry	VT	August 13, 1862	3464
Burlingame, Benjamin	Private	A, 47th Infantry	NY	July 9, 1865	3569
Burlingame, Zelotes	Private	H, U.S. Sharpshooters	US	October 7, 1862	3310
Burns, John	Private	I, 40th Infantry	NY	October 18, 1862	3282
Burnside, Frank	Private	A, 16th Heavy Artillery	NY	August 9, 1864	3474
Calhoun, John	Private	A, 7th Infantry	NJ	August 7, 1864	3441
Campbell, George W.	Private	K, 36th Infantry	WI	June 27, 1864	3390
Cassel, George A.	Private	B, 128 Infantry	IN	June 22, 1865	3553
Chamberlin, William A.	Private	I, 1st Cavalry	VT	April 28, 1865	3525
Chambers, Legrand	Corporal	D, 24th Cavalry	NY	July 25, 1864	3428
Charles, James H.	Private	14th Artillery	VT	June 26, 1864	3388
Christ, Petter	Private	K, 5th Infantry	MI	July 6, 1862	3318
Chroniger, Ephriam A.	Private	I, 102nd Infantry	PA	October 4, 1862	3365
Clark, Charles H.	Private	A, 8th New York Artillery	NY	June 27, 1864	3391
Clarry, Edward R.	Private	M, 1st Heavy Artillery	ME	July 11, 1864	3413
Clements, Lewis D.	Private	G, 29th Infantry	OH	September 7, 1862	3288
Coats, James A.	Private	M, 16th Heavy Artillery	NY	October 25, 1864	3504
Coffee, Jesse B.	Private	18th Infantry	WI	May 19, 1865	3538
Colby, Henry	Private	K, 2nd Infantry	CT	June 17, 1864	3404
Cole, John	Private	H, 7th Infantry	MI	October 12, 1863	3377
Colson, John A.	Private	B, 31st Infantry	ME	September 22, 1864	3469
Conklin, John	Private	K, 2nd Heavy Artillery	NY	July 15, 1864	3419
Cook, Moses	Private	B, U.S. 22nd Colored	US	December 17, 1864	3433
Corn, George	Private	E, 169th Infantry	NY	October 21, 1864	3496
Cornish, Thomas	Private	H, 4th U.S. Colored	US	October 16, 1864	3488
Cough, Bruce	Private	G, 94th Infantry	NY	December 5, 1862	3338
Cowles, Nathan G.	Private	G, 97th Infantry	NY	August 10, 1864	3443
Cox, Leander A.	Private	A, 37th Infantry	NC	July 9, 1862	3331
Coxey, James	Private	D, 76th Infantry	PA	June 26, 1865	3558
Coyne, Simon	Private	L, 6th Infantry	NY	August 9, 1864	3442
Croman, Jacob	Private	D, 104th Infantry	PA	August 24, 1862	3345
Cromer, George	Private	H, 22nd Infantry	IN	July 13, 1865	3571
Crowner, Ambrose	Private	H, 2nd Heavy Artillery	NY	June 26, 1864	3386
Culver, George W.	Private	F, 49th Infantry	NY	March 20, 1863	3361
Curtis, James	Private	G, 169th Infantry	NY	October 20, 1864	3499
Curtis, Joseph	Private	E, 12th Infantry	IN	July 5, 1865	3563
Curtis, Richard J.	Private	A, 16th Heavy Artillery	NY	October 14, 1864	3482
Dark, George	Private	E, 18th Infantry	WI	November 28, 1862	3339
Darling, Truman A.	Private	F, 5th Infantry	WI	October 17, 1862	3283
Datzius, Philip	Private	A, 47th Infantry	PA	November 9, 1864	3510
Daver, Patrick	Private	E, 8th Infantry	NJ	November 6, 1862	3506
Davis, Benjamin F.	Private	K, 81st Infantry	PA	August 15, 1862	3348
Davis, George Myron	Corporal	E, 37th Infantry	WI	September 21, 1864	3468
Dean, Horace A.	Private	H, 54th Infantry	PA	October 5, 1862	3311
Debaun, Jeremiah R.	Private	G, 109th Infantry	NY	August 19, 1864	3456
Deland, Alvin S.	Private	C, 9th Cavalry	NY	July 17, 1864	3423
Denald, Charles	Private	C, 142nd Infantry	NY	August 7, 1865	3575
Dickey, Madison	Corporal	L, 4th Cavalry	VT	December 1, 1864	3374
Dildine, John H.	Private	H, 55th Infantry	OH	May 22, 1865	3463
Dix, George	Private	A, 37th U.S. Colored	US	November 5, 1864	3509
Doran, James	Private	K, 8th Infantry	MI	October 21, 1864	3497
Dozier, Major	Private	I, 36th U.S. Colored	US	October 14, 1864	3481
Draper, Isaac T.	Private	E, 3rd Infantry	DE	July 12, 1864	3417
Eaton, Frederick	Private	E, 2nd Infantry	ME	July 7, 1862	3323

Name	Rank	Company and Regiment	State	Death of Death	Cypress Hills Plot Number
Ellis, Harrison	Sergeant	G, 42nd Infantry	NY	August 14, 1862	3347
Emery, M.A.	Private	E, 93rd Infantry	NY	July 7, 1862	3315
Evans, William, Jr.	Private	5th Ind. Ohio Battery	OH	April 24, 1865	3523
Fay, W.M.	Private	B, 85th Infantry	NY	July 7, 1862	3329
Fidget, Oswell	Private	B, 36th U.S. Colored	US	October 14, 1864	3486
Fogle, J.W.	Private	G, 4th Infantry	ME	July 7, 1862	3322
Fogle, Nicholas	Private	G, 101st Infantry	PA	July 7, 1862	3330
Ford, Lewis N.	Private	G, 93rd Infantry	NY	August 31, 1862	3368
Fought, Simon	Private	A, 33rd Infantry	OH	June 13, 1865	3550
Francis, John A.	Private	B, 38th U.S. Colored	US	October 12, 1864	3479
French, James	Private	K, 57th Infantry	PA	February 13, 1863	3359
Fuller, Amos L.	Private	E, 58th Infantry	VT	August 10, 1864	3472
Garnes, James	Private	H, 5th U.S. Colored	US	October 18, 1864	3490
Gaston, Theodore	Private	A, 46th Infantry	NY	July 5, 1864	3395
Gates, Jonathan	Private	H, 4th Infantry	MI	July 25, 1863	3383
Geohegan, John	Private	G, 16th Heavy Artillery	NY	October 9, 1864	3473
Gerald, George W.	Private	C, 1st Cavalry	ME	July 1, 1863	3381
Girton, Alfred	Private	F, 84th Infantry	PA	July 7, 1864	3411
Gleason, Thomas	Corporal	A, 5th Infantry	NY	July 30, 1864	3430
Good, Hazamiah	Private	L, 14th Heavy Art. (Col.)	RI	October 11, 1864	3478
Gove, George	Sergeant	I, 11th Infantry	ME	October 24, 1864	3501
Grandy, Stephen K.	Private	K, 118th Infantry	NY	August 20, 1864	3455
Gray, Francis	Private	C, 2nd Cavalry	ME	July 9, 1864	3414
Green, Samuel	Private	K, 76th Infantry	PA	June 24, 1865	3557
Gregor, Henry	Private	H, 1st Engineers	MI	October 30, 1862	3307
Griffin, Thomas H.	Private	A, 1st Heavy Artillery	ME	July 22, 1864	3401
Grindstaff, Green*	Private	D, 5th Cavalry	KY	May 25, 1865	3543
Groht, Henry	Private	C, 20th Infantry	VT	July 19, 1864	3424
Hall, Jacob	Private	K, 95th Infantry	PA	July 11, 1862	3290
Hall, John	Private	K, 10th Infantry	NY	January 10, 1863	3336
Hanna, Thomas	Private	E, 63rd Infantry	PA	March 22, 1863	3462
Hanscome, J. P.	Private	E, 1st Infantry	MN	November 17, 1862	3340
Harris, Albert F.	Corporal	G, 52nd Infantry	NY	June 27, 1864	3400
Harvey, James R.	Private	K, 2nd Heavy Artillery	PA	June 26, 1864	3387
Haskins, James D.	Corporal	D, 27th Infantry	VT	September 26, 1865	3576
Heath, Charles	Private	H, 4th Infantry	MI	February 23, 1863	3357
Hendrick, George O.	Private	A, 53rd Infantry	PA	July 18, 1864	3422
Hendricks, Mordecai	Corporal	D, 4th Infantry	DE	July 2, 1864	3398
Hickman, James W.	Private	H, 2nd Infantry	PA	June 26, 1864	3385
Hild, George	Private	Buell's Battalion	WI	November 11, 1862	3341
Hoag, Judson	Private	G, 169th Infantry	NY	October 27, 1864	3370
Hoard, Lorenzo	Private	C, 142nd Infantry	NY	October 14, 1864	3485
Holmes, Hugh P.	Private	I, 7th Infantry	ME	July 14, 1862	3302
Hopper, Edward M.	Private	G, 27th Infantry	MI	July 31, 1864	3432
Horseman, James	Private	B, 62nd Infantry	OH	October 20, 1864	3493
Howard, Wilson	Private	E, 22nd U.S. Colored	US	December 28, 1864	3517
Hozier, Andrew	Private	I, 64th Infantry	IL	May 20, 1865	3537
Hughes, Martin	Sergeant	C, 5th Infantry	ME	June 5, 1864	3405
Imboden, Eli	Private	I, 91st Infantry	IN	June 4, 1865	3546
Ingraham, Alexander	Private	F, 101th Infantry	NY	August 1, 1862	3352
Ingram, Robert L.	Private	A, 39th Infantry	OH	May 25, 1865	3541
Irving, Abraham	Private	D, 37th Infantry	NC	July 6, 1862	3319
Jackson, Abram	Private	F, 29th Infantry (Col.)	CT	October 24, 1864	3502
Jackson, James	Private	D, 6th Infantry	WI	August 7, 1864	3439
Jackson, John L.	Private	G, 29th Infantry (Col.)	CT	October 12, 1864	3477
Johnson, Augustus	Private	I, 7th U.S. Colored	US	October 20, 1864	3495

Appendix B

Name	Rank	Company and Regiment	State	Death of Death	Cypress Hills Plot Number
Johnson, John	Private	L, 14th Heavy Art. (Col.)	RI	March 10, 1864	3407
Jones, Michael	Private	C, 38th U.S. Colored	US	October 11, 1864	3476
Jones, Willis	Corporal	D, 84th Infantry	IL	June 6, 1865	3548
Joy, Granville W.	Private	E, 17th Infantry	ME	August 18, 1864	3454
Juan, Antonio	Private	A, 7th Infantry	NH	April 24, 1865	3522
Kimball, Jeremiah B.	Private	H, 6th Infantry	NJ	October 24, 1862	3280
Kinshaw, Jacob	Private	C, 17th Infantry	WI	May 17, 1865	3533
Kirkpatrick, Newton	Sergeant	C, 3rd Cavalry	IN	July 20, 1864	3425
Koch, David	Private	C, 3rd Infantry	MD	September 8, 1862	3313
Laheon, William M.	Private	A, 81st Infantry	NY	July 7, 1862	3326
Lake, George W.	Private	K, 16th Heavy Artillery	NY	October 10, 1862	3448
Lamback, William S.	Musician	D, 57th Infantry	PA	July 7, 1864	3409
LaRue, Joseph	Private	K, 11th Cavalry	PA	February 1, 1865	3518
Lemereaux, Squire	Private	D, 17th Infantry	PA	February 28, 1863	3372
Letson, J.W.	Private	K, 81st Infantry	NY	July 7, 1862	3327
Lloyd, Charles	Private	C, 22nd Artillery (Col.)	NY	October 27, 1864	3528
Long, Reuben	Sergeant	H, 24th Infantry	NC	July 23, 1864	3427
Loper, Luther M.	Sergeant	G, 115th Infantry	NY	July 5, 1865	3564
Lowell, Joseph	Private	D, 142nd Infantry	NY	May 9, 1865	3531
Mackie, John W.	Private	B, 51st Infantry	NY	September 11, 1864	3466
Magaw, William C.	Private	H, 101st Infantry	PA	July 27, 1862	3298
Maha, William	Private	D, 112 Infantry	NY	May 27, 1865	3544
Maine, Charles	Private	D, 11th U.S. Colored	US	September 18, 1862	3312
Maines, Henry S.	Private	E, 32nd Infantry	ME	May, 15, 1864	3281
Maloney, Daniel	Private	H, 97th Infantry	PA	October 11, 1864	3475
Mason, L.	Private	C, 9th Infantry	NY	October 8, 1862	3284
Matott, Victor	Sergeant	115th Infantry	NY	May 22, 1865	3540
McCabe, Alexander	Private	I, 3rd Infantry	NY	June 28, 1865	3560
McGrath, James	Private	E, 88th Infantry	NY	June 29, 1864	3393
McIntire John	Private	E, 3rd Infantry	NY	June 23, 1865	3555
McIsaac, Daniel	Private	D, 102nd Infantry	PA	October 23, 1862	3308
McKiernan, Edward	Private	G, 8th Infantry	NJ	July 13, 1862	3293
McKinney, Samuel	Private	K, 47th Infantry	NY	May 23, 1865	3536
McNeal, E.R.	Corporal	A, 13th Cavalry	OH	August 23, 1864	3457
McPherson, Wright	Private	A, 140th Infantry	IN	April 21, 1865	3521
Medare, Joseph	Private	D, 7th Infantry	NJ	July 14, 1862	3301
Merrick, John	Private	L, 14th Heavy Art. (Col.)	RI	January 26, 1864	3375
Michaels, Zina	Private	I, 1st Infantry	ME	July 27, 1864	3429
Miller, David	Private	I, 102nd Infantry	PA	July 17, 1862	3300
Miller, Frank	Private	G, 8th U.S. Colored	US	January 20, 1865	3471
Miller, T.	Private	K, 49th Infantry	NY	July 7, 1862	3325
Mills, Floyd T.	Private	G, 29th Infantry (Col.)	CT	October 20, 1864	3494
Moore, Guy	Private	K, 183rd Infantry	PA	October 14, 1864	3487
Moore, Thomas	Private	A, 6th U.S. Colored	US	October 19, 1864	3491
Morton, E.D.	Private	G, 9th Infantry	NY	September 18, 1862	3286
Mouse, Alexander	Private	E, (unit unknown)	US	February 18, 1863	3358
Moyer, A.	Private	I, 7th Infantry	MI	August 5, 1862	3353
Murch, Charles	Private	11, U.S. Infantry	US	August 5, 1862	3351
Murphy, James	Private	E, 5th Infantry	NJ	July 19, 1862	3299
Neil, John F.	Private	C, 56th Infantry	VT	November 24, 1864	3513
Neiman, John A.	Private	H, 51st Infantry	PA	August 5, 1864	3436
Newman, Benjamin	Private	A, 110th Infantry	PA	July 12, 1864	3416
Nichols, Joseph	Private	E, 1st Sharpshooters	MI	September 8, 1864	3460
O'Hara, Patrick	Private	A, 52nd Infantry	NY	July 25, 1864	3426
Oliver, George	Private	B, 13th Infantry	IN	May 24, 1865	3542

Name	Rank	Company and Regiment	State	Death of Death	Cypress Hills Plot Number
Owens, James	Private	B, 22nd U.S. Colored	US	October 21, 1864	3500
Partridge, William H.	Private	H, 33rd S.V.	NY	August 8, 1862	3349
Peck, Alpheus	Private	K, 142nd Infantry	NY	June 15, 1865	3552
Pedley, James	Private	G, 76th Infantry	NY	July 31, 1864	3434
Pendell, Benjamin D.	Private	H, 15th Infantry	MI	May 22, 1865	3539
Pennington, James	Private	B, 7th U.S. Colored	US	December 24, 1864	3516
Phipps, Joseph	Private	E, 8th Heavy Artillery	NY	August 9, 1864	3445
Pierson, Frank	Private	H, 4th Infantry	ME	August 8, 1862	3354
Ponet, James H.	Private	H, 13th Cavalry	OH	August 11, 1864	3447
Pouler, Joseph	Private	A, 1st Heavy Artillery	ME	July 14, 1864	3418
Quigley, Joseph B.	Private	D, 116th Infantry	PA	July 2, 1864	3399
Reynolds, Leonard	Private	C, 115th Infantry	NY	July 5, 1865	3565
Rice, Orson E.	Sergeant	B, 37th Infantry	WI	August 15, 1864	3450
Rivers, Alfred	Private	C, 38th Infantry	WI	July 6, 1864	3397
Robb, Charles H.	Private	E, 93rd Infantry	PA	July 10, 1862	3334
Roberts, George H.	Private	A, 44th Infantry	NY	February 1, 1863	3360
Roberts, George J.	Private	A, 11th Infantry	PA	July 23, 1862	3320
Robin, Augustus	Private	B, 7th Infantry	NH	October 30, 1864	3508
Robinson, John	Private	F, 88th Infantry	NY	July 8, 1862	3333
Rowe, Eli	Private	H, 3rd Infantry	ME	September 3, 1862	3367
Rows, H.	Private	E, 9th Infantry	MI	August 18, 1862	3346
Rubner, Andrew(s)	Private	B, 74th Infantry	NY	July 27, 1862	3314
Rudolph, Emmor E.	Private	E, 203rd Infantry	PA	June 21, 1865	3554
Sadowski, Frank	Private	B, 4th Heavy Artillery	NH	July 8, 1864	3412
Sailor, S.W.	Private	H, 69th Infantry	PA	July 26, 1862	3289
Sargent, Aaron	Private	G, 98th Infantry	NY	October 22, 1864	3498
Sargent, William	Private	I, 27th Infantry	NJ	February 28, 1863	3373
Scott, Alexander	Private	E, 25th Infantry	OH	December 10, 1862	3337
Sears, Benjamin	Private	G, 17th Infantry	NY	July 6, 1865	3567
Seigel, Noah W.	Private	A, 23rd Infantry	NC	July 12, 1862	3321
Shampine, J.	Private	I, 60th Infantry	NY	September 22, 1862	3343
Sharp, Joseph	Private	E, 14th Heavy Artillery	NY	September 8, 1864	3461
Simpkins, Silvanus	Private	D, 7th Infantry	NJ	July 10, 1862	3332
Smith E.	Private	F, 105th Infantry	NY	September 15, 1862	3287
Smith, Frederick E.	Private	H, 37th Infantry	VT	April 14, 1863	3384
Smith, John	Private	B, 11th Infantry	NJ	November 14, 1863	3376
Spear, Samuel	Private	I, 113th Infantry	IN	July 12, 1865	3570
Speckman, John	Private	G, 27th Infantry	MI	July 16, 1864	3420
Stacy, Thomas	Private	C, 3rd Infantry	MD	September 11, 1862	3364
Stearns, Oscar R.	Private	I, 76th Infantry	PA	May 10, 1865	3532
Stevens, Victor	Private	H, 57th Infantry	PA	July 24, 1862	3297
Stewart, James	Private	28th Infantry	MI	May 2, 1865	3529
Strunk, William C.	Private	G, 56th Infantry	PA	August 12, 1864	3446
Sullivan, Willis	Private	A, 83rd Infantry	IN	May 2, 1865	3506
Sutton, Jones	Private	15th Battery	IN	June 2, 1865	3545
Swallow, William	Private	F, 74th Infantry	OH	July 6, 1865	3566
Sweet, Joseph L.	Private	D, 11th Infantry	ME	July 7, 1862	3324
Swingle, David M.L.	Private	A, 62nd Infantry	OH	December 1, 1864	3514
Tarbox, William S.	Private	A, 32nd Infantry	ME	August 17, 1864	3453
Taylor, J.W.	Private	G, 4th Infantry	ME	July 7, 1862	3328
Taylor, Joseph	Bugler	E, Berdan's 1st U.S.S.S.	US	June 17, 1864	3403
Thompson, Henry	Private	A, 1st U.S. Colored	US	October. 14, 1864	3480
Tiffany, J.	Private	H, 31st Infantry	NY	August 12, 1862	3356
Tilson, Sylvester	Private	C, 109th Infantry	NY	August 7, 1864	3437
Tindale, Michael	Private	E, 1st Light Artillery	NJ	October 22, 1864	3503
Tolman, Moses B.	Private	G, 1st Heavy Artillery	ME	July 31, 1864	3431
Tucker, Andrew J.	Private	F, 7th Infantry	IN	September 24, 1864	3470

Appendix B

Name	Rank	Company and Regiment	State	Death of Death	Cypress Hills Plot Number
Tuttle, Michael	Private	5th Battery	NJ	October 22, 1864	3503
VanValkinburg, Jacob	Private	K, 169th Infantry	NY	July 29, 1865	3574
Van Zandt, Jacob	Private	C, 16th Heavy Artillery	NY	May 16, 1865	3534
Vaughn, Robert	Corporal	G, 134th Infantry	NY	August 2, 1863	3380
Vickery, Thomas W.	Private	C, 24th Cavalry	NY	June 30, 1864	3394
Vinet, Fabien	Private	B, 7th Heavy Artillery	NY	July 6, 1864	3408
Vopper, Francis	Private	F, 6th Infantry	NJ	October 12, 1862	3309
Wagner, Jacob	Private	I, 97th Infantry	PA	July 20, 1865	3573
Walsh, Michael	Corporal	G, 164th Infantry	NY	September 15, 1864	3484
Walther, Phillip	Musician	E, 151st Infantry	NY	August 18, 1863	3378
Waltman, Sylvanus	Private	A, 97th Infantry	PA	April 29, 1865	3526
Ward, Ebenezer	Private	B, 31st Infantry	ME	September 9, 1864	3465
Webster, James	Private	H, 123rd Infantry	IN	June 29, 1865	3561
Wentworth, John C.	Private	E, 11th Infantry	NH	August 17, 1864	3452
Wescott, Asa	Private	F, 147th Infantry	NY	July 25, 1863	3382
Wheeler, Ethan A.	Private	K, 4th Infantry	VT	October 8, 1862	3285
Wheeler, John R.	Private	A, 81st Infantry	NY	July 12, 1862	3291
Whitaker, Edward W.	Sergeant	F, 10th Heavy Artillery	NY	August 2, 1864	3435
White, Edward	Private	F, 22nd U.S. Colored	US	April 6, 1865	3520
White, William C.	Private	D, 6th Cavalry	MI	June 21, 1864	3402
Whitmore, Alonzo	Private	K, 22nd Cavalry	NY	August 21, 1864	3444
Whitmore, David	Private	D, 12th Infantry	MI	November 13, 1862	3342
Wiggins, Charles R.	Private	I, 104th Infantry	PA	July 16, 1862	3303
Wilcox, William	Private	I, 56th Infantry	NY	August 24, 1862	3366
Wilcox, William	Private	A, 2nd Heavy Artillery	NY	August 15, 1864	3451
Wilkerson, Lewis	Private	K, 74th Infantry	OH	June 8, 1865	3549
Williams, D.C.	Private	E, 35th Infantry	NC	June 26, 1864	3389
Williams, Edward	Private	G, 150th Infantry	NY	June 11, 1865	3547
Williams, John	Private	D, 12th Infantry	NY	July 7, 1864	3410
Williams, S.	Private	A, 49th Infantry	NY	July 6, 1862	3317
Williams, William	Corporal	K, 6th U.S. Colored	US	January 18, 1865	3438
Wilson, Henry	Private	B, 11th Infantry	PA	July 5, 1864	3396
Wilson, John	Private	B, 1st Infantry	MI	September 13, 1862	3363
Wisbaugh, Henry	Private	F, 76th Infantry	PA	October 30, 1864	3507
Wolfe, Frederick	Private	E, 72nd Infantry	PA	July 22, 1862	3295
Wright, John G.	Private	B, 7th Infantry	VT	July 7, 1862	3316
Yeoman, Samuel F.G.	Private	G, 2nd M.R.	NY	July 11, 1864	3415
Yorlet, Henry	Private	F, 93rd Infantry	PA	July 10, 1862	3335

Notes

1. The following civilians were buried at Portsmouth Grove and were removed to Cypress Hills National Cemetery:

Cassiedo, William F.L.	Citizen	Occupation unknown	July 17, 1865	3572
Emerson, John	Citizen	Construction corps	July 1, 1865	3562
Hastie, John	Citizen	Son of Thomas, soldier	March 19, 1865	3278

2. Three unknown soldiers of the 11th U.S. Colored were listed as buried at Portsmouth Grove in October 1865, although four unknown gravesites (3369, 3440, 3505, and 3551) were found amongst the Portsmouth Grove Hospital soldiers now interred at Cypress Hills National Cemetary.

3. Green Grindstaff remains somewhat of a mystery. His name appears as Co. L, 3rd RI Cavalry in the Adjutant General Report of the State of RI, but there is no corroborating evidence, including census records, to support this entry. Grindstaffs were in the Kentucky area at the time of the Civil War.

Source: Records of the Adjutant General — Roll of Honor / Burials, Nov. 14, 1865, Box 337 — RISA, located at the Office of the Secretary of State, A. Ralph Mollis State Archives Division. Plot numbers of gravesites obtained by author's visual inspection on April 23 and 24, 2010. Glenn Russell assisted with researching the soldiers and their names, but the author takes full responsibility for final name decisions.

Appendix C

Map of Cypress Hills National Cemetery

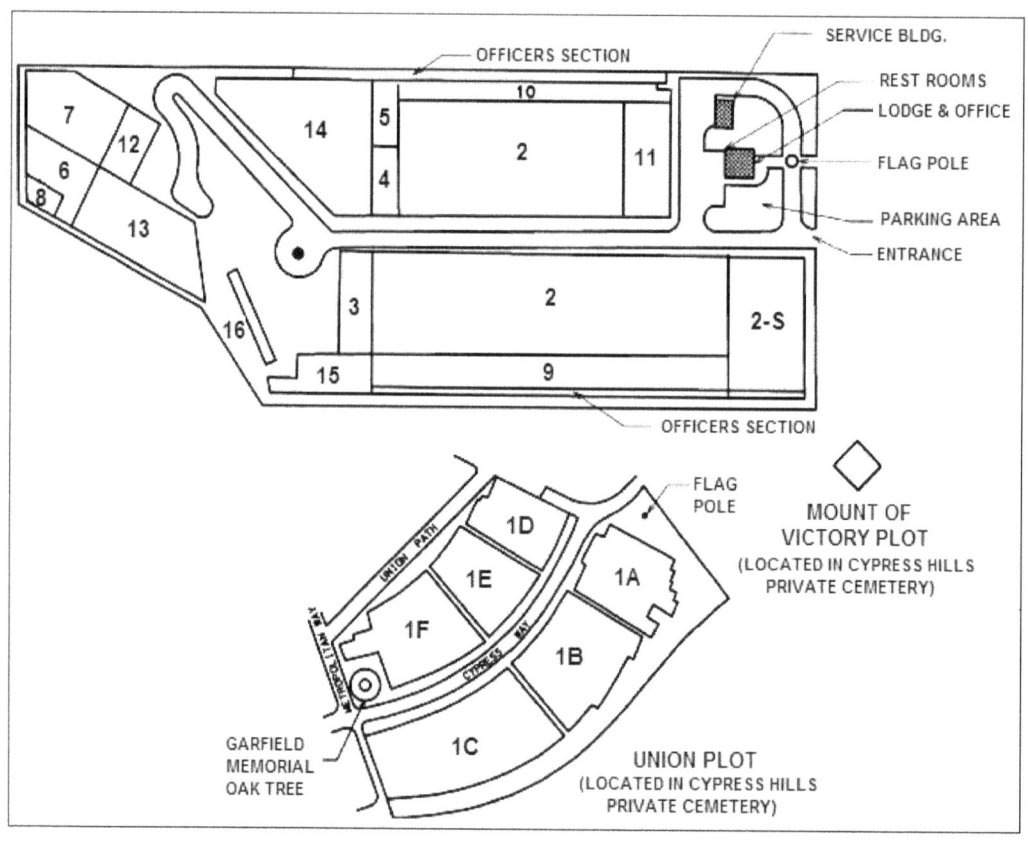

Source: United States Department of Veterans Affairs; Cypress Hills National Cemetery, Jamaica Avenue, Brooklyn, New York.

Notes

Chapter 1

1. See http://www.ri.net/schoolsPortsmouth/Admin/town.htm.
2. Seebert J. Goldowsky, M.D., "The Hospital at Portsmouth Grove," November 1959, 739 (paper presented before the Providence Medical Historical Society and the Benjamin Waterhouse Medical History Society at Boston, MA, on March 16, 1959, and later published in the *Rhode Island Medical Journal*).

Chapter 2

1. George Worthington Adams, *Doctors in Blue: The Medical History of the Union Army in the Civil War* (New York: Henry Schuman, 1952), 149.
2. Ibid.
3. Stephen O. Rogers, Letters, letter to his father and mother from Portsmouth Grove (PG), January 3, 1864, Abraham Lincoln Presidential Library & Museum.
4. James I. Robertson, Jr., and the Editors of Time-Life Books, *Tenting Tonight: The Soldier's Life* (Alexandria, VA: Time-Life Books, 1984), 97.
5. *Newport Advertiser*, October 25, 1862.
6. Noah Brooks, *Washington, D.C. in Lincoln's Time* (Chicago: Quadrangle Books, 1971), 17.
7. Page Smith, *Trial by Fire: A People's History of the Civil War and Reconstruction* (New York: McGraw-Hill, 1982), 409.
8. Alfred Jay Bollet, M.D., *Civil War Medicine: Challenges and Triumphs* (Tucson: Galen Press, 2002), 28; Samuel Wiessell Gross, M.D., *A Manual of Military Surgery; or, Hints on the Emergencies of Field Camp, and Hospital Practice* (Philadelphia: J.B. Lippincott, 1862; reprinted by Applewood Books, Bedford, MA), 3–5; Adams, *Doctors in Blue*, 47, 175.
9. Gross, *A Manual of Military Surgery*, 21.
10. See http://www.civilwarhome.com/civilwarmedicine.htm.
11. James M. McPherson, *Battle Cry of Freedom: The Civil War Era* (New York: Oxford University Press, 2003), 415.
12. Reid Mitchell, *Civil War Soldiers: Their Expectations and Their Experiences* (New York: Viking Penguin, 1988), 61.
13. See http://www.civilwarhome.com/civilwarmedicine.htm; McPherson, *Battle Cry of Freedom*, 415.
14. See http://www.history.com/topics/women-in-the-civil-war.
15. Adams, *Doctors in Blue*, 159–160.
16. Ibid., 161.
17. See http://www.wtv-zone.com/civilwar/dysentery.html.
18. See http://civilwarlibrarian.blogspot.com/2010/03news-did-doctors-perscription-cause.html. In his book *Did Lincoln Own Slaves?*, Gerald J. Prokopowicz stated that the pill contained "about nine thousand times more mercury than is now considered safe to ingest." His source datum was not provided; therefore this astounding number was not mentioned in the text.
19. See http://vermontcivilwar.org/medic/medicine2.php. An excellent summation by Ms. King that provides not only the Civil War physician's understanding of the illness and their prescribed treatments but also current knowledge and revised treatment for the conditions outlined.
20. See http://www.ncbi.nlm.nib.gov/pmc/articles/PMC2526887/pdf/tacca200101-0287.pdf.
21. Michael J. Varhola, *Everyday Life during the Civil War: A Guide for Writers, Students and Historians* (Cincinnati: Writer's Digest Books, 1999), 171–172.
22. Bollet, *Civil War Medicine*, 365.
23. Gross, *A Manual of Military Surgery*, 169.
24. Ibid., 49.
25. George Winston Smith, *Medicines for the Union Army: The United States Army Laboratories during the Civil War* (New York: Pharmaceutical Products Press, 2001), 130.
26. Ibid., 136.
27. Ibid.
28. Adams, *Doctors in Blue*, 140.
29. Whitman W. Bosworth, Letters, letter to his parents from Portsmouth Grove (PG), August 21, 1863, author's collection.
30. Bosworth, Letters, letter to his parents from PG, June 26, 1863, author's collection.
31. Bollet, *Civil War Medicine*, 91.
32. See http://www.civilwarhome.com/civilwarmedicine.htm.
33. Adams, *Doctors in Blue*, 168.
34. Ibid., 144.

35. Stephen B. Oates, *A Woman of Valor: Clara Barton and the Civil War* (New York: Free Press, 1994), 45.
36. Ibid.
37. See http://www.emedicinehealth.com/gangrene/article_em.htm.
38. See http://www.civilwarhome.com/civilwarmedicine.htm.
39. Adams, *Doctors in Blue*, 145.
40. Ibid., 141.
41. Robertson, *Tenting Tonight*, 97.
42. Bollet, *Civil War Medicine*, 236.
43. Bosworth, Letters, letter to his parents from Hammond General Hospital (HGH), January 25, 1863, author's collection.
44. Adams, *Doctors in Blue*, 147.
45. David Williams, *A People's History of the Civil War: Struggles for the Meaning of Freedom* (New York: New Press, 2005), 235–236.
46. Julian E. Kuz, M.D., and Bradley P. Bengtson, M.D., *Orthopaedic Injuries of the Civil War: An Atlas of Orthopaedic Injuries and Treatments during the Civil War* (Kennesaw, GA: Kennesaw Mountain Press, 1996), 16.

Chapter 3

1. The land previously occupied by the Marine Hospital on the Providence-Cranston boarder became the site of Rhode Island Hospital. Rhode Island Hospital has expanded immensely since the original building was demolished in 1956.
2. John T. Pierce, Sr., *Historical Tracts of the Town of Portsmouth, Rhode Island* (Portsmouth, RI: Hamilton Printing, 1991), 70.
3. Goldowsky, "The Hospital at Portsmouth Grove," 735.
4. *Newport Daily News*, July 9, 1862.
5. Richard M. Bayles, ed., *History of Newport County, Rhode Island* (New York: L.E. Preston, 1888), 614.
6. Thomas Williams Bicknell, LL.D., *The History of the State of Rhode Island and Providence Plantations*, vol. 3 (New York: American Historical Society, 1920), 1190.
7. Bayles, *The History of Newport County*, 615.
8. Ibid.
9. Ibid.
10. Ibid.
11. Pierce, *Historical Tracts*, 34.
12. "Historic and Architectural Resources of Portsmouth, Rhode Island: A Preliminary Report," Rhode Island Historical Preservation Commission, 1979, page 4.
13. Ibid.
14. Pierce, *Historical Tracts*, 61.
15. Rhode Island Black Heritage Society, ed., *African-Americans in Newport: An Introduction to the Heritage of African-Americans in Newport, Rhode Island [1700–1945]* (Rhode Island Historical Preservation & Heritage Commission, c. 1995), 3.
16. John M. Lovejoy, Letters, letter to his mother from Portsmouth Grove (PG), May 3, 1863, author's collection.
17. *Newport Daily News* editors, *Newport, and How to See It, with List of Summer Residents* (Newport: Davis & Pitman, 1873), 3.

18. Town Records, Office of the Town Clerk, Portsmouth, RI, *Land Evidence Book No. 14*, May 15, 1862, 360.
19. Thomas Coggeshall, Jr., Letter to unknown recipient from Middletown, RI, July 9, 1862, Newport Historical Society. *Newport Daily News*, July 9, 1862.
20. Joseph K. Barnes, Surgeon General, USA, by direction, *The Medical and Surgical History of the War of the Rebellion* (1861–1865) (Washington: Government Printing Office [Second Issue, 1875]), 939.
21. Russell F. Weigley, *Quartermaster General of the Union Army* (New York: Columbia University Press, 1959), 271.

Chapter 4

1. Geoffrey C. Ward with Ric Burns and Ken Burns, *The Civil War: An Illustrated History* (New York: Alfred A. Knopf, 1990), 90.
2. John C. Waugh, *Lincoln and McClellan: The Troubled Partnership between a President and His General* (New York: Palgrave Macmillan, 2010), 83.
3. *The Civil War Society's Encyclopedia of the Civil War* (New York: Portland House, 1997), 273.
4. Oates, *A Woman of Valor*, 45.
5. Ward and Burns, *The Civil War*, 139.
6. Stephen A. Wynalda, *366 Days in Abraham Lincoln's Presidency: The Private, Political, and Military Decisions of America's Greatest President* (New York: A Herman Graf Book, Skyhorse Publishing, 2010), 176.
7. *Warren Gazette*, October 11, 1899.
8. Colonel H. Crandall, *Annual Report of the Adjutant General of the State of Rhode Island, for the Year 1865* (Providence: Providence Press, Printers of the State, 1866), 722.
9. Richard Wheeler, *Sword Over Richmond: An Eyewitness History of McClellan's Peninsula Campaign* (New York: Harper & Row, 1986), 308.
10. National Archives and Records Administration, Alfred Luther Pension File Certificate No. 11,055.
11. Wheeler, *Sword Over Richmond*, 308.
12. NARA, Luther Pension File.
13. The First Rhode Island Light Artillery suffered the second highest casualty rate for a Rhode Island unit during the war. Only the 7th Regiment Rhode Island Volunteers could claim a higher number.
14. Goldowsky, "The Hospital at Portsmouth Grove," 736.
15. *Newport Mercury*, July 12, 1862.
16. William S. Dennett, Transcription, May 3 and July 4, 1862, Special Collections, University of Virginia Library. This account and those that follow were taken from a transcription likely originating from a diary.
17. Marjorie Barstow Greenbie, *Lincoln's Daughters of Mercy* (New York: Putnam's, 1944), 140–141.
18. Dennett, Transcription, UVL, May 3, 1862.
19. Goldowsky, "The Hospital at Portsmouth Grove," 736–737.
20. Ibid., 733.
21. Ibid., 736. Goldowsky writes that "two died en route and were buried at sea." Another account, which appears more credible, states that one was buried at Yorktown before departure while another was buried at sea.
22. See http://www.arlingtoncemetery.net/gmsternb.htm.
23. *Newport Daily News*, July 7, 1862.

24. Oates, *A Woman of Valor*, 47.
25. *Providence Journal*, July 7, 1862, and *Newport Daily News*, July 7, 1862.
26. *Newport Daily News*, July 7, 1862.
27. Ibid.; Goldowsky, "The Hospital at Portsmouth Grove," 737.
28. Coggeshall, Letter, July 7, 1862, NHS.
29. *Newport Daily News*, July 7, 1862.
30. Goldowsky, "The Hospital at Portsmouth Grove," 733.
31. *Newport Daily News*, July 7, 1862.
32. Goldowsky, "The Hospital at Portsmouth Grove," 733.
33. *Newport Daily News*, July 7, 1862.
34. Ibid.
35. Goldowsky, "The Hospital at Portsmouth Grove," 733.
36. *Newport Daily News*, July 7, 1862.
37. The Coggeshall surname is prominent on the Island today. Decedents can be traced back prior to Colonial days.
38. Coggeshall, Letter, July 9, 1862, NHS.
39. St. Paul's Episcopal Church, *Record Journal, Burials by G.W. Chevers, Rector, 1862, July 7- 9.*
40. Goldowsky, "The Hospital at Portsmouth Grove," 735.
41. In the second half of the twentieth century, writers confused Dr. Francis L. Wheaton with his son General Frank Wheaton, erroneously publishing the son's picture with the father's story. Both men served in the Second Rhode Island Volunteers, and their similar first names may have lead to the confusion. Frank's career was more illustrious, as he rose through the ranks during the war and afterward was hailed as a hero in his home state of Rhode Island.
42. *Newport Daily News*, July 14, 1862.
43. Ibid., July 9, 1862.
44. *Newport Mercury*, July 12, 1862.
45. Goldowsky, "The Hospital at Portsmouth Grove," 737.
46. Coggeshall, Letter, July 9, 1862, NHS.
47. See http://www.mayoclinic.com/health/typhoid-fever/DS00538.
48. See http://www.civilwarhome.com/civilwarmedicine.htm.
49. Ward, *The Civil War*, 132.
50. *Providence Journal*, July 10, 1862.
51. Ibid.; also, Goldowsky, "The Hospital at Portsmouth Grove," 737.
52. Dennett, Transcription, July 10, 1862, UVL.
53. Pierce, *Historical Tracts*, 70.
54. Crandall, *Annual Report*, 822–827.
55. *Newport Daily News*, July 22, 1862.
56. Ibid.
57. *Bristol Phenix*, July 19, 1862.
58. *Newport Daily News*, July 29, 1862.
59. Daniel Henry Austin, Diary, August 16, 1864, Rhode Island Civil War Round Table (RICWRT) monthly newsletter *Monthly Return* 11, no. 1 (June 2002) and no. 2 (September 2002).
60. George H. Peck, Diary, June 27, July 8, 18, August 5, 14, October 19, 1863, George H. Peck Miscellaneous Manuscripts, MSS 9001-P, Rhode Island Historical Society.
61. Drew Gilpin Faust, *This Republic of Suffering: Death and the American Civil War* (New York: Alfred A. Knopf, 2008), 92.
62. *Providence Journal*, September 15, 1862.
63. Crandall, *Annual Report*, 325.
64. Goldowsky, "The Hospital at Portsmouth Grove," 737.
65. Rhode Island State Archives, Records of the Adjutant General, Special Requisitions, Portsmouth Grove Hospital, 1862, documents dated July 12 and 19, 1862; *Bristol Phenix*, July 19, 1862.
66. *Bristol Phenix*, July 12, 1862.
67. Dennett, Transcription, July 10, 1862, UVL.

Chapter 5

1. Pierce, *Historical Tracts*, 70.
2. Ibid.
3. *Newport Daily News*, July 9, 1862.
4. Ibid.
5. Ibid.
6. Ibid.
7. Ibid.
8. Ibid.
9. *Newport Daily News*, July 7, 1862.
10. *Newport Daily News*, July 9, 1862.
11. *Providence Journal*, September 12, 1862.
12. D.C. Denham, "Lovell General Hospital as I Remember It," *Newport Mercury*, March 26, 1898.
13. *Newport Daily News*, July 26, 1862.
14. Ibid., July 10, 1862.
15. Ibid., July 26, 1862.
16. Ibid., July 14, 1862.
17. Ibid.
18. Ibid., July 14, 18 and 19, 1862.
19. Ibid., July 14, 1862.
20. Ibid.
21. *Bristol Phenix*, July 12, 1862.
22. James Campi, Jr., *Civil War Battlefields, Then and Now* (Berkeley, CA: Thunder Bay Press, 2008), quotation taken from inside flyleaf of dust jacket.
23. *Newport Daily News*, July 14, 1862.
24. Ibid., July 15, 1862.
25. *Bristol Phenix*, July 19, 1862.
26. Francis T. Miller, ed., *The Photographic History of the Civil War*, vol. 4, *Soldier Life and Secret Service: Prisons and Hospitals* (Secaucus, NJ: Blue & Grey Press, 1987), 295.
27. *Newport Advertiser*, July 24, 1862.
28. Ibid.
29. *Bristol Phenix*, July 26, 1862.
30. Whitman W. Bosworth, Letters, letter to his parents from PG, July 12, 1863, author's collection.
31. Ibid. Various letters were used to obtain the stated information. All are in the author's collection.
32. *Providence Journal*, July 12, 1862.
33. Peck, Diary, MSS 9001-P, August 2, 1864, RIHS.
34. Rogers, Letters, letter to his father and mother from PG, January 2, 1864, ALPLM.
35. Varhola, *Everyday Life*, 87–89.
36. Bosworth, Letters, letter to his parents from PG, July 15, 1863, author's collection.
37. Ibid., July 22, 1863.
38. Bosworth, Letters, letter to his parents from PG, August 30 and September 9, 1863, author's collection.
39. *Newport Daily News*, July 30, 1862.
40. *Bristol Phenix*, September 13, 1862.
41. Ibid.
42. *Providence Journal*, July 10, 1862. The full con-

tent of Bishop Clark's letter makes informative reading. Though one man's opinion, it certainly offers a significant defense in consideration of Dr. Wheaton's choices and leadership that infamous day.
43. *Newport Daily News*, July 14, 1862.
44. Goldowsky, "The Hospital at Portsmouth Grove," 738. The full content of Surgeon General Vanderpool's letter was published in the *Providence Journal*, July 14, 1862.
45. *Newport Daily News*, July 16, 1862.
46. Ibid.
47. *Providence Evening Press*, July 26, 1862.
48. Ibid., July 24, 1862; *Newport Daily News*, July 27, 1862.
49. Goldowsky, "The Hospital at Portsmouth Grove," 738.
50. Francis L. Wheaton, 1862, Francis L. Wheaton Miscellaneous Manuscripts, MSS 9001-W, Rhode Island Historical Society. Dr. Seebert Goldowsky's account states that Dr. Wheaton spent the remaining three years in the Washington, D.C., area as a brigade surgeon and mustered out of the service at war's end. No documentation was found to support this contention, but a reference to Dr. Wheaton's discharge on September 12, 1862, was found in the aforementioned file.
51. *Newport Daily News*, August 1, 1862.
52. *Newport Advertiser*, August 14, 1862; Goldowsky, "The Hospital at Portsmouth Grove," 738.
53. *Newport Daily News*, August 12, 1862.

Chapter 6

1. *Newport Daily News*, July 15, 1862.
2. Ibid., July 28, 1862.
3. Dennett, Transcription, July 10, 1862, UVL.
4. *Bristol Phenix*, August 9, 1862.
5. Georgeanna Woolsey Bacon and Eliza Woolsey Howland, *Letters of a Family during the War for the Union, 1861–1865* (Charleston, SC: Bibliolife, 2010), 498. The Woolsey ladies served as nurses during the war, except for Abby, who worked tirelessly for the U.S. Sanitary Commission.
6. Robert Grandchamp, *From Providence to Fort Hell: Letters from Company K, Seventh Rhode Island Volunteers* (Westminster, MD: Heritage Books, 2008), 34–35.
7. John F. Austin, Letters, letter to his wife Emily from Portsmouth Grove (PG), January 27, 1863, John F. Austin Collection, MSS 272, Rhode Island Historical Society.
8. *Newport Daily News*, July 7 and 22, 1862.
9. Peck, Diary, MSS 9001-P, November 27, 1864, RIHS.
10. Ibid., January 1, 1864.
11. Ibid.
12. Ibid., January 11, 1864.
13. Ibid., March 18, 1864.
14. Rogers, Letters, letter to his father and mother from PG, January 3, 1864, ALPLM.
15. Seth H. Alden, Letters, letter to his sister from Portsmouth Grove (PG), March 28, 1863, Hamilton College Library.
16. Peck, Diary, MSS 9001-P, February 22, 1864, RIHS.
17. Bacon and Howland, *Letters of a Family*, 498.
18. Peck, Diary, MSS 9001-P, January 11, 1864, RIHS.
19. Ibid., February 20, 1864.
20. Dennett, Transcription, December 5, 1861, UVL.
21. Denham, "Lovell General Hospital."
22. John Hill Merrill, letter to his wife Mollie from Camp Barry, Washington, D.C., December 27, 1862.
23. Peck, Diary, MSS 9001-P, May 28, 1864, RIHS.
24. Ibid., August 13, 1864.
25. Ibid., May 3, 1864.
26. Ibid., May 30, 1864.
27. Ibid., January 29, 1865.
28. Bosworth, Letters, letter to his parents from PG, August 7, 1863, author's collection.
29. Ibid., January 25, 1863.
30. Peck, Diary, MSS 9001-P, November 13, 1864, RIHS.
31. Peck, Diary, listed on end pages after February 28, 1865, final diary entry, MSS 9001-P, RIHS.
32. Rogers, Letters, letter to his father and mother from PG, January 2, 1864, ALPLM.
33. Bacon and Howland, *Letters of a Family*, 498.
34. See http//www.civilwarhome.com/sanitarycommission.htm.
35. *The U.S. Sanitary Commission of the United States Army: A Succinct Narrative of its Works and Purposes* (New York: Published for the Benefit of the United States Sanitary Commission, 1864), 83.
36. Oates, *A Woman of Valor*, 32.
37. *Newport Advertiser*, March 26, 1863.
38. Because of resource limitations, the State of Rhode Island and Providence Plantations, Office of the Secretary of State (Archives), still has cardboard boxes of historical documents to sift through. Someday the building contractor's name may surface and clear up this slight mystery.
39. Margaret E. Wagner, Gary W. Gallagher, and Paul Finkelman, eds., *The Library of Congress Civil War Desk Reference* (New York: Grand Central Press Book/Simon & Schuster, 2002), 628.
40. Bollet, *Civil War Medicine*, 219.
41. U.S. Sanitary Commission, extracted from footnotes at bottom of page.
42. Bollet, *Civil War Medicine*, 219.
43. Barnes, *The Medical and Surgical History*, 938.
44. Bacon and Howland, *Letters of a Family*, 501.
45. *Newport Daily News*, August 18, 1862.
46. Adams, *Doctors in Blue*, 161.
47. Rhode Island State Archives, Records of the Adjutant General, Portsmouth Grove Hospital, Quarter Master General Correspondence, 1862, Box 4, document dated August 20, 1862.
48. RISA, PG, Q.M. General Correspondence, document dated August 21, 1862.
49. Ibid., August 23, 1862.
50. Ibid., September 11, 1862.
51. Ibid., August 21-November 1862.
52. Ibid., September 6, 1862.
53. Goldowsky, "The Hospital at Portsmouth Grove," 739; Barnes, *The Medical and Surgical History*, 953.
54. RISA, PG, Q.M. General Correspondence, document dated September 16, 1862.
55. Ibid., November 27, 1862.
56. Ibid., December 11, 1862.
57. Goldowsky, "The Hospital at Portsmouth Grove," 739.
58. RISA, PG, Q.M. General Correspondence, document dated October 20, 1862.

59. Pierce, *Historical Tracts*, 71; Thomas E. Greene, "The Post Office at Portsmouth Grove, Rhode Island," *Rhode Island Postal History Journal* 12, no. 3 (July–October 2000).
60. *Newport Daily News*, August 18, 1862.
61. Goldowsky, "The Hospital at Portsmouth Grove," 739.
62. Pierce, *Historical Tracts*, 73.
63. Barnes, *The Medical and Surgical History*, 939.
64. *Providence Journal*, September 27, 1862.

Chapter 7

1. Crandall, *Annual Report*, 353.
2. *Providence Journal*, July 12, 1862. Chartered on February 1, 1741, by King George II, the Newport Artillery Company is the oldest military organization in America.
3. Crandall, *Annual Report*, 354.
4. Ibid.
5. Peck, Diary, MSS 9001-P, April 19, 1864, RIHS.
6. Ibid., October 20–21, 1864.
7. Crandall, *Annual Report*, 354.
8. Peck, Diary, MSS 9001-P, June 24, 1864, RIHS.
9. Ibid., September 22, 1864.
10. Alden, Letters, letter to his cousin from PG, March 27, 1863, HCL.
11. Peck, Diary, May 17, 1864, MSS 9001-P, RIHS.
12. Rogers, Letters, letter to his father and mother from PG, February 9, 1864, ALPLM.
13. Peck, Diary, MSS 9001-P, February 26, 1864, RIHS.
14. Ibid., February 24, 1864.
15. Patients detailed to dry scrub used sand as an abrasive rather than cleaning the traditional way with soap and water because wet scrubbing was thought to increase the risk of tetanus.
16. Peck, Diary, MSS 9001-P, February 27, 1864, RIHS.
17. See http://footnote.com/page/3094_charles_william_cole_soldier/.
18. Bacon and Howland, *Letters of a Family*, 497.
19. Peck, Diary, MSS 9001-P, August 8, 1864, RIHS.
20. D.H. Austin, Diary, August 9, 1864, RICWRT.
21. Bollet, *Civil War Medicine*, 430.
22. Alden, Letters, letter to his sister from PG, June 8, 1863, HCL.
23. Ibid., June 14, 1863.
24. Bosworth, Letters, letter to his parents from PG, July 27, 1963, author's collection.
25. Ibid.
26. Ibid., August 21, 1863.
27. Ibid., July 27, 1863.
28. Ibid., August 14, 1863.
29. J. Lovejoy, Letters, letter to his cousin Cynthia from PG, June 18, 1863, author's collection.
30. Goldowsky, "The Hospital at Portsmouth Grove," 742. Goldowsky's account is taken from Circular No. 6, War Department, Surgeon General's Office, Washington, November 1, 1865: *Reports on the Extent and Nature of the Materials Available for the Preparation of a Medical and Surgical History of the Rebellion*, prepared by George Alexander Otis and Joseph Janvier Woodward of the U.S. Surgeon General's Office. The entire circular has been digitized and made available online by Google Books.
31. Ibid.
32. *Newport Daily News*, July 14, 1863.
33. Crandall, *Annual Report*, 722. *Newport Advertiser*, July 15, 1863.
34. Bosworth, Letters, letter to his parents from PG, August 4, 1863, author's collection.

Chapter 8

1. Ward, *The Civil War*, 190; Darryl Lyman, *Civil War Wordbook: Including Sayings, Phrases and Expletives* (Conshohocken, PA: Combined Books, 1994), 119, 141, 142, and 164.
2. Jane Stuart Woolsey, *Hospital Days: Reminiscence of a Civil War Nurse* (Rosedale, Minnesota: Edinborough Press, 2001), 32.
3. Gross, *A Manual of Military Surgery*, 142–143.
4. Goldowsky, "The Hospital at Portsmouth Grove," 741.
5. Ibid. This reference is cited in footnote of Goldowsky's article.
6. Peck, Diary, MSS 9001-P, January 9, 1865, RIHS.
7. *Newport Daily News*, July 26, 1862.
8. Ibid.
9. Ibid.
10. Bosworth, Letters, letter to his parents from PG, August 14, 1863, author's collection. Not to give away the story, the subtitle was not included. It said: "One Dog Killed."
11. Peck, Diary, MSS 9001-P, March 30, 1864, RIHS.
12. Ibid., April 28, 1864.
13. Ibid., May 1, 1864.
14. Ibid., May 30, 1864.
15. Ibid., September 25, 1864.
16. Ibid., September 4, 1864.
17. Ibid., October 12, 1864.
18. *Newport Daily News*, October 21, 1864.
19. Rogers, Letters, letter to his father and mother from PG, January 2, 1864, ALPLM.
20. Peck, Diary, January 5, 25, April 29, May 26, July 13, 23, August 29, September 25, October 15, 17, 26, 27, November 7, 8, 12, December 1 and 10, 1864, MSS 9001-P, RIHS.
21. Ibid., January 3, 1865.
22. Peck, Diary, MSS 9001-P, January 10, 1865, RIHS.
23. Ibid.
24. Ibid., January 9, 1865.
25. Ibid., January 24, 1865.
26. Ibid., February 9 and 10, 1865.
27. John D. Billings, *Hardtack and Coffee or the Unwritten Story of Army Life* (Boston: George M. Smith, 1887), 144.
28. See http://www.civilwarhome.com/discipline.htm.
29. Peck, Diary, MSS 9001-P, April 19, 1864, RIHS.
30. Ibid., June 13, 1864.
31. Ibid., June 7 and 9, 1864.
32. Ibid., September 1, 1864.
33. Ibid., October 23, 1864.
34. Ibid., December 12, 1864.
35. Ibid., January 19, 1865.
36. Maud Howe Elliott, *This was My Newport* (Cambridge, MA: Mythology, 1944), 60–62 (hereafter cited as Elliott, *This was My Newport*).
37. Pierce, *Historical Tracts*, 71.

Chapter 9

1. *Newport Daily News*, August 20, 1862; Elliott, *This was My Newport*, 149.
2. Designated as a national historic landmark, the country's oldest Jewish synagogue is also located on Touro Street. Built in 1759, it is known as Touro Synagogue.
3. Goldowsky, "The Hospital at Portsmouth Grove," 741.
4. *Newport Mercury*, August 4, 1866.
5. *Newport Daily News*, July 13, 1864.
6. Ibid., September 23, 1864.
7. The information was written on poster board and affixed to it a carte de visite of Mrs. Charity Slocum. The display is a possession of the Military Order of the Loyal Legion of the United States-Massachusetts Commandery Photograph Album Collection (MOLLUS-MASS Albums), vol. 82, page 4131, the U.S. Army Military History Institute, Carlisle Barracks, Pennsylvania. The note said: "She gave herself without stint for aid and relief from the beginning of the Rebellion to its close; a constant visitor at Portsmouth Grove Hospital."
8. The story was extracted from a handwritten undated account given to the author on March 3, 2010, by Ed Regan from stories told to his family by his great-grandmother, Agnes Wilbour Richardson, a nurse at the hospital.
9. *Newport Advertiser*, August 10 and September 3, 1862, and *Providence Journal*, September 2, 1862.
10. *Newport Daily News*, June 28, 1864.
11. Gross, *A Manual of Military Surgery*, 37.
12. *Newport Advertiser*, November 27, 1862.
13. Peck, MSS 9001-P, Diary, November 23, 1864, RIHS.
14. Ibid., November 24, 1864.
15. Ibid.
16. *Newport Daily News*, December 21, 1864.
17. *Newport Advertiser*, October 22, 1863.
18. Ibid., December 4, 1862.
19. *Bristol Phenix*, July 12, 1862.
20. *Newport Daily News*, January 7, 1863. Though impossible to substantiate, with a German accent and a reference to General Franz Sigel, the Union soldier may have been a member of the all–German 41st New York Infantry led by the general himself.
21. Ibid.
22. Nancy Jensen Devin and Richard V. Simpson, *Images of America: Portsmouth, Rhode Island* (Dover, NH: Arcadia Publishing, 1997), 6.

Chapter 10

1. *Bristol Phenix*, September 27, 1862.
2. See http://www.congressionalcemetery.org/PDF/Obits/E/Obits_Edwards.pdf.
3. Goldowsky, "The Hospital at Portsmouth Grove," 740.
4. *Providence Journal*, September 27, 1862.
5. Research documentation provided by Dr. Stephen Altic, D.O., extracted from the following source material: Ezra S. Stearns, *History of Rindge, New Hampshire, from the Date of the Rowley Canada or Massachusetts Charter to the Present time, 1739–1874, with a Genealogical Register of the Rindge Families* (Boston: Press of George H. Ellis, 1875), 369–370; Carded Medical File, Dr. E. Seyffarth, in custody of National Archives and Records Administration; and Barnes, *The Medical and Surgical History*, which includes multiple references to Dr. Seyffarth (vol. 7, 22; vol. 10, 647, 693, 768, 785, 791; vol. 11, 286; vol. 12, 459, 527, 532–533, 547, 549, 554, 672, 683).
6. *Newport Daily News*, July 30 and August 1, 1862.
7. Denham, "Lovell General Hospital."
8. J. Lovejoy, Letters, letter to his cousin Cynthia from PG, February 2, 1863, author's collection.
9. Crandall, *Annual Report*, 731.
10. NARA, Luther Pension File.
11. Walter K. Schroder, *Images of America: Dutch Island and Ft. Greble* (Dover, NH: Arcadia Publishing, 1998), 19.
12. See http://www.acwv.info/1-files-veterans/M/mceachern/mceachern.htm.
13. Charlotte F. Dailey, *Report upon the Disabled Rhode Island Soldiers; Their Names, Condition, and in What Hospital They Are* (Providence: Alfred Anthony, Printer to the State, 1863), 1–6.
14. Ibid., 6–24.
15. *Newport Daily News*, "The Grist Mill," taken from clippings consolidated in a folder at the Portsmouth Public Library.
16. *Providence Evening Press*, December 12, 1862, and initially reported in the *Boston Journal*.
17. J. Lovejoy, Letters, letter to his cousin Cynthia from PG, February 19, 1863, author's collection.
18. Bosworth, Letters, letter to his parents from PG, August 7, 1863, author's collection.
19. J. F. Austin, Letters, letter to his wife Emily from PG, January 27, 1863, MSS 272, RIHS.
20. See http://emergency.cdc.gov/agent/smallpox/overview/disease-facts.asp.
21. Goldowsky, "The Hospital at Portsmouth Grove," 740; Denham, "Lovell General Hospital."
22. Goldowsky, "The Hospital at Portsmouth Grove," 740.
23. J.F. Austin, Letters, letter to his wife Emily from PG, January 27, 1863, MSS 272, RIHS.
24. See http://www.who.int/mediacentre/factsheets/smallpox/en/; Bollet, *Civil War Medicine*, 291–292.
25. J. Lovejoy, Letters, letter to his cousin Cynthia from PG, February 2, 1863, author's collection.
26. Alden, Letters, letter to an unidentified recipient from PG, undated, HCL.
27. Alden, Letters, letter to his sister from PG, April 1, 1863, HCL; NARA, Seth H. Alden Pension File Certificate No. 384,990.
28. *Newport Advertiser*, January 29, 1863.
29. *Newport Daily News*, February 17, 1863.
30. Denham, "Lovell General Hospital"; see also http://www.whale.to/vaccines/tilden6.html.
31. *Newport Advertiser*, January 8, 1863.
32. Ibid., May 14, 1863. Several decades ago, smallpox was eradicated from the face of the earth after the World Health Organization instituted a massive program of inoculation to contain and eradicate the disease. Until then, the disease still existed in Africa and India. Only the United States and Russia are known to have laboratory samples for study in case of an unforeseen outbreak.
33. Peck, Diary, MSS 9001-P, December 8, 1864, RIHS.

34. Ibid., December 22, 1864, RIHS. Crandall, *Annual Report*, 356.
35. *Newport Daily News*, February 16, 1863.

Chapter 11

1. *Newport Daily News*, July 14, 1862; Goldowsky, "The Hospital at Portsmouth Grove," 741.
2. L.P. Brockett, M.D., and Mary C. Vaughan, *Woman's Work in the Civil War: A Record of Heroism, Patriotism and Patience* (Philadelphia: Zeigler, McCurdy, 1867), 318.
3. Laura L. Behling, ed., *Hospital Transports* (New York: State University of New York Press, 2005), 22.
4. Brockett and Vaughan, *Woman's Work in the Civil War*, 319.
5. Katherine Prescott Wormeley, *The Other Side of War with the Army of the Potomac* (Boston: Ticknor, 1889), 111.
6. Nancy Scripture Garrison, *With Courage and Delicacy — Civil War on the Peninsula: Women and the U.S. Sanitary Commission* (Cambridge, MA: Da Capo Press, 2003), 174.
7. Ibid., 175.
8. Brockett and Vaughan, *Woman's Work in the Civil War*, 322; Garrison, *With Courage and Delicacy*, 176.
9. Bacon and Howland, *Letters of a Family*, 480–482.
10. Garrison, *With Courage and Delicacy*, 175.
11. Bacon, *Letter of a Family*, 498.
12. Ibid., 495.
13. Ibid., 502.
14. *Providence Journal*, September 27, 1862.
15. *Newport Daily News*, November 13, 1862.
16. Katherine P. Wormeley, Letters, letter to "My dear friend," from Portsmouth Grove (PG), November 30, 1862, Special Collections and University Archives, Wichita State University Libraries, Kantor Collection of the U.S. Sanitary Commission.
17. Ibid.
18. Wormeley, Letters, letter to Mr. Knapp from PG, December 5, 1862, WSUL.
19. Garrison, *With Courage and Delicacy*, 177; Bacon and Howland, *Letters of a Family*, 503.
20. Bacon and Howland, *Letters of a Family*, 503–504.
21. Brockett and Vaughan, *Woman's Work in the Civil War*, 316–317.
22. Garrison, *With Courage and Delicacy*, 177.
23. *U.S. Sanitary Commission*, 268.
24. Brockett and Vaughan, *Woman's Work in the Civil War*, 323.
25. Goldowsky, "The Hospital at Portsmouth Grove," 740.
26. Denham, "Lovell General Hospital."
27. The image is from a photograph album presented by G.T. Clark to A.A. Brewster, 1865, now in the custody of Dr. Stephen Altic, D.O. Additional research by Dr. Altic extracted from Military Service Records, Rufus Messenger, 50th Pennsylvania Volunteers, in custody of the National Archives and Records Administration; Carded Medical File, Rufus Messenger, 5th Pennsylvania Volunteers, in custody of U.S. National Archives and Records Administration; *History of Pennsylvania Volunteers*, in custody of Samuel P. Bates; and Historical Data Systems, Inc.. Duxbury, MA.
28. See http://www.wickedlocal.com/Kingston/fun/entertainment/books/ x359572517/Library-news.
29. *Newport Mercury*, November 10, 1866.
30. Denham, "Lovell General Hospital."
31. Brockett and Vaughan, *Woman's Work in the Civil War*, 322.
32. See http://www.historynet.com/northern-volunteer-nurses-of-americas-civil-war.htm.
33. Varhola, *Everyday Life*, 38.
34. *Newport Advertiser*, November 13, 1862.
35. *Newport Mercury*, December 27, 1862.
36. Bacon and Howland, *Letters of a Family*, 499.
37. *Providence Journal*, September 27, 1862.
38. Ibid., October 29, 1862.
39. Goldowsky, "The Hospital at Portsmouth Grove," 740.
40. Rogers, Letters, letter to his father and mother from PG, January 2 and 3, 1864, ALPLM.
41. Oliver A. Ricker, Diary, April 23, 1863, *Civil War Correspondence, Diaries, and Journals at the Massachusetts Historical Society*, microfilm edition, reel 7, Massachusetts Historical Society, MHS (hereafter cited as Ricker, Diary, MHS).
42. Peck, Diary, MSS 9001-P, December 4 and 5, 1864, RIHS.
43. *Newport Daily News*, July 29 and August 4, 1862.
44. Alden, Letters, letter to his sister from PG, April 1, 1863, HCL.
45. Peck, Diary, MSS 9001-P, February 2, and 7, 1864, RIHS.
46. Ibid., December 4–5, 1864.
47. Denham, "Lovell General Hospital."
48. Alden, Letters, letter to his sister from PG, April 12, 1863, HCL.
49. Bacon and Howland, *Letters of a Family*, 500 and 501; *Newport Daily News*, November 4, 1864. The Reverend Proudfit's first name was found in articles published in the *Providence Journal*.
50. J. Lovejoy, Letters, letter to his cousin Cynthia from PG, April 30, 1863, author's collection.
51. Rogers, Letters, letter to his father and mother from PG, February 21, 1864, ALPLM.
52. Denham, "Lovell General Hospital."

Chapter 12

1. Bacon, *Letter of a Family*, 494.
2. Ibid., 495–496.
3. Oates, *A Woman of Valor*, 232–234.
4. *Newport Daily News*, January 12, 1862.
5. Ibid., January 10, 1863.
6. See http://rayscorner.ca/the_history_of_seth_c_vickery.htm.
7. Bacon, *Letter of a Family*, 495–496.
8. Ibid., 496.
9. Ibid., 498.
10. Andrew Jacobs, Letter, to Lieutenant Cottle from Portsmouth (PG), January 27, 1863, Special Collections & Archives [United States. Army. New Jersey Infantry Regiment. 1861–1864) Letters, 1862–1864], Ralph B. Draugton Library, Auburn University.
11. Ricker, Diary, February 17, 1863, MHS.
12. Alden, Letters, letter to his cousin from PG, March 31, 1863, HCL.
13. Bosworth, Letters, letter to his parent from PG, July 22, 1863, author's collection.

14. Ibid.
15. Bosworth, Letters, letter to his parents from HGH, January 25, 1863, author's collection.
16. *Newport Advertiser*, May 7, 1863.
17. Thomas M. Aldrich, *The History of Battery A, First Regiment Rhode Island Light Artillery in the War to Preserve the Union, 1861–1865* (Providence: Snow & Farnham, 1904), 393 and 401.
18. Pierce, *Historical Tracts*, 71.
19. Salvatore G. Cilella, Jr., *Upton's Regulars: The 121st New York Infantry in the Civil War* (Lawrence, KS: University Press of Kansas, 2009), 479; J. Lovejoy, Letters, letter to his cousin, Cynthia from PG, July 20, 1863, author's collection.
20. J. Lovejoy, Letters, letter to his cousin Cynthia from PG, March 18, 1863, author's collection.
21. Ibid., June 6, 1863.
22. Ibid., Letters, letter to "Boys, Jonathan, & Henry" from PG, June 23, 1863, author's collection.
23. Ibid., Letters, letter to his cousin Cynthia from PG, June 18, 1863, author's collection.
24. Ibid.
25. Bosworth, Letters, letter to his parents from PG, July 27, 1863, author's collection.
26. *Newport Advertiser*, May, 7, 1863.
27. Ibid., July 16, 1863.
28. Bosworth, Letters, letter to his parents from PG, August 30, 1863, authors collection.
29. Julian E., Kuz, M.D., and Bradley P. Bengtson, M.D. *Orthopaedic Injuries of the Civil War: An Atlas of Orthopaedic Injuries and Treatments During the Civil War* (Kennesaw, GA: Kennesaw Mountain Press, 1996), 14.
30. Bollet, *Civil War Medicine, 151–152*.
31. Gordon E. Dammann, DDS, and Alfred Jay Bollet, M.D., *Images of Civil War Medicine: A Photographic History* (New York: Demos Medical Publishing, 2008), 171.
32. Research documentation provided by Dr. Stephen Altic, D.O., as extracted from Barnes, *The Medical and Surgical History*, vol. 4, 693.
33. Goldowsky, "The Hospital at Portsmouth Grove," 742; *Providence Journal*, October 27, 1862.
34. *Providence Journal*, October 22, 1862.
35. A town poor farm was located less than a mile from the Portsmouth Grove Hospital on land that is now occupied by a defense contractor.
36. Goldowsky, "The Hospital at Portsmouth Grove," 739.
37. J. Lovejoy, Letters, letter to his cousin Cynthia from PG, February 2, 1863, author's collection.
38. Ibid.
39. Ricker, Diary, March 29, 1863, MHS.
40. J. Lovejoy, Letters, letter to his cousin Cynthia from PG, March 18, 1863, author's collection.
41. John W. Warner, Letters, letter to his parents from Portsmouth Grove (PG), May 22, 1864, Milne Special Collections and Archives Department, University of New Hampshire Library, Durham, NH.
42. *Newport Daily News*, November 27, 1862.
43. J. Lovejoy, Letters, letter to his cousin Cynthia from PG, August 12, 1863, author's collection.
44. Ibid., August 18, 1863.
45. J. Lovejoy, Letters, letter to his brother Jonathan from PG, August 12, 1863, author's collection. Listed and printed in eBay and used with permission of Lovejoy's great-great-granddaughter.
46. Bollet, *Civil War Medicine*, 321–322.
47. Bosworth, Letters, Letter to his parents from PG, August 14, 1863, author's collection.
48. J. F. Austin, Letters, letter to his wife from PG, February 8 and 11, 1863, MSS 272, RIHS.
49. J. F. Austin, Letters, letter to his wife from PG, February 8, 1863, MSS 272, RIHS.
50. Jacobs, Letter, to his friend Lieutenant Cottle from PG, January 27, 1863, AU.
51. Ricker, Diary, April 8, 1863, MHS.
52. Ibid., April 11, 1863.
53. Ibid., April 25, 1863.
54. Goldowsky, "The Hospital at Portsmouth Grove," 740. Portraits of Dr. Lovell and his wife hang in Newport's Redwood Library, the oldest circulating library still in existence in America.
55. Ricker, Diary, May 5, 1863, MHS.
56. Ibid., May 6, 1863. Secretary Salmon P. Chase may have been in the area to satisfy his future son-in-law, William Sprague IV of Cranston, RI, who was courting and would soon marry Chase's daughter, Kate, considered the belle of Washington.
57. *New York Times*, March 9, 1863. After an illustrious career, Brig. General Wool retired on August 1, 1863.
58. *Newport Daily News*, May 19, 1863.
59. Ibid., May 9, 1863.
60. Ibid., July 18, 1863.
61. *Hospital Register*, September 26, 1863. An original copy of the newspaper is in the author's possession.
62. Rogers, Letters, letter to his father and mother from PG, January 2, 1864, ALPLM.
63. D.H. Austin, Diary, August 11, 1864, RICWRT.
64. Ricker, Diary, April 17, 1863, MHS.
65. Peck, Diary, MSS 9001-P, May 2 and 4, 1864, RIHS.
66. J. Lovejoy, Letters, letter to his mother from PG, June 25, 1863, author's collection.
67. Goldowsky, "The Hospital at Portsmouth Grove," 740; Bollet, *Civil War Medicine*, 219.
68. Bosworth, Letters, letter to his parents from PG, July 12, 1863, author's collection.
69. J. Lovejoy, Letters, letter to his mother and sister Mary, July 10, 1863, author's collection.
70. Bosworth, Letters, letter to his parents from PG, July 12, 1863, author's collection.
71. Ricker, Diary, April 22, 1863, MHS.
72. Robert Roper, *Walt Whitman and his Brothers in the Civil War: Now the Drum of War* (New York: Walker, 2008), 213. John and Allen Lovejoy's brother, Jonathan, was a patient at Armory Square Hospital and quite possibly could have met Walt Whitman during his stay.
73. Peck, Diary, MSS 9001-P, April 23 and 28, 1864, RIHS.
74. Goldowsky, "The Hospital at Portsmouth Grove," 741.
75. Heman Packard Kingman, Letters, letter to his cousin Martin Kingman, from Eckington Hospital, June 8, 1862, Little Compton Historical Society.
76. Bosworth, Letters, letter to his parents from PG, August 7, 1863, authors collection.
77. Ibid., July 22, 1863.
78. Ricker, Diary, May 18, 1863, MHS.
79. *Providence Journal*, September 12, 1862.
80. Bosworth, Letters, letter to his parents from PG, July 27, 1863, author's collection.

81. Ibid., September 15, 1862.
82. Peck, Diary, MSS 9001-P, August 1 and April 19, 1864, RIHS.
83. Bacon and Howland, *Letters of a Family*, 497.
84. J. Lovejoy, Letters, letter to his cousin Cynthia from PG, June 25, 1863, author's collection.
85. Bacon and Howland, *Letters of a Family*, 499.
86. Lydin McKeen, Letter from Patten, Maine, July 12, 1863, to Hiram Keay, a patient at Portsmouth Grove Hospital. Letter is from author's collection. Hiram served in the same regiment as Medal of Honor recipient Lt. Col. Joshua Chamberlain. The award was given to Lt. Chamberlain for his valorous actions at Little Round Top, Gettysburg, PA.
87. Rogers, Letters, letter to his father and mother from PG, February 9, 1864, ALPLM.
88. J. Lovejoy, Letters, letter to his mother and sister Mary, July 10, 1863, author's collection.
89. Ricker, Diary, April 9, 1863, MHS.
90. Ibid., May 11, 1863. Ricker's entries become progressively difficult to read, as if he accomplished the writing in a prone position, which may have been because of his failing health.
91. Ibid., Letters, letter to his cousin Cynthia from PG, August 9, 1863, author's collection.
92. Ibid., August 12, 1863.
93. Adin B. Thayer, Letters, letter to his sister from PG, January 20, 1863, Special Collections/Musselman Library, Gettysburg College, Gettysburg, PA.
94. Ibid., March 16, 1863.
95. Allen Lovejoy, Letters, letter to his mother from Portsmouth Grove (PG), March 23, 1863, author's collection.
96. A. Lovejoy, Letters, letter to his sister Mary from PG, June 25, 1863, author's collection.
97. A. Lovejoy, Letters, letter to his mother from PG, July 20, 1863, author's collection.
98. Bosworth, Letters, letter to his parents from FSH, June 26, 1863, author's collection.
99. George D. Phillips, Letters, letter to Emma from Portsmouth Grove (PG), December 20, 1863, Connecticut Historical Society Museum & Library.
100. Bosworth, Letters, letter to his parent from PG, July 15, 1863, author's collection.
101. Ibid., August 14, 1863.
102. J.F. Austin, Letters, letter to his wife from PG, January 27, 1863, MSS 272, RIHS.
103. Bosworth, Letters, letter to his parents from PG, August 14, 1863, author's collection.
104. Warner, Letters, letter to parents from PG, April 8, 1864, MSC&AD/UNH.
105. Peck, Diary, MSS 9001-P, October 12, 1864, RIHS.
106. Ibid., November 11, 1864.
107. Ricker, Diary, May 14, 1863, MHS.
108. Bosworth, Letters, letter to his parents from FSH, June 29, 1863, author's collection.
109. J. Lovejoy, Letters, letter to his mother and sister Mary, July 10, 1863, author's collection.
110. Rogers, Letters, letter to his father and mother from PG, February 9, 1864, ALPLM.
111. Phillips, Letters, letter to Emma from PG, December 20, 1863, CHS.
112. Dennett, Transcription, January 26, 1862 (visited Washington sites); February 12, 1862 (saw Gen. McClellan); March 11, 1862 (guarding Gen. McClellan's quarters); March 28, 1862 (saw *Monitor*); April 19, 1862 (viewed Professor Lowe's flight); and June 15, 1862 (saw Negro shot), UVL.
113. Dennett, Transcription, April 24, 1862, UVL.
114. Thayer, Letters, letter to his father from PG, January 20, 1862, SC/ML, GC.
115. Ibid., March 16, 1862.
116. Warner, Letters, letter to his parents from PG, May 2, 1864, MSC&AD/UNH.
117. John B. Glenn, Letters, letter to his sister Callie from Portsmouth Grove (PG), February 23, 1863 and October 7, 1862, author's collection.
118. Ricker, Diary, March 30, 1863, MHS.
119. Ibid., April 20, 1863.
120. Warner, Letters, letter to his parents from PG, May 2, 1864, MSC&AD/UNH.
121. Peck, Diary, MSS 9001-P, July 22, 1864, RIHS.
122. Rogers, Letters, letter to his father and mother from PG, January 2, 1864, ALPLM.
123. Ibid., January 3, 1864.
124. Bosworth, Letters, letters to his parents from PG, August 30, 1863 and September 9, 1863, authors collection.
125. Rogers, Letters, letter to his father and mother from PG, February 24, 1864, ALPLM.
126. Ricker, Diary, April 30, 1863, MHS.
127. Goldowsky, "The Hospital at Portsmouth Grove," 741.
128. *Newport Advertiser*, September 10, 1862.
129. Ibid., October 25, 1862.
130. Peck, Diary, MSS 9001-P, October 12, 1864, RIHS.
131. J. Lovejoy, Letters, letter to his mother from PG, June 12, 1863, author's collection.
132. A. Lovejoy, Letters, letter to his mother from PG, June 12, 1863, author's collection.
133. Ibid., July 20, 1863.
134. Ibid., July 29, 1863.
135. Rogers, Letters, letter to his father and mother from PG, February 9, 1864, ALPLM.
136. *American Medical Times*, January 30, 1864, 60.
137. Bosworth, Letters, letter to his parent from PG, September 9, 1863, author's collection.
138. Ibid., January 2, 1864.
139. Phillips, Letters, letter to Emma from PG, November 24, 1863, CHS.
140. Ibid., December 20, 1863.
141. Rogers, Letters, letter to his father and mother from PG, January 2, 1864, ALPLM.
142. Peck, Diary, MSS 9001-P, March 26, 1864, RIHS.
143. Rogers, Letters, letter to his father and mother from PG, January 2, 1864, ALPLM.
144. Ibid., November 2, 3 and 7, 1864.
145. P.C. Headley, *Massachusetts in the Rebellion: A Record of the Historical Position of the Commonwealth and the Services of the Leading Statesmen, the Military, the Colleges, and the People, in the Civil War of 1861–65* (Boston: Walker, Fuller, 1866), 376–377.
146. Peck, Diary, November 7–8, 1864, MSS 9001-P, RIHS.
147. Ibid., November 2, 1864.
148. Ella Lonn, Ph.D., *Desertion during the Civil War* (Gloucester, MA: Appleton-Century-Crofts, 1966), 234.
149. Glenn Shirley, *Buckskin Joe* (Lincoln: University of Nebraska Press, 1966), 59 (hereafter cited as, Shirley, *Buckskin Joe*).

150. Shirley, *Buckskin Joe*, 65–66.
151. Peck, Diary, MSS 9001-P, May 15, 1864, RIHS.
152. Ibid., May 19, 1864.
153. Ibid., August 15, 1864.
154. Ibid., December 13, 1864.
155. Ibid., January 13, 1865.
156. Ibid., August 14, 1864.
157. Ibid., January 1, 1865.
158. Ibid., March 9, 1864. Interesting to note, the first battle of King Philip's War took place in Bristol back in 1675, where an Indian sachem named Metacomet used high ground along the Narragansett Bay as his main base of operation. The rise was called Mount Hope, a name that remains to this day.
159. *Newport Advertiser*, May 19, 1864.
160. *Newport Daily News*, April 28, 1864 and November 21, 1864.
161. Varhola, *Everyday Life*, 101.
162. Phillips, Letters, letter to Emma from PG, November 24, 1863, CHS.
163. Peck, Diary, January 1, 1864, MSS 9001-P, RIHS.
164. Dennett, Transcription, December 25, 1862, UVL.
165. Bosworth, Letters, letter to his parents from PG, September 27, 1863, author's collection. The man Bosworth traveled with most likely was a civilian doctor contracted by the government, as fraternization between military doctors and enlisted men was frowned upon.
166. Peck, Diary, October 24 and April 16, 1864, RIHS.
167. Ibid., January 22, 1865.
168. Charles H. Gowsley, letter to Ruth M. Whitman from Portsmouth Grove (PG), May 3, 1863, author's collection.
169. J. Lovejoy, Letters, letter to his sister Mary from PG, June 25, 1863, author's collection.
170. Ibid., June 6, 1863.
171. Rogers, Letters, letter to his father and mother from PG, January 3, 1864, ALPLM.
172. Alden, Letters, letter to his sister from PG, June 14, 1863, HCL.
173. Peck, Diary, MSS 9001-P, May 26, 1864, RIHS.
174. Ibid., November 6, 1864.
175. Phillips, Letters, letter to Emma from PG, November 24, 1863, CHS.
176. Bosworth, Letters, letter to his parents from PG, August 7, 1863, author's collection.
177. J.F. Austin, Letters, letter to his wife Emily from PG, February 27, 1863, MSS, 272, RIHS.
178. Rogers, Letters, letter to his father and mother from PG, February 21, 1864, ALPLM.
179. Ibid., February 9, 1864.
180. Cilella, *Upton's Raiders*, 90.
181. Thayer, Letters, letter to his father from PG, January 20, 1863, SC/ML, GC.
182. Private Thayer's service record was extracted from a biographical sketch prepared by Christopher Gwinn in June 2006 at Gettysburg College.
183. Phillips, Letters, letter to Emma from PG, November 24, 1863, CHS. Information on the death of Phillips's brother Alonzo was provided by Glenn Russell and obtained from 1890 Veterans Schedule found on Ancestry.com. Slightly less than fifteen acres, Bedloe's Island is now called Liberty Island, site of the Statue of Liberty. The eleven-point star foundation, upon which the Statue of Liberty is constructed, is all that remains of Ft. Wood.

184. Dennett, Transcription, December 1–3, 1862, UVL.
185. Denham, "Lovell General Hospital."
186. Ibid., March 19, 1898.
187. Ibid.
188. Ibid.
189. J. Lovejoy, Letter, letter to his cousin Cynthia from PG, June 25, 1863, author's collection.
190. J. Lovejoy, Letters, letter to his cousin Cynthia from Camp Distribution, near Alexandria, Virginia, August 24, 1863, author's collection.
191. Ibid., August 24, 1863. The same comment is cited in Cilella, *Upton's Raiders*, 212.
192. Jacobs, Letter, letter to Lieutenant Cottle, January 27, 1863, AU.
193. Robert Grandchamp, *The Seventh Rhode Island Infantry in the Civil War*. (Jefferson, NC: McFarland, 2007), 117.
194. Crandall, *Annual Report*, 355 and 356.
195. Bacon and Howland, *Letters of a Family*, 504.
196. Dammann and Bollet, *Images of Civil War Medicine*, 132.

Chapter 13

1. Rogers, Letters, letter to his father and mother from PG, January 3, 1864, ALPLM.
2. Peck, Diary, MSS 9001-P, January 2, 1864, RIHS.
3. Ibid., December 21, 1864.
4. Ibid., November 7, 1864.
5. Ibid., January 8, 1864.
6. Ibid., February 18, 1864.
7. *Newport Daily News*, March 30, 1864.
8. Peck, Diary, MSS 9001-P, February 26, 1864, RIHS.
9. Crandall, *Annual Report*, 355.
10. Peck, Diary, MSS 9001-P, August 12, 1864, RIHS.
11. Ibid., March 24, 1864.
12. Crandall, *Annual Report*, 356.
13. *Evening Press*, September 1, 1862.
14. *Bristol Phenix*, c. August 1862.
15. Peck, Diary, MSS 9001-P, April 8, 1864, RIHS.
16. Ibid., April 11, 1864.
17. Rogers, Letters, letter to his father and mother from PG, February 9, 1864, ALPLM.
18. From the collection of Dr. Stephen Altic, D.O.
19. Peck, Diary, MSS 9001-P, April 16, 1864, RIHS.
20. Warner, Letters, letter to his parents from PG, May 22, 1864, MSC&AD/UNH.
21. *Newport Advertiser*, June 9, 1864.
22. Peck, Diary, MSS 9001-P, June l0, 1864, RIHS.
23. *Newport Advertiser*, June 30, 1864.
24. *Newport Daily News*, May 26, 1864.
25. Ibid., June 27, 1864.
26. Ibid.
27. Peck, Diary, MSS 9001-P, June 27, 1864, RIHS.
28. Ibid.
29. *Newport Daily News*, June 28, 1864.
30. Ibid., June 29, 1864.
31. William C. Wardwell, *Grand Army of the Republic, Department of Rhode Island, Personal War Sketches of the Members of Babbitt Post No. 15, Bristol* (Philadelphia: L.H. Everts, 1890), 47. This book is part of the diverse collection of the Bristol Historical & Preservation Society.
32. Research documentation provided by Dr.

Stephen Altic, D.O., extracted from the following source material: Historical Data Systems, Inc., Duxbury, MA; Barnes, *The Medical and Surgical History*, vol. 2, 329; Michael S. Caldwell's Genealogy Database as of 17 January 2011; and *Tyrone Daily Herald*, April 10, 1920.

33. Andrew McIlwaine Bell, *Mosquito Soldiers: Malaria, Yellow Fever, and the Course of the American Civil War* (Baton Rouge: Louisiana State University Press, 2010), 33.
34. Peck, Diary, MSS 9001-P, July 4, 1864, RIHS.
35. Ibid., July 18, 1864.
36. See http://www.bpmlegal.com/76NY/rosterp.html. Crandall, *Annual Report*, 824.
37. D.H. Austin, Diary, June 2, 7, 9, 12, 14, 15, and 28, 1864, RICWRT.
38. Ibid., July 29–30, 1864.
39. Ibid., August 5, 1864.
40. Ibid., August 7, 1864.
41. *Newport Daily News*, August 7, 1864.
42. Ibid., October 11, 1864.
43. See http://americancivilwar.com/statepic/va/va075.html and http://www.homeofheroes.com/photos/1_civilwar/pinn_robert.html. The lead about First Sergeant Pinn's heroics and award were provided by Ron Coddington.
44. Research documentation provided by Dr. Stephen Altic, D.O., extracted from the following source material: Military Service and Medical Record, P.A. Hopkins, 1st Rhode Island Light Artillery, in custody of National Archives and Records Administration; Barnes, *The Medical and Surgical History*, vol. 10, 973; Historical Data Systems, Inc., Duxbury, MA; and Crandall, *Annual Report*, 768. Interestingly, Crandall reports the loss of six horses during the battle as easily as he does the wounding of several men.
45. Rogers, Letters, letter to his father and mother from PG, January 3, 1864, ALPLM.
46. Alden, Letters, letter to his sister from PG, March 28, 1863, HCL.
47. *Newport Daily News*, November 25, 1864.
48. Goldowsky, "The Hospital at Portsmouth Grove," 742.
49. Wardwell, *Grand Army*, 97.
50. *Newport Daily News*, November 18, 1864.
51. Peck, Diary, MSS 9001-P, December 24, 1864, RIHS.
52. Ibid., December 23, 1864.
53. *Newport Daily News*, July 8, 1865. This account was extracted from a previously published article in the *Providence Bulletin* (n.d.) and assumed to be written by someone from Portsmouth Grove Hospital.
54. Peck, Diary, MSS 9001-P, December 25, 1864, RIHS.
55. *Newport Daily News*, December 27, 1864.
56. Ibid.
57. The information about Sherman's nephew was inscribed on the reverse of a carte-de-visite from the collection of Dr. Stephen Altic, D.O. Though the first name of the soldier was not listed, the name was later identified from research by Dr. Altic, Glenn Russell, and the author.

Chapter 14

1. Peck, Diary, January 8–9, 1865, MSS 9001-P, RIHS. Peck's diary entry did not disclose the soldier's name, but an image of Rapp from the collection of Dr. Stephen Altic, D.O., briefly mentions the death on the reverse of the image. Two years previous (February 11, 1863), the *Newport Daily News* reported that a body "of an Irishman" was found at Ferry Neck, the northern end of Portsmouth. The newspaper reported that the deceased was last seen in an intoxicated state. Identifying the victim by nationality helped to perpetuate the stereotype of the "drunken Irishman." Today, such reporting would lead to slander litigation by the family of the deceased.
2. Ibid., January 18, 1865.
3. Ibid., January 20, 1865.
4. Goldowsky, "The Hospital at Portsmouth Grove," 739.
5. Peck, Diary, January 28, 1865, MSS 9001-P, RIHS.
6. Ibid., February 13, 1865.
7. Phillips, Letters, letter to Emma from PG, November 24, 1863, CHS.
8. Peck, Diary, December 1, 1864, MSS 9001-P, RIHS.
9. Ibid., February 15, 1865.
10. Denham, "Lovell General Hospital."
11. James L. Swanson, *Bloody Crimes: The Chase for Jefferson Davis and the Death Pageant for Lincoln's Corpse* (New York: William Morrow, 2010), 240.
12. Denham, "Lovell General Hospital."
13. Army of the United States: Certificate of Disability for Discharge, Private Hugh Finnegan at Lovell General Hospital, Portsmouth Grove, RI, May 2, 1865. Document provided to author by Hugh's descendant, John Finnegan.
14. Carte-de-visite with identification of soldier on reverse in the collection of Dr. Stephen Altic, D.O. Research documentation also provided by Dr. Altic, extracted from the following source material: Military Service and Pension Records, P. Baggett, 3rd Rhode Island Cavalry, National Archives and Records Administration.
15. Research documentation provided by Dr. Stephen Altic, D.O., extracted from the following source material: Historical Data Systems, Inc., Duxbury, MA; Military Service Record, Rufus Messenger, 50th Pennsylvania Volunteers, in custody of National Archives and Records Administration; and Carded Medical File, Rufus Messenger, 50th Pennsylvania Volunteers, in custody of National Archives and Records Administration.
16. Goldowsky, "The Hospital at Portsmouth Grove," 742.
17. See http://www.1stalabamacavalryusv.com/roster/stories.asp?trooperid=2163.
18. Goldowsky, "The Hospital at Portsmouth Grove," 742 and 743.
19. Greenbie, *Lincoln's Daughters of Mercy*, 143.
20. William H. Price, *The Civil War Handbook* (Fairfax, VA: L.B. Prince, 1961), 13.
21. See http://www.pa-roots.com/pacw/hospitals/hospitallist.htm.
22. Goldowsky, "The Hospital at Portsmouth Grove," 739.
23. Ibid., 743.
24. *Newport Mercury*, June 2, 1866.
25. Goldowsky, "The Hospital at Portsmouth Grove," 742.
26. See http://www.congressionalcemetery.org/PDF/Obits/E/Obits_Edwards.pdf.

27. See http://congressionalcemetery.org/HCC_Home.html.
28. See http://www.si.edu/oahp/nmaidig/cemetery.htm. Today, questions remain whether Dr. Edwards's body was removed and reinterred in another cemetery.
29. *Coast Artillery Journal*, February 1926, 196–197.
30. Research documentation provided by Dr. Stephen Altic, D.O., extracted from the following source material: Historical Data Systems, Inc., Duxbury, MA; various U.S. Federal Census Records most recent in the Kempsville District, Princess Anne County, VA; and http://www.carolshouse.com/cemeteryrecords/emmanuel/.
31. Crandall, *Annual Report*, 631. See http://jhmas.oxfordjournals.org/cgi/pdf_extract/XXXIII/4/551.
32. See http://en.wikipedia.org/wiki/Robert_Pinn.
33. PPL, NDN, "The Grist Mill," clippings.
34.. R. Lee Parks, great-great-grandson of Peyton S. Rhyne, electronic mail messages to author, October 10–12, 2011, and a telephone conversation on October 14, 2011.
35. http://www.acwv.info/1-files-veterans/M/mceachern/mceachern.htm.
36. See http://freepages.military.rootsweb.ancestry.com/~pa91/pwilss4.html.
37. See http://freepages.military.rootsweb.ancestry.com/~pa91/pcoopw1.html.
38. National Archives and Records Administration, Hugh Finnegan Pension File Certificate No. 54,802. (Circular No. 7.), Department of the Interior Pension Office, August 9, 1865; and [3–405.] (Pensioner Dropped.) U.S. Pension Agency, Boston, Mass., January 31, 1896, Hugh Finnegan. Copies of pension documents provided to the author by John Finnegan, descendant of Hugh Finnegan.
39. Dr. William Condon, DVM, of Portsmouth, RI, a descendant of Isaiah Stauffacher, provided copies of a discharge, muster rolls and other pertinent documents that are currently in the family's possession. Additional information was obtained by Glenn Russell extracted from the 1890 Veterans' Schedule found on Ancestry.com.
40. Shirley, *Buckskin Joe*, 68–70.
41. The reader is encouraged to learn more about Buckskin Joe's adventures in Glenn Shirley's fascinating and quick-read book, *Buckskin Joe*, from which this closing paragraph was extracted.
42. Ricker, Diary, May 14, 1863, MHS.
43. Ibid., circa May 21, 1863 (exact date is undistinguishable).
44. Dennett, Transcription, January 16 and 21, 1863, UVL.
45. The certificate of promotion was found in the manuscript collection (MSS 272) of John F. Austin at the Rhode Island Historical Society.
46. Grandchamp, *From Providence to Fort Hell*, 35.
47. See http://rayscorner.ca/the_history_of_seth_c_vickery.htm.
48. *Bristol Phenix*, September 8, 1914. Peck passed away at 8:40 A.M. and his obituary appeared in the afternoon edition of the local newspaper. Additional details of Peck's postwar years were obtained from the Rhode Island Historical Society and taken from notes written by Delia Kovac in 2008. Information on the date of George Peck's death and the burial grounds that contain his remains was obtained by Glenn Russell at the Bristol Town Clerk's Office. In his research, Mr. Russell also made frequent use of the 1890 *Veteran's Schedule (Nation-wide census of Civil War Veterans)*.
49. Editors, *Representative Men and Old Families of Rhode Island*, vol. 3 (Chicago: J. H. Beers, Chicago, 1908) 1660–1662.
50. NARA, Luther Pension File.
51. Ibid.
52. See http://www.ric.edu/whatsnews/details.php?News_ID=390.
53. *Proceedings, Department of Rhode Island, Grand Army of the Republic, 1898–1900*, 33rd Annual Encampment, 1900," 99.
54. NARA, Luther Pension File.
55. *Warren Gazette*, October 11 and 13, 1899.
56. See www.civilwardata.com. Addition information about Whitman W. Bosworth was provided by Glenn Russell from information found in the 1890 Veterans Schedule posted on Ancestry.com.
57. Cilella, *Upton's Raiders*, 331.
58. Information was taken from written accounts provided by Peggy McGuire, great-granddaughter of John Lovejoy.
59. Cilella, *Upton's Raiders*, 479.
60. Peggy McGuire, great-granddaughter of John Lovejoy, email message to author, May 27, 2010.
61. J. Lovejoy, Letters, letter to his cousin Cynthia from PG, April 14, 1863, author's collection.
62. Cilella, *Upton's Raiders*, 32.
63. Lovejoy, Letter, letters to his cousin Cynthia from Albany, NY, July 2, 1865, author's collection.
64. Ibid.
65. Cilella, *Upton's Raiders*, 391 and 479. Coincidentally, Cynthia's maiden name was the same first name as John's brother Allen.
66. Ibid., 479. Lovejoy's son's full name may have been Emory Upton, as John's obituary lists the name as E. Upton.
67. Ibid.
68. Obituary of John M. Lovejoy, undated newspaper clipping most likely taken from the *Ostego Republican* in the county where John lived. A copy of the obituary notice was provided by Peggy McGuire, great-great-granddaughter of John M. and Allen Lovejoy.
69. Peggy McGuire, great-great-granddaughter of John Lovejoy, email message to author on June 23, 2010.
70. Research documentation provided by Dr. Stephen Altic, D.O., extracted from the following source material: Historical Data Systems, Inc., Duxbury, MA; Barnes, The *Medical and Surgical History*, vol. 2, 329; *Tyrone Daily Herald*, John Shelow's obituary, Tyrone, PA.; and Ancestry.com
71. Extracted from a biographical sketch prepared by Christopher Gwinn at Gettysburg, College. Price, *Civil War Handbook*, 13.
72. Price, *Civil War Handbook*, 14.
73. Woolsey, *Hospital Days*, 1.
74. Ibid., 10.
75. Ibid., 10 and 13.
76. Ibid., 13.
77. *Newport Mercury*, November 3 and 6, 1866.
78. See http://www.lifespan.org/Newport/about/history.htm.
79. Goldowsky, "The Hospital at Portsmouth Grove," 740. Details of Mrs. Richardson's later life and that of her husband were excerpted from an untitled

typewritten copy of their life researched by Ed Regan, a great-grandson. In its collection, the Newport Historical Society has an incomplete boxed set of George H. Richardson's diaries (1868–1916). They contain both personal and business notations along with rough sketches of many of his carpentry projects. Only a few indirect references are made to his war years. The Richardsons lived on Whitfield Street in a three-story house just off fashionable Bellevue Avenue, only a few blocks from the Newport Historical Society.

80. See http://www.wickedlocal.com/Kingston/fun/entertainment/books/x359572517/Library-news.

81. Ibid.

82. *The Brockton Hospital Cook Book, 1910 Edition* (The Brockton Hospital Ladies' Aid Association, 1910), 111 and 200.

83. Adams, *Doctors in Blue*, 154.

84. *Providence Journal*, July 10, 1862.

85. Denham, "Lovell General Hospital."

86. Wheaton, File MSS 9001-W, RIHS.

87. *Providence Journal*, October 20, 1862.

88. *Newport Mercury*, August 4, 1866. The property was recently offered for sale and listed at $1.425 million.

89. See http://www.arlingtoncemetery.net/gmsternb.htm.

90. Pierce, *Historical Tracts*, 73.

91. *Newport Mercury*, January 27, 1866.

92. Ibid., May 26, 1866.

93. Pierce, *Historical Tracts*, 73.

94. Town Records, Office of the Town Clerk, Portsmouth, RI, *Land Evidence Book No. 15*, 39–42, August 4–5, 1865.

95. Pierce, *Historical Tracts*, 73. A carpenter who worked at the residence on two separate occasions provided renovation details to the author.

96. Electronic mail message of July 12, 2010, from property owners.

97. *Newport Daily News*, May 1, 1866.

98. The actual number of interments was confirmed by a visual audit conducted by the author on April 23–24, 2010. Previous accounts listed far fewer burials at Cypress Hills National Cemetery, a number that was factually accepted for over half a century.

99. See http://www.cem.va.gov/CEMs/nchp/cypresshills.asp.

100. Ibid.

101. See http://19thindianaironbrigade.com/Heath_William_B_.html.

102. *U.S. Sanitary Commission*, 106.

103. Ibid., 105.

104. St. Paul's, *Burials, 1862*, July 6–9.

105. Records of the Adjutant General, Letters to the Governor/Secretary of State, Vol. 42, #140, C#00257 — RISA.

106. Information about the Portsmouth Grove Hospital Library Association was extracted from several folders maintained by Special Collections, Providence Public Library, Providence, RI.

107. *Newport Daily News*, September 19, 1898.

108. Goldowsky, "The Hospital at Portsmouth Grove," 733–743. The sketch is shown on page 739.

109. Rhode Island State Archives, *1862-Plan of Grounds*, File Box 304 — RISA. The only enclosure in the file was the aforementioned drawing.

110. Price, *Civil War Handbook*, 14.

111. PPL, NDN, "The Grist Mill," clippings.

112. Pierce, *Historical Tracts*, 73.

113. See http://www.nuwc.navy.mil/hq/history/0002.html.

114. Ibid.

115. Alden, Letters, letter to his sister from PG, June 14, 1863, HCL.

Bibliography

Books

Adams, George Worthington. *Doctors in Blue: The Medical History of the Union Army in the Civil War.* New York: Henry Schuman, 1952.
Aldrich, Thomas M. *The History of Battery A, First Regiment Rhode Island Light Artillery in the War to Preserve the Union, 1861–1865.* Providence: Snow & Farnham, 1904.
Bacon, Georgeanna Woolsey, and Eliza Woolsey Howland. *Letters of a Family during the War for the Union, 1861–1865.* Charleston, SC: Bibliolife, 2010.
Barnes, Joseph K., Surgeon, U.S. Army (by direction of). *Medical and Surgical History of the War of the Rebellion (1861–1865).* Washington, DC: Government Printing Office, 1888.
Bayles, Richard M., ed. *History of Newport County, Rhode Island.* New York: L.E. Preston, 1888.
Behling, Laura L., ed. *Hospital Transports.* New York: State University of New York Press, 2005.
Bell, Andrew McIlwaine. *Mosquito Soldiers: Malaria, Yellow Fever, and the Course of the American Civil War.* Baton Rouge: Louisiana State University, 2010.
Bicknell, Thomas Williams, LL.D. *The History of the State of Rhode Island and Providence Plantations.* New York: American Historical Society, 1920.
Billings, John D. *Hardtack and Coffee, or the Unwritten Story of Army Life.* Boston: George M. Smith, 1887.
Bollet, Alfred Jay, M.D. *Civil War Medicine: Challenges and Triumphs.* Tucson: Galen Press, 2002.
Brockett, L.P., M.D., and Mary C. Vaughan. *Woman's Work in the Civil War: A Record of Heroism, Patriotism and Patience.* Boston: R.H. Curran, 1867.
Brooks, Noah. *Washington, D.C. in Lincoln's Time.* Chicago: Quadrangle Books, 1971.
Campi, James, Jr. *Civil War Battlefields, Then and Now.* Berkeley, CA: Thunder Bay Press, 2008.
Cilella, Salvatore G., Jr. *Upton's Regulars: The 121st Infantry in the Civil War.* Lawrence: University Press of Kansas, 2009.
The Civil War Society's Encyclopedia of the Civil War. New York: Portland House, 1997.
Coffin, Charles Carleton. *The Boys of '61; or, Four Years of Fighting.* Boston: Estes and Lauriat, 1881.
Dammann, Gordon E., DDS, and Alfred Jay Bollet, M.D. *Images of Civil War Medicine: A Photographic History.* New York: Demos Medical Publishing, 2008.
Devin, Nancy Jensen, and Richard V. Simpson. *Images of America: Portsmouth, Rhode Island.* Dover, NH: Arcadia Publishing, 1997.
Elliott, Maud Howe. *This Was My Newport.* Boston: Mythology, 1944.
Faust, Drew Gilpin. *This Republic of Suffering: Death and the American Civil War.* New York: Alfred A. Knopf, 2008.
Garman, James E. *A History of Portsmouth, Rhode Island, 1638–1978.* Newport, RI: Franklin Printing House, 1978.
Garrison, Nancy Scripture. *With Courage and Delicacy—Civil War on the Peninsula: Women and the U.S. Sanitary Commission.* Cambridge, MA: Da Capo Press, 1999.
Grandchamp, Robert. *From Providence to Fort Hell: Letters from Company K, Seventh Rhode Island Volunteers.* Westminster, MD: Heritage Books, 2008.
_____. *The Seventh Rhode Island Infantry in the Civil War.* Jefferson, NC: McFarland, 2007.
Greenbie, Marjorie Barstow. *Lincoln's Daughters of Mercy.* New York: Putnam's, 1944.
Gross, Samuel Wiessell, M.D. *A Manual of Military Surgery; or, Hints on the Emergencies of Field, Camp and Hospital.* Philadelphia: J.B. Lippincott, 1862. Reprinted by Applewood Books, Bedford, MA.

Headley, P.C. *Massachusetts in the Rebellion: A Record of the Historical Position of the Commonwealth and the Services of the Leading Statesmen, the Military, the Colleges, and the People, in the Civil War of 1861–65*. Boston: Walker, Fuller, 1866.
Kuz, Julian E., M.D., and Bradley P. Bengtson, M.D. *Orthopaedic Injuries of the Civil War: An Atlas of Orthopaedic Injuries and Treatments during the Civil War*. Kennesaw, GA: Kennesaw Mountain Press, 1996.
Lonn, Ella, Ph.D. *Desertion during the Civil War*. Gloucester, MA: Appleton-Century-Crofts, 1966.
Lyman, Darryl. *Civil War Wordbook: Including Sayings, Phrases and Expletives*. Conshohocken, PA: Combined Books, 1994.
McPherson, James M. *Battle Cry of Freedom: The Civil War Era*. New York: Oxford University Press, 2003.
Miller, Francis T., ed. *The Photographic History of the Civil War*. Vol. 4, *Soldier Life and Secret Service: Prisons and Hospitals*. Secaucus, NJ: Blue & Grey Press, 1987.
Mitchell, Reid. *Civil War Soldiers: Their Expectations and Their Experiences*. New York: Viking Penguin, 1988.
Mottelay, Paul, F., ed. *The Soldier in Our Civil War: A Pictorial History of the Conflict, 1861–1865*. Boston: J.H. Brown, 1884.
Newport Daily News editors. *Newport, and How to See It, with List of Summer Residents*. Newport: Davis & Pitman, 1873.
Oates, Stephen B. *A Woman of Valor: Clara Barton and the Civil War*. New York: Free Press, 1994.
Pierce, John T. Sr. *Historical Tracts of the Town of Portsmouth, Rhode Island*. Portsmouth, RI: Hamilton Printing, 1991.
Price, William H. *The Civil War Handbook*. Fairfax, VA: L.B. Prince, 1961.
Prokopowicz, Gerald J. *Did Lincoln Own Slaves? And Other Frequently Asked Questions about Abraham Lincoln*. New York: Pantheon Books, 2008.
Representative Men and Old Families of Rhode Island. Chicago: J.H. Beers, 1908.
Rhode Island Black Heritage Society, ed. *African-Americans in Newport: An Introduction to the Heritage of African-Americans in Newport, Rhode Island [1700–1945]*. Rhode Island Historical Preservation & Heritage Commission, c. 1995.
Robertson, James I., Jr., and the Editors of Time-Life Books. *Tenting Tonight: The Soldier's Life*. Alexandria, VA: Time-Life Books, 1984.
Roper, Robert. *Walt Whitman and his Brothers in the Civil War: Now the Drum of War*. New York: Walker, 2008.
Schroder, Walter K. *Images of America: Dutch Island and Ft. Greble*. Dover, NH: Arcadia, 1998.
Shirley, Glenn, ed. *Buckskin Joe*. Lincoln: University of Nebraska Press, 1966.
Smith, George Winston. *Medicines for the Union Army: The United States Army Laboratories during the Civil War*. New York: Pharmaceutical Products Press, 2001.
Smith, Page. *Trial by Fire: A People's History of the Civil War and Reconstruction*. Vol. 5. New York: McGraw-Hill, 1982.
Spicer, William A. *History of the Ninth and Tenth Regiments, Rhode Island Volunteers, and the Tenth Rhode Island Battery, in the Union Army in 1862*. Providence, RI: Snow & Farnham, 1892.
Stearns, Ezra S. *History of the Town of Rindge, New Hampshire, from the Date of the Rowley Canada or Massachusetts Charter to the Present Time, 1736–1874, with a Genealogical Register of the Rindge Families*. Boston: Press of George H. Ellis, 1875.
Swanson, James L. *Bloody Crimes: The Chase for Jefferson Davis and the Death Pageant for Lincoln's Corpse*. New York: William Morrow, 2010.
The U.S. Sanitary Commission of the United States Army: A Succinct Narrative of its Works and Purposes. New York: Published for the Benefit of the United States Sanitary Commission, 1864.
VanDenBossche, Kris, ed. *"Pleas Excuse All Bad Writing": A Documentary History of Rhode Island during the Civil War Era (1854–1865)*. Peace Dale, RI: Rhode Island Historical Document Transcription Project, 1993.
Varhola, Michael J. *Everyday Life during the Civil War: A Guide for Writers, Students and Historians*. Cincinnati: Writer's Digest Books, 1999.
Wagner, Margaret E., Gary W. Gallagher, and Paul Finkelman, eds. *The Library of Congress Civil War Desk Reference*. New York: Simon & Schuster, 2002.
Walter, John F. *The Confederate Dead in Brooklyn*. Bowie, MD: Heritage Books, 2003.
Ward, Geoffrey C., with Ric Burns and Ken Burns. *The Civil War: An Illustrated History*. New York: Alfred A. Knopf, 1990.
Wardwell, William C., ed. *Grand Army of the Republic: Personal War Sketches of the Members of Babbitt Post No. 15, Bristol*. Philadelphia: L.H. Everts, 1890.
Waugh, John C. *Lincoln and McClellan: The Troubled Partnership between a President and His General*. New York: Palgrave Macmillan, 2010.
Weigley, Russell F. *Quartermaster General of the Union Army*. New York: Columbia University Press, 1959.
Wheeler, Richard. *Sword Over Richmond: An Eyewitness History of McClellan's Peninsula Campaign*. New York: Harper & Row, 1986.
Williams, David. *A People's History of the Civil War: Struggles for the Meaning of Freedom*. New York: New Press, 2005.

Woolsey, Jane Stuart. *Hospital Days: Reminiscence of a Civil War Nurse*. Roseville, MN: Edinborough Press, 2001.
Wormeley, Katherine Prescott. *The Other Side of War with the Army of the Potomac*. Boston: Ticknor, 1889.
Wynalda, Stephen A. *366 Days in Abraham Lincoln's Presidency: The Private, Political, and Military Decisions of American's Greatest President*. New York: A Herman Graf Book, Skyhorse Publishing, 2010.
Young, Jesse Bowman. *What a Boy Saw in the Army*. New York: Hunt and Eaton, 1894.

Electronic Sources

About Physicians. "Lifespan: History." http://www.lifespan.org/Newport/about/history.htm.
"American Civil War Veterans of Australia & New Zealand: Duncan McEachern." http://www.acwv.info/1-files-veterans/M/mceachern/mceachern.htm.
Arlington National Cemetery Website. George Miller Sternberg, Brigadier General, United States Army. http://www.arlingtoncemetery.net/gmsternb.htm.
Centers for Disease Control and Prevention. "Smallpox Disease Overview." http://emergerncy.cdc.gov/agent/smallpox/overview/disease-facts.asp.
"Chaffin's Farm, New Market Heights, Virginia: American Civil War, September 29–30, 1864." http://americancivilwar.com/statepic/va/va075.html.
"Charles William Cole — Soldier: Story, Pictures and Information." http://www.footnote.com/page/3094_charles_william_cole_soldier/.
Civil War Librarian. "News — Did Doctor's Prescription Cause the Civil War?" http://civilwarlibrarian.blogspot.com/2010/03/news-did-doctors-perscription-cause.html.
"Civil War Medical Care, Battle Wounds, and Disease." Author credits *The Civil War Society's Encyclopedia of the Civil War*. http://www.civilwarhome.com/civilwarmedicine.htm.
Congressional Cemetery. http://www.si.edu/oahp/nmaidig/cemetery.htm.
Curtin, Roland G., M.D. "Phenolic Substances: Nascent Phenic Acid, Carbolic Acid, Creosote, Guaiacol, and Benzoyl of Guaiacol." http://www.ncbi.nlm.nib.gov/pmc/articles/PMC2526887/pdf/tacca200101-0287.pdf.
"Discipline in the Civil War Armies." http://www.civilwarhome.com/discipline.htm. Source of article cited as *Historical Times Encyclopedia of the Civil War*, edited by Patricia L. Faust.
Dr. and Mrs. Algernon Coolidge and the Cotuit Library Association of Cape Cod, Massachusetts. http://jhmas.oxfordjournals.org/cgi/pdf_extract/XXXIII/4/551.
"Dysentery & Diarrhea." http://www.wtv-zone.com/civilwar/dysentery.html. Source of article cited as *Atlas Editions: Civil War Cards*.
1890 Veterans Schedule. Ancestry.com.
Emedicinehealth. "Gangrene Causes, Symptoms, Treatment, Types and Prevention." http://www.emedicinehealth.com/gangrene/article_em.htm.
Emmanuel Episcopal Church Cemetery, Virginia Beach, VA, Old Princess Anne County. http://www.carolshouse.com/cemeteryrecords/emmanuel/.
Grandchamp, Robert. "RIC (Rhode Island College) students who served in the Civil War." http://www.ric.edu/whatsnews/details.php?News_ID=390.
"Heath, William B." http://19thindianaironbrigade.com/Heath_William_B_.html.
Historic Congressional Cemetery. "Congressional Cemetery: History Comes Alive." http://congressionalcemetery.org/HCC_Home.html.
Historical Data Systems, Inc., Duxbury, MA. www.civilwardata.com.
"The History of Seth C. Vickery. A Summary from the Record of the History of Seth C. Vickery, Stepfather to Timothy W. Riley Jr." http://rayscorner.ca/the_history_of_seth_c_vickery.htm.
"Interments in the Historic Congressional Cemetery." http://www.congressionalcemetery.org/PDF/Obits/E/Obits_Edwards.pdf.
King, Janet, RN, BSN, CCRN. "Civil War Medicine." http://vermontcivilwar.org/medic/medicine2.php.
Library News, Kingston, MA. "Wicked Local Kingston." http://www.wickedlocal.com/Kingston/fun/entertainment/books/x359572517/ Library-news.
Massachusetts Civil War Research Center. massachusettscivilwar.com. Also see research@massachusetttscivilwar.com.
Naval Undersea Warfare Center. "The Navy & Rhode Island: A History." http://www.nuwc.navy.mil/hq/history/0002.html.
91st PA. "Samuel Wilson II." http://freepages.military.rootsweb.ancestry.com/~pa91/pwilss4.html.
_____. "William R. Cooper." http://freepages.military.rootsweb.ancestry.com/~pa91/pcoopw1.html.
Reports on the Extent and Nature of the Materials Available for the Preparation of a Medical and Surgical History of the Rebellion. http://books.google.com/.
"Robert A. Pinn": Photo of Medal of Honor Recipient Robert A. Pinn. http://www.homeofheroes.com/photos/1_civilwar/pinn_robert.html.

"Robert Pinn." http://en.wikipedia.org/wiki/Robert_Pinn.
76th NYSV — Roster (P). *76th NY Roster-P.* http://www.bpmlegal.com/76NY/roster-p.html.
Smith, Carl S. "Stories about Troopers from the 1st Alabama: Jonathan M. Stewart." http://www.1stalabama cavalryusv.com/roster/stories.asp?trooperid=2163.
Tilden, John, MD. "Smallpox (*Variola*)." http://www.whale.to/vaccines/tilden6.html.
Town of Portsmouth, Rhode Island. "Portsmouth Schools." http://www.ri.net/schools/Portsmouth/Admin/town.htm.
"Typhoid fever." http://mayoclinic.com/health/typhoid-fever/DS00538.
United States Department of Veterans Affairs. Arlington National Cemetery, Arlington, VA. www.arlingtoncemetery.org/.
_____. Cypress Hills National Cemetery, Brooklyn, NY. http://www.cem.va.gov/CEMs/nchp/cypresshills.asp.
_____. Salisbury National Cemetery, Salisbury, NC. http://www.cem.va.gov/CEMs/nchp/salisbury.#gi.
"The U.S. Sanitary Commission and Other Relief Agencies." Author credits article by Holland Thompson, *The Photographic History of the Civil War.* http://civilwarhome.com/sanitarycommission.htm.
"Woman in the Civil War." http://www.history.com/topics/women-in-the-civil-war.
World Health Organization (WHO). "Smallpox: Historical Significance." http://www.who.int/mediacentre/factsheets/smallpox/en/.

Historical Societies

Bristol Historical & Preservation Society, Bristol, RI.
Little Compton Historical Society, Little Compton, RI.
Newport Historical Society, Newport, RI.
Rhode Island Historical Society, Providence, RI.

Libraries (Personal Visits)

Brown University Archives, John Hay Library, Brown University, Providence, RI.
Cotuit Library, Cotuit, MA.
Middletown Public Library, Special Collections, Middletown, RI.
Newport Public Library, Special Collections, Newport, RI.
Portsmouth Free Public Library, Special Collections, Portsmouth, RI.
Providence Public Library, Special Collections (C. Fiske Harris Collection on American Civil War and Slavery), Providence, RI.
Redwood Library and Athenaeum, Newport, RI.
Rhode Island College James P. Adams Library, Special Collections, Providence, RI.
Rogers Public Library, Special Collections, Bristol, RI.
U.S. Naval War College, Henry E. Eccles Library, Newport, RI.
University of Rhode Island, University Libraries, Special Collections and Archives, Kingston, RI.
Warren Public Library, Warren, RI.

Manuscript Collections (Archival)

Alden, Seth H. Letters. Hamilton College Library Special Collections, Clinton, NY.
Alden, Seth H. Pension File Certificate No. 384,990. National Archives and Records Administration, Washington, DC.
Austin, John F. Letters. Rhode Island Historical Society, Providence, RI.
Blanding, Christopher. Enlistment broadside. The Library Company of Philadelphia, Philadelphia, PA.
Coggeshall, Thomas, Jr. Letter. Newport Historical Society, Newport, RI.
Dennett, William S. Letters. Albert and Shirley Small Special Collections Library, Alderman Library of the University of Virginia Libraries, Charlottesville, VA.
Finnegan, Hugh. Pension File Certificate No. 54,802. National Archives and Records Administration, Washington, DC.
Hoyt, Edward Jonathan (Buckskin Joe). Photograph. Dickinson Research Center, National Cowboy & Western Heritage Museum, Oklahoma City, OK.
Jacobs, Andrew. Letter. Special Collections & Archives, Ralph B. Draughon Library, Auburn University, Auburn, AL.

Lopes, Isaac. Letter. Office of the Secretary of State, A. Ralph Mollis State Archives Division, Providence, RI.
Luther, Alfred. Pension File Certificate No. 11,055. National Archives and Records Administration, Washington, DC.
Massachusetts Commandery, Military Order of the Loyal Legion and the U.S. Army Military History Institute, Department of the Army, U.S. Army War College and Carlisle Barracks, Carlisle, PA.
Office of the Secretary of State, A. Ralph Mollis State Archives Division, Providence, RI.
Peck, George H. Diary (1864–65). Rhode Island Historical Society, Providence, RI.
Phillips, George D. Letters. Connecticut Historical Society Museum & Library, Hartford, CT.
Rhode Island State Archives, Records of the Adjutant General, Portsmouth Grove Hospital, Quarter Master General Correspondence, 1862.
Rhode Island State Archives, Records of the Adjutant General, Special Requisitions, Portsmouth Grove Hospital, 1862.
Richardson, George H. Diaries (1868–1916, incomplete set). Newport Historical Society, Newport, RI.
Ricker, Oliver A. Diary (January–September 1863). *Civil War Correspondence, Diaries, and Journals at the Massachusetts Historical Society*, microfilm edition, reel 7 of 29 reels. Boston: Massachusetts Historical Society, 1985.
Rogers, Stephen O. Letters. Abraham Lincoln Presidential Library & Museum, Springfield, IL.
St. Paul's Episcopal Church, Portsmouth, RI.
Thayer, Adin B. Letters. Special Collections/Musselman Library, Gettysburg College, Gettysburg, PA.
Warner, John W. Letters. Milne Special Collections and Archives Department, University of New Hampshire Library, Durham, NH.
Wheaton Francis L. Miscellaneous Manuscripts, Rhode Island Historical Society.
Wormeley, Katherine P. Letters. Special Collections and University Archives, Wichita State University Libraries, Wichita, KS.

Manuscript Collections (Private)

Austin, Daniel Henry. Excerpts from his diary. Rhode Island Civil War Round Table (RICWRT) monthly newsletter *Monthly Return* 11, no. 1 (June 2002) and no. 2 (September 2002). Furnished to the author by Mark Dunkelman. (The diary is in the possession of Austin's great-granddaughter Kirsten Austin. Copies of the diary were forwarded to the editor of the RICWRT's *Monthly Return* editor through William Woodward Farlee.)
Baggett, Patrick. Photograph. Ron Coddington collection. The same image is also found in the Dr. Stephen Altic collection.
Bosworth, Whitman W. Letters. Author's collection.
Crofton, James. Copy of discharge provided by Richard A. Rupp.
Finnegan, Hugh. Copy of discharge and other pertinent military and genealogy documents provided by John Finnegan, a descendent of Hugh Finnegan.
Glenn, John B. Letters. Author's collection.
Gowsley, Charles H. Letters. Author's collection.
Lovejoy, Allen, and John M. Lovejoy. Letters originally owned by the great-great-granddaughter of Allen and John Lovejoy, now in the possession of the author.
McKeen, Lydin. A letter from Patten, Maine, dated July 12, 1863, to Hiram Keay. Letter is in author's collection.
Various photographs taken from a presentation album from a nurse to a patient at Portsmouth Grove Hospital and accompanying research material relating to several images. Dr. Stephen Altic, D.O. collection.

Newspapers

Bristol Phenix, Bristol, RI. Accessed at Rogers Public Library, Bristol, RI.
Hospital Register, Satterlee U.S. Army General Hospital, West Philadelphia, PA.
New York Times, New York, NY.
Newport Advertiser, Newport, RI. Accessed at the U.S. Naval War College, Henry E. Eccles Library, Newport, RI.
Newport Daily News, Newport, RI. Accessed at the Newport Public Library, Newport, RI.
Newport Mercury, Newport, RI.
Providence Evening Press, Providence, RI. Taken from newspaper clippings in author's possession.
Providence Journal, Providence, RI.
Sakonnet Times, Tiverton, RI.
Tyrone Daily Herald, Tyrone, PA.

Wall Street Journal, New York, NY.
Warren Gazette, Warren, RI.

Bulletins, Periodicals, Reports, and Newspaper Columns

"American Medical Intelligence." *Army Medical Times*, January 30, 1864.
The Brockton Hospital Cookbook, 1910 Edition. The Brockton Hospital Ladies' Aid Association, 1910.
"Defenses of Key West, Florida." *Coast Artillery Journal*, February 1926.
Denham, D.C. "Lovell General Hospital as I Remember It." *Newport Mercury*.
Goldowsky, Seebert J., M.D. "The Hospital at Portsmouth Grove." *Rhode Island Medical Journal*, 1959.
Greene, Thomas E. "The Post Office at Portsmouth Grove, Rhode Island." *Rhode Island Postal History Journal* 12, no. 3 (July–October 2000).
"Historical and Architectural Resources of Portsmouth, Rhode Island: A Preliminary Report." Rhode Island Historical Preservation Commission, January 1979.
Proceedings, Department of Rhode Island, Grand Army of the Republic, 1898–1900. 33rd Annual Encampment, 1900.

State Publications

Crandall, H., Colonel. *Annual Report of the Adjutant General of the State of Rhode Island, for the Year 1865*. Providence: Providence Press, 1866.
Dailey, Charlotte F. *Report upon the Disabled Rhode Island Soldiers; Their Names, Condition, and in What Hospital They Are*. Providence: Alfred Anthony, Printer to the State, 1863.

Town Records

Office of the Town Clerk, *Land Evidence Books*, Portsmouth, RI.

Index

absent without leave (AWOL) 63, 66, 113, 119, 124, 135
Adams, George Worthington 10, 11
African American 95, 116, 125, 130, 140
alcohol 10, 11, 61
Alden, Seth H. 43, 56, 78, 89, 92, 117, 160
Alexandria, VA 35, 74, 76
America (steamer) 21, 22, 23
American Medical Association 151
amputations 11, 12, 25, 27, 76, 90, 95, 96, 126, 129, 156
Andrew, John A. 98, 111
Annapolis, MD 16, 118, 126
Annual Report of the Adjutant General of the State of Rhode Island for the Year 1865 59, 124
Antietam, battle of 93, 99, 136
Aquidneck Island 5, 17, 30, 37, 71, 80, 85, 141, 149, 151, 160
Aquidneck Islanders 23, 33, 34, 40, 45, 150
Arlington National Cemetery 26, 151, 152, 154
Armstrong, William A. 96, 156
Army Medical Department 45
Army Medical Museum 59
Army Medical School 151
Arnold, Samuel G. 23
artillery: Massachusetts (13th Regiment Massachusetts Light Artillery) 75; Pennsylvania (2nd Regiment Pennsylvania Heavy Artillery) 134; Rhode Island (1st Regiment Rhode Island Light Artillery) 20, 28, 44, 52, (3rd Regiment Rhode Island Heavy Artillery) 52, 131, (14th Regiment Rhode Island Heavy Artillery [Colored]) 75, 102, 139, (Battery B Rhode Island Detached Militia) 20
Ashley, Herbert 152
Atlantic (steamer) 21, 22, 23, 24, 25, 31
Austin, Daniel H. 55, 100, 129, 130
Austin, John F. 42, 55, 77, 78, 98, 106, 118, 142

bacillus tetani 12
Bacon, Cyrus, Jr. 28
Baker, J. 50, 158
bakery 31, 42, 51, 101, 130
Baltic (steamer) 130
Baltimore, MD 23, 46, 76, 145
Bancroft, George 16
bandages 12, 69, 70, 126; lint for 69, 70, 126
Barili, Signor A. 68
Barnard, John 19
Barnstable, MA 140
Barton, Clara 90
baseball 114
Battle Cry of Freedom 8
Bay State (steamer) 93, 127
Bedloe's Island 119, 121
Bell, Andrew McIlwine 128
Billings, John D. 65
Blacks 22, 44, 64, 89, 107, 116, 125
blacksmith 9, 51
Blanding, Christopher 52
blood poisoning 12, 78, 95
Bolding, William 124
Booth, Edwin 17
Booth, John Wilkes 17, 136, 139
Boston, MA 14, 17, 18, 47, 57, 75, 85, 96, 104, 120, 125, 136, 142
Bosworth, Whitman W. 35, 37, 44, 56, 57, 59, 60, 62, 63, 77, 93, 94, 98, 101, 102, 106, 107, 109, 110, 116, 118, 144
Bradford Coaling Station 159
Brady, Mathew 34, 138
bread 26, 31, 32, 34, 42, 43, 44, 45, 47, 62, 104, 110, 132
Brewster, Ada 84, 85, 86, 125, 149
Bristol, RI 15, 27, 37, 40, 111, 114, 127, 131, 143, 144
Bristol Phenix 29, 33, 41, 71, 124
Bristol Train of Artillery 143
Brooklyn, NY 154, 156
Brooks, Erastus 138
Brooks, Nathaniel G. 100
Brooks, Noah 8
Brown, Harry E. 99
Brown University 25, 115, 139, 150, 151

Browning, Orville 19
Buckingham, William A. 111
Bureau of Refugees, Freedmen and Abandoned Lands 73
burial yard 9, 26, 50, 129, 155, 158
Burnside, Ambrose E. 61, 91
Burnside Corps 130
Butler, Benjamin 98

Camp Meigs, MA 75
Cape Hatteras, NC 131
Cargill, Charles 93
carpenter 9, 27, 51, 149
Carpenter, Benoni 39, 73, 139
Carr, Stephen A. 121
Carver General Hospital 42, 84
cavalry: Alabama (1st Alabama Cavalry, U.S. Volunteers) 137; Massachusetts (4th Regiment of Cavalry, Massachusetts Volunteers) 111; New Hampshire (1st Regiment New Hampshire Volunteer Cavalry) 97; Rhode Island (3rd Regiment Rhode Island Cavalry) 124, 136
cemetery see burial yard
Certificate of Disability 75, 98, 142, 143
Chace, William S. 52, 55, 64
chapel 51, 86, 87, 89, 94, 98, 131
chaplain 9, 26, 87, 89, 100
Charlestown, MA 142
Charlestown, WV 145
Chase, Mrs. Borden 24
Chase, Salmon 98
Chesapeake Bay 27
Chestnut Hill, Philadelphia, PA 247
Chevers, George W. 24, 156
Christmas 69, 71, 87, 89, 116, 131, 132, 145
City of Newport (steamer) 71, 126
City Point, VA 96, 111, 130
Clark, Thomas M. 37, 157
cleanliness 11, 38, 55, 82
Clift, Samuel E. 26
clothing 32, 34, 41, 48, 54, 68, 69, 80, 102, 126, 142
coal 48, 123, 132, 135, 152, 159
coal mines 152
Coatzacoalcos (steamer) 23
Coddington, William 14, 15
Coggeshall, Thomas, Jr. 23, 24, 25
Cold Harbor, battle of 129
Cole, Edmund 49, 134, 135
Cole, Olive M. 152
Collins, Timothy 64, 65, 134
Colvin, Charles 121
Confederacy 19, 26, 32, 68, 69, 70, 107
Confederates 20, 21, 23, 32, 35, 54, 61, 71, 73, 107, 119, 130, 138, 142, 147
Congressional Cemetery 138
conscription/draft 56, 57, 58
Constitution 29, 40
cooks 9, 43, 44
Coolidge, Algernon 73, 139, 140
Cooper, William R. 141

copperheads 107
cotton 70, 103
Cotuit, MA 139, 140
Cranston, William H. 23, 35, 39, 40, 99, 126
Crater, Battle of the 61, 137
Cristy, Peter 26
Cypress Hills Cemetery 156
Cypress Hills National Cemetery 154, 155, 156, 157

Dailey, Charlotte F. 75, 76
Daniel Webster (steamer) 89, 90, 91
Davis, John W. 99
Davis, William 54, 73
Denham, C.R. 86
Denham, D.C. 89, 119, 120, 121
Dennett, William 22, 26, 41, 43, 107, 108, 116, 119, 142
Dennis, Sarah C. 85, 86, 148
deserters 112, 124, 142, 146
Dexter's Photograph Rooms 110
diarrhea 7, 10, 22, 25, 76, 92, 96, 147
Dix, John A. 111
doctors 8, 9, 10, 11, 12, 13, 22, 23, 24, 25, 33, 39, 59, 60, 61, 73, 74, 75, 78, 82, 92, 93, 94, 95, 96, 97, 113, 116, 127, 128, 136, 138, 144, 145
Doctors in Blue 10
draft see conscription
Drewry's Bluff, VA 156
drinking/drunkenness 17, 58, 59, 61, 62, 63, 64, 65, 66, 106, 134, 139
Dutch Island 75
dysentery 10, 147

East Greenwich, RI 28, 156
Eckington Hospital 101
Edwards, Lewis A. 64, 73, 74, 119, 121, 131, 135, 136, 138
Elliott, Maud Howe 66, 150
embalming 28
erysipelas 12
Evans, Abraham 26
Evening Press 39, 74

Fair Oaks, VA 20, 27, 52
Fairfax County Court House 125
Fairfax Seminary (hospital) 35, 74, 97
Fall River, MA 17, 34, 54, 71, 72, 86, 136
Fall River Herald 71
field hospital 7, 8, 21, 95, 104, 129, 131
Finnegan, Hugh 136, 141
First Bull Run 8, 20, 23, 35, 39, 112
Follett, John F. 79
Fort Adams 14, 29, 31, 52
Fort Monroe 19, 21, 54, 73, 74, 107, 128, 130
Fort Schuyler Hospital 93
Fort Sumter 8
Fort Towson 73
Fort Wood 119, 121
Fourth of July (Independence Day) 22, 23, 63, 69, 107, 128

Frederick, MD 12
Fredericksburg, VA 28, 42, 78, 90, 91, 92, 99, 105, 143
Freemasons 68

Gaines' Mill 20, 74, 131, 143
Galligan, John 124
gangrene 11, 12, 129, 140
Garrett Farm 139
General Assembly (State of Rhode Island) 68, 76, 154
Geneva Convention 138
Gettysburg, Battle of 93, 94, 105, 107, 119, 148
Gibson, William 97
Goldowsky, Seebert J. 158
Goldsmith, Middleton 11
Gowsley, Charles H. 116
Grand Division of the Sons of Temperance 63
Grant, Ulysses S. 61, 147
Grapevine Bridge 21
Grassdale-Digby, district of Victoria Australia 140
Griswold, John N.A. 152

Haley, Michael 66
Hammond, John H. 52, 64
Hammond, William A. 15, 39, 81, 82
Hammond General Hospital 35, 44, 93
Hampton, NH 97
hardtack 22, 25, 32
Hardtack and Coffee 65
Harrison's Landing, VA 20, 23
Harvard Medical School 139
Heath, William B. 156
hemorrhagic smallpox 78
Hentzelman, Dr. 74
Higgins, John 58
Hill, Edwin 131
Hingham, MA 111
Hodgkinson, Pvt. 76, 77
Holmes, Obadiah 17
Hoover, J. Edgar 138
Hopkins, Perez A. 130, 131
hospital guards 27, 52–67, 71, 77, 79, 109, 111, 113, 114, 121, 138, 143
Howe, Julia Ward 15, 150
Hoyt, Edward Jonathan (Buckskin Joe) 112, 113, 141, 142
Hutchinson, Anne 15

infantry: Connecticut (17th Regiment Connecticut Infantry) 106; Maine (16th Regiment Maine Volunteer Infantry) 43, 105, (20th Regiment Maine Volunteer Infantry) 103, (31st Regiment Maine Volunteer Infantry) 96, 156; Maryland (5th Regiment Maryland Volunteer Infantry) 85; Massachusetts (18th Regiment Massachusetts Volunteer Infantry) 91, 94, (21st Regiment Massachusetts Volunteer Infantry) 92, (25th Regiment Massachusetts Volunteer Infantry) 104, 156, (28th Regiment Massachusetts Volunteer Infantry) 139, (36th Regiment Massachusetts Volunteer Infantry) 7, 76, 77, (40th Regiment Massachusetts Volunteer Infantry) 87; Michigan (5th Michigan Volunteer Infantry) 26, (7th Michigan Volunteer Infantry) 28, (8th Michigan Volunteer Infantry) 155; New York (26th Regiment New York Infantry) 94, (49th Regiment New York Infantry) 112, (76th Regiment New York Infantry) 129, (81st Regiment New York Infantry) 55, (88th Regiment New York Infantry) 27, 155, (115th Regiment New York Infantry) 157, (121st Regiment New York Infantry) 58, 93, 147; North Carolina (37th North Carolina Infantry) 23, 26, 140; Pennsylvania (25th Pennsylvania Infantry) 141, (50th Pennsylvania Infantry) 137, (61st Pennsylvania Infantry) 26, (72nd Pennsylvania Infantry) 27, (91st Pennsylvania Infantry) 141, (101st Pennsylvania Infantry) 23, (102nd Pennsylvania Infantry) 33, 154; Rhode Island (2nd Regiment Rhode Island Volunteers) 25, 27, 114, 127, 149, (4th Regiment Rhode Island Volunteers) 52, 76, 99, 136, (7th Regiment Rhode Island Volunteers) 42, 67, 90, 96, 98, 121, 136, (9th and 10th Regiment Rhode Island Volunteers) 32, (12th Regiment Rhode Island Volunteers) 28, 139, 143; Wisconsin (31st Regiment Wisconsin Volunteers) 141
International Red Cross 138
Invalid Corps 56
Irving, Abraham 26
Ishland (steamer) 129, 130
Island Cemetery 148, 151

Jackson, Rev. 27
Jackson, Stonewall 107
Jackson, NH 148
Jacobs, Andrew 92, 98, 121
James River 20
Jamestown, RI 75, 140
Johnson, Agustus 130
Johnston, Joseph E. 19, 20

Keay, Hiram 103
Keen, W.W. 11
Knowles, H.B. 73

Ladies' Union Aid Society 80, 94
Larned, R.M. 87
laundry 47, 48, 51, 56, 82, 101, 130
Lee, Robert E. 20, 94, 138
Lincoln, Abraham 8, 9, 17, 19, 20, 91, 107, 109, 135, 136, 139, 145, 146
Lincoln Industrial School 148
liquor 35, 61–67,71,150
Little Compton, RI 15
Livermore, H.B. 73
Loper, Isaac 157
Loper, Luther M. 157
Lovejoy, Allen 93, 94, 96, 97, 104, 105, 106, 110, 119, 145, 147

Lovejoy, John M. 57, 58, 74, 78, 93, 94, 96, 97, 98, 100, 101, 103, 104, 105, 107, 109, 110, 116, 117, 118, 119, 121, 145, 146, 147, 160
Lovejoy, Jonathan 93, 97, 110, 145
Lovell, Joseph 98
Lowe, Thadeous 107
Luther, Alfred 20, 21, 74, 74, 131, 143, 144

Magee, James 127
Magruder, John B. 20
Manassas Junction, VA 19
Marine Hospital 14, 67
Markey, John 64, 124
Marsh, James E. 73
Marye's Heights 91
Masterson, James 140
Mauran, Edward C. 29, 124
McClellan, George B. 19, 20, 60, 68, 107, 111, 138
McEachern, Duncan 75, 140
McKeen, Lydin 103, 104
McKibben, D.J. 39, 40, 47, 73
McKim, William M. 17, 47, 48
McKim's Mansion 145
McNaughten, Philip 73
McPherson, James M. 8
Mechanicsville, Battle of 21
Medal of Honor 130, 140, 156
Medical and Surgical History of the War of the Rebellion 17, 50, 58, 96, 128, 147
medical perscriptions and treatments: ammonia 10; blue mass 9; brandy 10, 11, 86, 150; bromine 12, 95; calomel 10, 128; castor oil 59, 128; chalk 9; cinnamon 10; cloves 10; creosote 10; distilled water 10; eggnog 10; lead acetate 10; maggots 12, 129, 140; mercury 9, 10; mustard plaster 10, 94; nutmeg 10; opium 9, 10, 119; porter 11; punch 10; quinine 10, 11, 12, 128; sherry wine 10; silver nitrate 10; sodium chloride 10; Spiritus Frumenti 10; Spiritus Lavandulae Compositus 10; Spiritus Vini Gallici 10; strychnine 10; sulfuric acid 10; turpentine 10; vaccination 78; Vinum Album 10; whiskey 10, 64, 65
Melville, George 160
Melville Boat and Marina District 6, 159, 160
Messinger, Rufus 137
Mexican War 25, 73
Middletown, RI 5, 15, 17, 23, 24, 79, 131
Miller, David 33, 154
minstrel show 115, 116
Monroe Crossroads, NC 137
Morton, Lloyd 75, 76
mosquito 55, 104
Mosquito Soldiers 128
Mount Hope 15
Mt. Pleasant Hospital 92

Narragansett Bay 5, 14, 15, 16, 23, 40, 50, 51, 54, 55, 75, 111, 112, 114, 117, 121, 123, 127, 135, 138, 142, 152, 154, 159
New Bedford, MA 71
New England Women's Auxiliary Association 85

New Market Heights, VA (Battle of Chaffin's Farm) 130
New York, NY 23, 49, 54, 57, 75, 77, 96, 112, 119, 121, 129, 130, 137, 149, 154
New York Herald 102
New York Times 39, 98
Newport, RI 5, 14, 15, 16, 17, 23, 24, 27, 29, 30, 31, 35, 39, 40, 46, 50, 66, 68, 71, 78, 79, 80, 81, 92, 97, 99, 110, 116, 120, 124, 126, 131, 135, 136, 140, 148, 149, 150, 151, 152, 157
Newport Advertiser 34, 59
Newport Artillery Company 52, 159
Newport Daily News 27, 30, 38, 59, 78, 102, 132
Newport Dinner Train 5, 160
Newport Historical Society 39, 56, 149
Newport Mercury 85, 151
nurses 9, 23, 41, 42, 43, 47, 51, 59, 67, 69, 80–89, 90, 92, 94, 97, 99, 138, 148, 149, 150

Ocean Hall 68
Office of the Secretary of State, A. Ralph Mollis State Archives Division 36, 48, 50, 146, 157
O'Leary, Charles 96, 131
Oshkosh, WI 157
osteomyelitis 12

Paine, A.M. 73
Palmer & Co. 96
Patten, ME 103
Pawtucket, RI 65, 139
Pawtucket Guard 42
paymaster 108, 109, 132
Peck, George H. 27, 28, 43, 44, 45, 54, 55, 62, 63, 64, 65, 66, 71, 87, 89, 98, 103, 107, 109, 111, 114, 116, 117, 123, 124, 125, 126, 131, 132, 135, 143, 144
Peckham, Amos 79
Pedley, James 129
Pemberton Square Hospital 75
Peninsula Campaign 25, 26, 42, 45, 81, 85, 112, 131, 138
Pennsylvania 94, 112, 128, 145, 147
pension 137, 140, 141, 143, 144
Perry (steamer) 26, 29, 47, 71, 78, 79, 93, 99, 130, 154
Petersburg, VA 61, 85, 96, 126, 128, 129, 130, 136, 137, 141, 145, 149
Phelps, Thaddeus 73
Philadelphia, PA 10, 12, 27, 39, 46, 53, 76, 99, 100, 138, 141, 145, 147
Phillips, George 106, 107, 111, 116, 117, 118, 119, 135
physicians *see* doctors
Pittsburgh, PA 33
Plymouth, MA 85
Plympton, MA 91
pneumonia 10, 13, 151
Pomeroy, Elijah 28
Portsmouth, RI 5, 6, 14, 15, 16, 17, 18, 23, 24, 25, 28, 29, 30, 31, 34, 35, 37, 38, 41, 42, 43, 46, 47, 48, 49, 56, 57, 58, 59, 60, 61, 62, 65, 66, 67, 68, 69, 70, 71, 73, 74, 75, 76, 77, 78, 79, 80, 81, 83, 85, 87, 89, 90, 92, 93, 95, 96, 97, 98, 100, 101,

105, 107, 108, 110, 111, 112, 113, 116, 118, 119, 127, 129, 130, 131, 132, 133, 134, 135, 138, 139, 140, 141, 142, 143, 144, 145, 147, 148, 149, 150, 152, 153, 154, 155, 156, 157, 158, 159, 160
Portsmouth Grove Estate 14, 17
Portsmouth Grove Hospital Library Association 87, 157
Post (Providence newspaper) 52
post exchange 135
post office 49, 63, 99, 120, 154
Prescott, O.S. 87
Princeton University 73
prisoners 21, 23, 32, 35, 54, 71, 74, 126, 140
Proudfit, Alexander 89, 131
Providence, RI 14, 15, 17, 18, 26, 28, 31, 32, 36, 37, 39, 47, 48, 49, 50, 52, 54, 63, 67, 70, 71, 73, 76, 77, 88, 91, 92, 93, 94, 97, 101, 110, 114, 115, 116, 117, 124, 125, 127, 129, 130, 131, 139, 141, 142, 146, 150, 151, 157
Providence Evening Press 39, 74
Providence Journal 74
Providence Public Library 88
pyemia 12

Quaker Hill 87
Quartermaster Department 25, 92, 175
Quartermaster General's Office 17, 56, 101, 102

railroad 5, 17, 28, 31, 41, 50, 62, 124, 125, 135, 141, 147, 159
Rappahannock 19
rations 11, 25, 29, 41–45, 90, 98, 114, 121
Readville, MA 75
Rhode Island Colony 15
Rhode Island Historical Cemetery No. 9 157
Rhode Island Historical Society 91, 150
Rhyne, Peyton S. 140
Richardson, Agnes Wilbour 85, 149
Richardson, George H. 252, 149
Richmond, VA 19, 20, 35, 60, 74, 119, 136, 144
Ricker, Oliver A. 87, 92, 94, 97, 98, 100, 101, 102, 104, 107, 108, 109, 142
Robinson, John 27, 154, 155
Rogers, Stephen O. 7, 35, 43, 54, 63, 87, 89, 100, 104, 107, 109, 110, 111, 117, 118, 123, 125
Russell, Albert 124
Russell, James 76

St. Marks (steamer) 77
St. Paul's Episcopal Church 24, 157
Salisbury National Cemetery 105
Salisbury Prison 143
salted beef 25
sanitation 13, 32, 80
Santa Fe, NM 73
Satterlee U.S. Army General Hospital 99, 100, 147
Savannah, GA 133
Sawtell, Walter H. 156
Scituate, RI 27, 142
Seven Days' Battles 20
Seville, David R. 85, 86

Seyffarth, Edmund 73, 74, 75, 96
Sheldon, H. Lawrence 73
Shelow, John M. 127, 128, 147
Sherman, William Tecumseh 132
Sherwood, Isaac T. 23
Silvie, Cpt. 73
Simmons, George W. 143
singing 116, 125
skating 114
Slocum, Charity 697
smallpox 75, 76, 77, 78, 79, 83, 84, 152
Smith, Eliza 23
Smith, James 154
Smith, John 66
Smith, William H. 94
Smithfield, RI 58
Snow, Byron D. 93
Society of Friends 87
Soldiers' and Sailors' Monument 143, 144
Sons of Temperance 63, 68, 151
Sousa, John Philip 138
South Hingham, MA 92
Spanish-American War 156, 157
Spaulding, J. 27
Sprague, Byron B. 152
Sprague, William 14, 75, 76, 77, 98, 124, 152
Stanton, Edwin 19, 39
Stauffacher, Isaiah 141
Sternberg, George Miller 23, 73, 151, 152
steward 9, 22, 23, 31, 78, 97, 108
Stewart, Isaac Newton 137
Stewart, Jonathan Milton 137
Stone, Albert H. 27
Striebling, G.C. 23, 24
substitutes 57
sunstroke 149
supplies 21, 24, 25, 31, 34, 35, 48, 55, 69, 71, 76, 82, 85, 90, 136, 139, 151
Surgeon General 13, 14, 15, 25, 32, 38, 39, 46, 69, 81, 98, 151, 152, 157
surgeons 7, 8, 9, 11, 12, 13, 14, 15, 21, 23, 24, 25, 27, 28, 29, 30, 32, 33, 38, 39, 44, 46, 48, 58, 61, 63, 67, 69, 73, 74, 75, 78, 81, 82, 85, 90, 92, 93, 95, 96, 98, 99, 100, 128, 136, 137, 138, 139, 142, 143, 151, 152, 156, 157
sutlers 22, 35, 37, 100
Sylph (steamer) 31

Taber, J.M., Jr. 158
Taylor, John 121
Taylor, Mrs. Thomas H.B. 148
tents 7, 25, 26, 29, 31, 32, 34, 38, 46, 52, 55, 66, 140
tetanus 12
Thanksgiving Day 43, 44, 69, 70, 71, 83, 111, 113, 116, 131
Thayer, Adin B. 105, 108, 118, 119, 147
This Is My Newport 66, 150
Tilley, Benjamin J. 68, 69, 126, 127, 131, 132, 151
Tiverton, RI 15
tobacco 35, 83, 100, 102, 103, 126

Town Council of Portsmouth 77
Trinity Church 87
typhoid/typhoid fever 10, 22, 25, 27, 42, 43, 76, 89, 92, 112, 152

U.S. Naval Academy 16, 83, 126
U.S. Navy 5
U.S. Sanitary Commission 22, 30, 42, 45, 46, 71, 80, 83, 85, 87, 138, 148
University of Pennsylvania 73, 97

Vallum (medical inspector) 35
Vanderpool, S. Oakley 38, 39
ventilation 11, 46, 138
Veteran Reserve Corps (previously called Invalid Corps) 56, 76, 136, 145
Vickery, Seth C. 91, 143

Walker, Daniel 99
War Department 30, 31, 54, 80, 110, 124, 156
Ward, Geoffrey C. 26
ward master 9, 26, 51, 59, 61, 78, 79, 83, 89, 97, 98, 119
Wareham, MA 143
Warner, John W. 97, 106, 107, 108, 119, 125, 126
Warren, RI 20
Washington, D.C. 7, 8, 18, 30, 32, 35, 39, 42, 44, 46, 47, 48, 49, 60, 73, 76, 84, 90, 92, 93, 96, 97, 101, 110, 126, 138, 151, 156, 157
Waterville, ME 105

Watson, Benjamin F. 109
Webster Times 36, 102
Weldon Railroad, Battle of 147
Western Metropolis (steamer) 121, 126, 127
Wheaton, Francis L. 21, 24, 25, 29, 30, 32, 34, 35, 37, 38, 39, 98, 150
Whetten, Harriet 82, 84, 86, 92
White House Landing, VA 82, 130
Whiting, Samuel S. 38, 156
Whitney, Moses 65, 89
Wilbour, Agnes Adams 85, 189
Wilbour, Mary Simmons 85
Wilderness, Battle of the 127, 155
Williams, Joshua Appleby 136
Williamsburg, VA 33, 111
Wilson, Samuel II 141
Wolfe, Frederick 27
Wool, John Ellis 98, 99
Woolsey, Georgeanna 42, 81, 82, 84, 87
Woolsey, Jane Stuart 46, 47, 61, 82, 86, 92, 148
Woolsey, Sarah Chauncey 83, 84, 86, 90, 92
Woonsocket, RI 136
World War II 5, 159
Wormeley, Katherine Prescott 42, 80, 81, 82, 83, 84, 85, 86, 148, 151

Yazoo fever 121
Yorktown, VA 20, 21, 23, 25, 29, 150
Young Ladies' Fair 71

www.ingramcontent.com/pod-product-compliance
Ingram Content Group UK Ltd.
Pitfield, Milton Keynes, MK11 3LW, UK
UKHW050526150426
5217IPUK00026B/1811

9 780786 468614